Diseases of the Chest and Heart 2015-2018

Diagnostic Imaging and Interventional Techniques

J. Hodler • R.A. Kubik-Huch • G.K. von Schulthess •
Ch.L. Zollikofer (Eds)

DISEASES OF THE CHEST AND HEART 2015-2018

DIAGNOSTIC IMAGING AND INTERVENTIONAL TECHNIQUES

**47th International Diagnostic Course
in Davos (IDKD)**
Davos, March 22-27, 2015

including the
Nuclear Medicine Satellite Course "Diamond"
Davos, March 21-22, 2015

Pediatric Radiology Satellite Course "Kangaroo"
Davos, March 21, 2015

Breast Imaging Satellite Course "Pearl"
Davos, March 21, 2015

and additional IDKD Courses 2015-2018

presented by the Foundation for the
Advancement of Education in Medical Radiology, Zurich

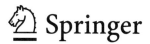 Springer

Editors

J. Hodler
Radiology
University Hospital
Zurich, Switzerland

R.A. Kubik-Huch
Radiology
Kantonsspital
Baden, Switzerland

G.K. von Schulthess
Nuclear Medicine
University Hospital
Zurich, Switzerland

Ch.L. Zollikofer
Kilchberg/Zurich, Switzerland

DOI 10.1007/978-88-470-5752-4

ISBN 978-88-470-5751-7   ISBN 978-88-470-5752-4 (eBook)

Springer Milan Dordrecht Heidelberg London New York

Library of Congress Control Number: 2015931953

Cover design: Massimiliano Pianta, Milan, Italy
Typesetting: Blu8, Cremona, Italy

Springer-Verlag Italia S.r.l., Via Decembrio 28, 20137 Milan

Springer is a part of Springer Science+Business Media (www.springer.com)

Preface

The International Diagnostic Course in Davos (IDKD) is a unique learning experience for imaging specialists. The course is useful for experienced radiologists, imaging specialists in training and clinicians wishing to be updated on the current state of the art and the latest developments in the fields of imaging and image-guided interventions.

This organ based and disease oriented course deals with imaging of the chest and heart, and includes pediatric imaging. In addition, there will be satellite courses covering pediatric radiology and nuclear medicine related to the chest and heart in more depth. In addition a breast imaging satellite course is offered.

During the last few years there have been considerable advances in this field driven by clinical as well as technological developments. These will be highlighted in the workshops given by internationally known experts in their field. The presentations encompass all the relevant imaging modalities including CT, MRI, PET, and conventional radiology.

This Syllabus contains condensed versions of the topics presented in the workshops. As a result, this book offers a comprehensive review of the state-of-the-art in imaging and intervention of chest and cardiac diseases as well as the breast.

This Syllabus was initially designed to provide the relevant information for the course participants in order to allow them to fully concentrate on the lectures and participate in the discussions without the need of taking notes. However, the Syllabus has developed into a convenient update for radiologists, radiology residents, nuclear physicians and clinicians interested in lung and heart diseases.

Additional information on IDKD courses can be found on the IDKD website: www.idkd.org

J. Hodler
R.A. Kubik-Huch
G.K. von Schulthess
Ch.L. Zollikofer

Table of Contents

Nuclear Medicine Satellite Course "Diamond"

Pediatric Radiology Satellite Course "Kangaroo"

Breast Imaging Satellite Course "Pearl"

List of Contributors

WORKSHOPS

Update in the Diagnosis and Staging of Lung Cancer

José Vilar[1], Jeremy J. Erasmus[2]

[1] Hospital Universitario Dr. Peset, Valencia, Spain
[2] Department of Radiology, MD Anderson Cancer Center, Houston, TX, USA

Introduction

Primary lung cancer is the leading cause of cancer mortality in the world and its incidence is expected to rise in the next several decades, especially in more recently industrialized countries such as China. This high mortality is largely explained by the fact that patients with lung cancer often present with advanced stage disease. Imaging is important in the early detection and clinical staging of lung cancer. Indeed, both the therapeutic options and the management of patients with lung cancer are to a considerable degree dependent upon disease stage at presentation. Detailed knowlegde and the appropriate use of imaging in the staging evaluation of patients with non-small cell lung cancer (NSCLC) are required to avoid unnecessary procedures, excess radiation, and redundant information. This is facilitated by the use of guidelines as well as the participation of multidisciplinary teams in which radiologists, pathologists, pulmonologists, surgeons, and medical and radiation oncologists discuss and reach a consensus on individualized imaging and treatment. The main objective of this chapter is to review the basic concepts related to the detection, staging, and follow-up of patients with NSCLC.

Detection of Lung Cancer

Preclinical Detection

The most common finding in an asymptomatic patient with NSCLC is the solitary pulmonary nodule (SPN), defined as a single intraparenchymal lesion ≤3 cm in diameter that is not associated with atelectasis or lymphadenopathy. When the lesion is >3 cm, it is defined as a mass. SPNs are detected incidentally on chest radiographs or computed tomography (CT) but can also be detected by screening programs for lung cancer. The chance of a pulmonary nodule being a cancer is directly related to the prevalence of the disease (pretest probability) and thus is much higher in high-risk groups such as heavy cigarette smokers.

Clinical Manifestations of NSCLC

Most patients are in their fifth and sixth decades of life and approximately three quarters of patients are symptomatic at presentation [1]. Many patients present with nonspecific systemic manifestations of malignancy, including anorexia, weight loss, or fatigue. Symptoms also depend on the local effects of the primary mass, the presence of regional or distant metastases, and the coexistence of paraneoplastic syndromes. While solitary peripherally located tumors tend to be asymptomatic, central endobronchial tumors can manifest as fever, dyspnea, hemoptysis, and cough. Symptoms that can occur as a result of local growth and the invasion of adjacent nerves, vessels, and mediastinal structures include chest pain, vocal cord paralysis and hoarseness, facial and upper truncal edema, headaches, neck vein distention, enlarged collateral chest wall vessels (superior vena cava obstruction), and dysphagia (esophageal involvement). Clinical signs and symptoms can also be caused by tumor excretion of a bioactive substance, or hormone, or as a result of immune-mediated neural tissue destruction caused by antibody- or cell-mediated immune responses. These paraneoplastic syndromes occur in 10–20% of lung cancer patients. Antidiuretic and adrenocorticotropin hormones are the more frequently excreted hormones and can result in hyponatremia and serum hypo-osmolarity and in Cushing's syndrome (central obesity, hypertension, glucose intolerance, plethora, hirsutism), respectively [1].

Role of Imaging in Detecting Lung Cancer

Imaging has an important role in screening for a lung malignancy because diagnosis at an early stage, before clinical presentation, is associated with an improved prognosis. Lung cancer screening is typically performed with low-dose CT (LDCT), as screening with chest radiography has been shown to have limited benefit. Randomized control trials have been or are being conducted to examine the role of screening in lung cancer management. The

Diseases of the Chest and Heart 2015-2018,
DOI: 10.1007/978-88-470-5752-4_1 © Springer-Verlag Italia 2015

National Lung Screening Trial (NLST), a randomized study comparing the effectiveness of LDCT vs. chest radiography in more than 50,000 participants, reported significant reductions in lung cancer (20%) and all-cause mortality (6.7%) [2]. Accordingly, LDCT is currently advocated as a screening tool for lung cancer. However, optimal screening strategies have not been determined. Thus, it is uncertain whether younger patients and/or smokers with fewer pack-years of smoking history than stated in the eligibility criteria used for individuals examined in the NLST (55- to 74-year-old patients with at least 30 pack-years of smoking history and still active smokers, or former smokers who stopped smoking within the previous 15 years) will also benefit from screening. It is hoped that contentious issues, including over diagnosis bias, whether detection of pre-clinical disease affects survival, and the cost-effectiveness of screening programs, will be resolved in the coming years [3-5].

The detection of lung cancer can be incidental, by screening, or when the lesion has caused symptoms. Low-dose CT is more sensitive than chest radiographs for detecting early lung cancer.

Characterization of a Pulmonary Nodule

Previous chest radiographs or CT images, if available, may suffice in characterizing a nodule as benign, i.e., if there is stability in size for >2 years. However, nodules, especially subsolid (pure ground glass or partly solid) nodules, can remain stable for >2 years due to their very slow growth rates and ultimately prove to be indolent adenocarcinomas. The absence of prior studies or the presence of signs of radiologic change are indications for CT evaluation to better characterize an SPN. Size, growth and morphology are the main parameters of an SPN that should be analyzed with CT. Positron emission tomography (PET) can provide useful information about the metabolic behavior of the nodule.

Growth

Growth can be estimated by evaluating prior imaging studies. Lung cancers typically double in volume (a 26% increase in diameter) between 30 and 400 days (average, 240 days). Very rapid duplication times are generally inconsistent with malignancy. Rather, volume doubling times <20–30 days are suggestive of an infectious or inflammatory etiology but they can also occur with lymphoma or rapidly growing metastases. Lung cancers can have long volume doubling times. In a CT screening study analyzing the growth rates of small lung cancers, the volume doubling time ranged from 52 to 1733 days (mean, 452 days) and approximately 20% of these malignancies had a volumetric doubling time >2 years [6]. These nodular opacities were typically well-differentiated adenocarcinomas. In contrast to the growth of solid nodules assessed only on the basis of size, in subsolid

nodules growth can manifest not only as an increase in size but also as an increase in attenuation and/or the development or increase in size of a solid component. These imaging features of growth are suspicious for an increased risk of malignancy [7]. The measurement of serial volumes, rather than diameters, together with the computer-calculated volume doubling time of small nodules has been suggested as an accurate and potentially useful method to assess growth [8, 9]. In an analysis of the growth rates of stage I lung cancers determined with serial volumetric CT measurements, the median time to a volume doubling was 207 days (50% of the tumors doubled in volume at 8 weeks and 75% at 14 weeks) [9]. Recently, nodule mass, defined as the combination of nodule volume and density, was proposed as a more accurate determination of the growth of partly solid nodules [10]. By multiplying nodule volume and density, mass measurements, which are subject to less variability than volume or diameter measurements, may allow earlier detection of the growth of partly solid nodules.

Morphology

Lung cancers typically have irregular or spiculated margins, although this finding can occasionally be seen with benign nodules as well (Fig. 1). A smooth margin, a feature typical of benign nodules, cannot be used to exclude lung cancer because malignant nodules may also have this appearance. The presence of fat (attenuation –40 to –120 Hounsfield units, HU) in a pulmonary nodule or mass indicates benignity, usually a hamartoma or, less frequently, lipoid aspiration pneumonia (Fig. 2). Characteristic patterns of benign calcification, whether central (involving >10% of the cross-sectional area of the nodule), diffuse, or laminated, are usually indicative of prior granulomatous disease. Popcorn-type calcification is typically due to the chondroid tissue in pulmonary hamartomas but can be

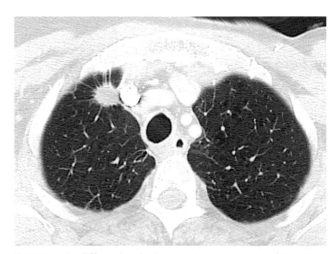

Fig. 1. Poorly differentiated adenocarcinoma. Computed tomography (CT) shows a nodule with a spiculated margin in the right upper lobe. Note that spiculation is typical for primary lung malignancy. At resection pleural invasion was present

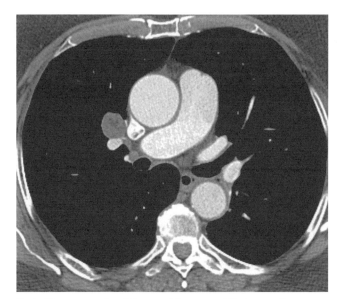

Fig. 2. Hamartoma in a 76-year-old woman. CT shows a 2-cm centrally located nodule in the right upper lobe containing focal low attenuation (−50 HU), consistent with a hamartoma

seen in carcinoid tumors. The presence of calcium does not exclude the diagnosis of cancer and has been reported to occur in up to 14% of lung cancers histologically. Generally, this calcification is amorphous or, if focal, is not central in location or it forms only a small portion of the nodule. The widespread use of thin-collimation CT images has increased the detection of nodules with low attenuation [11-13]. These subsolid nodules (pure ground glass nodules and partly solid) have a higher incidence of malignancy than solid nodules (Fig. 3). According to one study, 63% of partly solid nodules are malignant as opposed to 18% for ground glass opacities and 7% for solid nodules [11]. Importantly, with these nodules the likelihood of malignancy varies according to the size of the

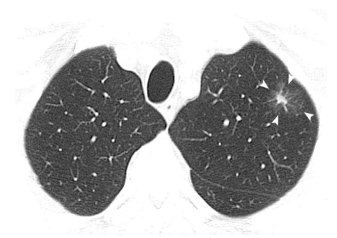

Fig. 3. Invasive adenocarcinoma in a 79-year-old man. CT shows a partly solid nodule in the left upper lobe with an 8-mm solid component (*arrowheads*). Note that the presence of a >5-mm soft-tissue component on CT makes the likelihood of malignancy high

soft-tissue component on CT [14, 15]. The frequencies of lobulation, spiculation, and pseudocavitation (small focal lucencies) are also significantly higher in malignant partly solid nodules.

Significant changes in the pathologic classification of lung adenocarcinoma were proposed in 2011 [16].The new adenocarcinoma classification now includes the terms adenocarcinoma in situ (AIS), a preinvasive lesion, minimally invasive adenocarcinoma (MIA), and invasive adenocarcinoma [16]. AIS was formerly classified as a bronchioloalveolar cell carcinoma and is a small (≤3 cm), localized adenocarcinoma that has no stromal, vascular, or pleural invasion and demonstrates lepidic growth [16]. MIA is a solitary adenocarcinoma (≤3 cm) with ≤5-mm invasion in any one focus and a predominantly lepidic pattern of growth [16]. MIA is excluded if the tumor invades the lymphatics, blood vessels, or pleura or contains necrosis. Invasive adenocarcinomas are composed of a complex heterogeneous mixture of histologic subtypes and are classified according to the most predominant one (lepidic, acinar, papillary, micropapillary, or mostly solid patterns) [16]. For mucinous malignancies, the term invasive mucinous adenocarcinoma has replaced mucinous bronchioloalveolar cell carcinoma. These tumors differ from mucinous AIS and MIA by a size >3 cm and/or showing invasion >0.5 cm and/or multiple nodules, or the lack of a circumscribed border with miliary spread into adjacent lung parenchyma. Invasive mucinous adenocarcinomas typically manifest as solid nodules or consolidative opacities.

Positron Emission Tomography (PET) Findings

The conventional radiologic assessment of an SPN is complemented by the use of PET and the radiopharmaceutical ^{18}F-2-deoxy-D-glucose (FDG), a D-glucose analog labeled with fluorine-18. The reported sensitivity and specificity of PET for malignant pulmonary lesions are 97% and 78%, respectively. The spatial resolution of PET scanners is in the range of 6 mm; therefore, smaller lesions should not be evaluated with PET. When FDG uptake by a solid nodule ≥1 cm in diameter is low, the likelihood of malignancy is generally considered to be low. However, in a study of 360 patients with lung nodules evaluated by FDG-PET, 43 patients had solid nodules with a standardized uptake value (SUV) <2.5, 16 of which were malignant [17]. False-negative results for malignancy include slow-growing cancers, especially adenocarcinomas with subsolid morphology and carcinoid tumors (Fig. 4). Nomori et al. reported that nine of ten well-differentiated adenocarcinomas manifesting as ground glass nodular opacities were falsely negative on FDG-PET [18]. The sensitivity (10%) and specificity (20%) for ground glass opacities in that study were significantly lower than for solid nodules (90% and 71%, respectively). False-positive results are most commonly caused by infections and inflammatory processes, including Wegener's granulomatosis, sarcoidosis, organizing pneumonia, amyloid, and rheumatoid nodules.

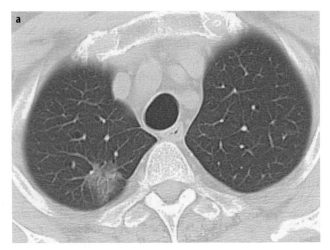
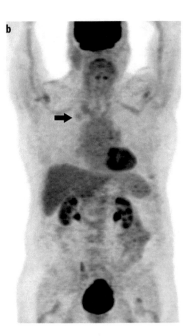

Fig. 4 a, b. Adenocarcinoma in situ in an 89-year-old man. CT shows a 3-cm pure ground glass nodular opacity in the right upper lobe. **b** Whole-body positron emission tomography (PET) maximum intensity projection image shows low-grade ^{18}F-2-deoxy-D-glucose (FDG) uptake in the nodule (*arrow*). Note that adenocarcinomas manifesting as ground glass nodular opacities are frequently falsely negative on FDG-PET

Pulmonary nodules can be characterized according to their growth, morphology, and metabolic activity. Standard imaging protocols based on the pretest probability (risk) should be used to rule out malignancy.

Guidelines for the Evaluation of an Incidentally Detected Pulmonary Nodule

The Fleischner Society guidelines for the evaluation of an incidentally discovered solid nodule in an adult patient integrate lesion morphology, growth rate, patient age, and smoking history (see below). In addition, to complement the recommendations for incidentally detected solid nodules, the Society recently published recommendations specifically aimed at the management of ground glass and partly solid nodules (see below) [19, 20]. Importantly, for both, risk factors such as smoking history, family history of lung cancer, or exposure to carcinogenic agents are not considered in the current guidelines due to a lack of sufficient data. Other issues to be aware of are that a slight temporary decrease in size can be seen with adenocarcinomas manifesting as ground glass or partly solid nodules, due to fibrosis or atelectasis, and enlargement and/or increasing attenuation with or without the new appearance of a solid component during follow up should be managed with a high degree of suspicion [20].

Recommendations for the Management of Incidentally Detected Solid Nodules

The Fleischner Society guidelines [19] are summarized in the following.

Low-Risk Populations (Little or No History of Smoking, and No Other Risk Factors)

1. Nodules ≤4 mm have a very small likelihood of malignancy such that re-assessment is not necessary.
2. Nodules >4-mm but ≤6-mm should be re-assessed using CT at 12 months; if stable, no further evaluation is required. The exception is the non-solid or partially solid nodule, for which re-assessment may need to be continued to exclude the risk of an indolent adenocarcinoma.
3. Nodules >6 mm but ≤8 mm should be re-assessed using CT at 6–12 months and, if stable, again at 18–24 months.
4. Nodules >8 mm should either be re-assessed using CT at 3, 9, and 24 months, to determine their size stability, or further evaluated with contrast-enhanced CT, CT-PET, biopsy, or resection.

High-Risk Populations (History of Smoking, or Other Exposure or Risk Factor)

1. Nodules ≤4 mm should be re-assessed at 12 months; if stable, no further evaluation is required. The exception is the non-solid or partially solid nodule, for which re-assessment may need to be continued to exclude the risk of an indolent adenocarcinoma.
2. Nodules >4 mm but ≤6 mm should be re-assessed using CT at 6–12 months and, if stable, again at 18–24 months.
3. Nodules >6 mm but ≤8 mm should be re-assessed using CT at 3–6 months and, if stable, again at 9–12 months and 24 months.
4. Nodules >8 mm should either be re-assessed using CT at 3, 9, and 24 months to assess stability or a contrast-enhanced CT, CT-PET, biopsy, or resection should be performed.

Recommendations for the Management of Incidentally Detected Solitary Ground Glass and Part Solid Nodules

The Fleischner Society guidelines [20] are summarized in the following.

1. Solitary pure ground glass nodules ≤5 mm require no CT follow-up.
2. Nodules >5 mm should be initially followed-up at 3 months using CT to confirm persistence, followed by annual surveillance CT for a minimum of 3 years.
3. Solitary, partly solid nodules should be initially followed-up at 3 months using CT to confirm persistence. If persistent, with a solid component <5 mm, yearly surveillance CT should be performed for a minimum of 3 years. If persistent with a solid component ≥5 mm, then biopsy or surgical resection is recommended. PET/CT should be considered for partly solid nodules >10 mm.

Recommendations for the Management of Incidentally Detected Multiple Ground Glass and Part Solid Nodules

1. Pure ground glass nodules ≤5 mm should be followed-up using CT at 2 and 4 years.
2. Pure ground glass nodules >5 mm without a dominant lesion(s) should be initially followed-up using CT at 3 months to confirm persistence, after which annual surveillance CT for a minimum of 3 years should be performed.
3. A dominant nodule(s) with a partly solid or solid component should be initially followed-up at 3 months using CT to confirm persistence. If persistent, biopsy or surgical resection is recommended, especially for lesions with a solid component >5 mm.

Staging of Lung Cancer

Staging, a standardized anatomic description of disease extent, is determined both clinically and pathologically and guides appropriate treatment. In general, the clinical stage underestimates the extent of disease compared with the pathologic stage. Radiologic imaging is an essential component of clinical staging and allows the assessment of disease manifestations that are important for surgical, oncological, and radiation therapy planning, including size of the primary tumor, its location and relationship to normal anatomic structures in the thorax, and the presence of nodal and or metastatic disease. The 7th edition of the tumor node metastasis (TNM) staging system allows a standardized definition of stage and, consequently, indicates the most appropriate treatment. While useful in ascertaining advanced disease, chest radiography is limited in accurately determining TNM descriptors in patients with potentially resectable disease, which typically requires imaging with CT and/or magnetic resonance imaging (MRI) and/or PET/CT. A contrast-enhanced CT of the chest is recommended for the evaluation of all patients with known or suspected primary lung cancer [21]. CT accurately assesses most characteristics of the primary tumor (T descriptor), including size and location, but locoregional invasion can be difficult to determine. CT is also useful in detecting nodal metastasis and determining the absence or presence of intra- and extrathoracic metastatic disease, including contralateral lung nodule(s), pleural and pericardial nodule(s) and effusions, bone metastases, and adrenal nodules/masses. CT of the chest alone is sufficient for the staging of patients with pure ground glass nodules and an otherwise normal study, and for patients with peripheral stage IA disease [21]. Otherwise, further imaging with FDG-PET is recommended for patients eligible for curative treatment. FDG-PET/CT has an increasing role in staging, particularly for detecting nodal (N descriptor) and distant (M descriptor) metastasis. When PET is unavailable or cannot be performed, a contrast-enhanced CT of the abdomen is recommended [21].

T Descriptor

The T descriptor defines the size, location, and extent of the primary tumor and is based on differences in survival (Fig. 5). However, although a T4 descriptor generally precludes resection, tumors with cardiac, tracheal, and vertebral-body invasion are designated in the 7th edition staging system as being potentially resectable in the absence of N2 and or N3 disease.

The following parameters must be analyzed regarding T descriptor determination: (1) size, (2) location, (3) extension.

1. *Tumor size* is a determinant of the T descriptor and essential to define surgical and radiotherapy strategies as well as to evaluate the response to treatment. In the 7th edition of the TNM classification, size is a significant parameter related to survival. T1 is subclassified as T1a (<2 cm) or T1b (>2 cm to <3 cm); T2 is subclassified as T2a (>3 cm to <5 cm or T2 by other factor and <5 cm) or T2b (>5 cm to <7 cm); tumors >7 cm are classified as T3. Size is usually measured on CT or MRI. On CT, lung window settings should be used, as mediastinal windowing may underestimate the size.
2. *Tumor location* is important in that it provides information to surgeons and radiation oncologists that can affect therapeutic management. For instance, centrally located tumors close to the spinal cord impose radiation dose-volume constraints, and determining tumor margins is important as they can affect radiotherapy delivery. This is especially important with the increasing use of conformal radiation therapy, in which multiple radiation beams are used to generate dose distributions that conform tightly to target volumes. The relation of the tumor to a fissure must be reported, as it may imply a change in surgical technique (pneumonectomy instead of lobectomy) when there is evidence that the lesion crosses the fissure (Fig. 6). The

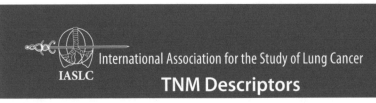

International Association for the Study of Lung Cancer
TNM Descriptors

T – Primary Tumour

TX   Primary tumour cannot be assessed, *or* tumour proven by the presence of malignant cells in sputum or bronchial washings but not visualized by imaging or bronchoscopy

T0   No evidence of primary tumour

Tis Carcinoma in situ

T1   Tumour 3 cm or less in greatest dimension, surrounded by lung or visceral pleura, without bronchoscopic evidence of invasion more proximal than the lobar bronchus (i.e., not in the main bronchus)

    T1a   Tumour 2 cm or less in greatest dimension[1]

    T1b   Tumour more than 2 cm but not more than 3 cm in greatest dimension

T2   Tumour more than 3 cm but not more than 7 cm; or tumour with *any* of the following features[2]:

    • Involves main bronchus, 2 cm or more distal to the carina

    • Invades visceral pleura

    • Associated with atelectasis or obstructive pneumonitis that extends to the hilar region but does not involve the entire lung

    T2a   Tumour more than 3 cm but not more than 5 cm in greatest dimension

    T2b   Tumour more than 5 cm but not more than 7 cm in greatest dimension

T3   Tumour more than 7 cm or one that directly invades any of the following: chest wall (including superior sulcus tumours), diaphragm, phrenic nerve, mediastinal pleura, parietal pericardium; *or* tumour in the main bronchus less than 2 cm distal to the carina[1] but without involvement of the carina; *or* associated atelectasis or obstructive pneumonitis of the entire lung or separate tumour nodule(s) in the same lobe as the primary.

T4   Tumour of any size that invades any of the following: mediastinum, heart, great vessels, trachea, recurrent laryngeal nerve, oesophagus, vertebral body, carina; separate tumour nodule(s) in a different ipsilateral lobe to that of the primary.

N – Regional Lymph Nodes

NX   Regional lymph nodes cannot be assessed

N0   No regional lymph node metastasis

N1   Metastasis in ipsilateral peribronchial and/or ipsilateral hilar lymph nodes and intrapulmonary nodes, including involvement by direct extension

N2   Metastasis in ipsilateral mediastinal and/or subcarinal lymph node(s)

N3   Metastasis in contralateral mediastinal, contralateral hilar, ipsilateral or contralateral scalene, or supraclavicular lymph node(s)

M – Distant Metastasis

M0   No distant metastasis

M1   Distant metastasis

    M1a   Separate tumour nodule(s) in a contralateral lung; tumour with pleural nodules or malignant pleural or pericardial effusion[3]

    M1b   Distant metastasis

Notes:

[1] The uncommon superficial spreading tumour of any size with its invasive component limited to the bronchial wall, which may extend proximal to the main bronchus, is also classified as T1a.

[2] T2 tumours with these features are classified T2a if 5 cm or less or if size cannot be determined, and T2b if greater than 5 cm but not larger than 7 cms.

[3] Most pleural (pericardial) effusions with lung cancer are due to tumour. In a few patients, however, multiple microscopical examinations of pleural (pericardial) fluid are negative for tumour, and the fluid is non-bloody and is not an exudate. Where these elements and clinical judgment dictate that the effusion is not related to the tumour, the effusion should be excluded as a staging element and the patient should be classified as M0.

Fig. 5. Descriptions of malignant lung tumors, nodes, and metastases for classification purposes. Reprinted with permission courtesy of the International Association for the Study of Lung Cancer. Copyright 2009 IASLC

proximity to a main pulmonary artery can also involve a change in surgical approach.

3. *Tumor extension* can be divided into local and distant. Local extension is included in the T descriptor, whereas distant metastases relate to the M descriptor. In the TNM staging system, additional pulmonary nodules in the same lobe are classified as T3, nodule/s in other ipsilateral lobes are T4 and nodule/s in the contralateral lung are M1a. The determination of the degree of pleural, chest-wall, and mediastinal invasion, as well as central airways, pulmonary veins, and artery involvement is important not only to radiation oncologists but also to surgeons evaluating the tumor for resectability. For instance,

pulmonary artery involvement may require a pneumonectomy rather than a lobectomy in order to obtain clear surgical margins. Additionally, involvement of the origin of the lobar bronchus or main bronchus may require a sleeve resection or pneumonectomy. Thoracic wall invasion does not preclude surgery but must be reported to the surgeon to ensure appropriate surgical resection, typically en bloc resection of the chest wall.

Role of Imaging in T Descriptor Determination

CT and MRI are useful in determining gross chest wall or mediastinal invasion (Fig. 7). However, limited loco-

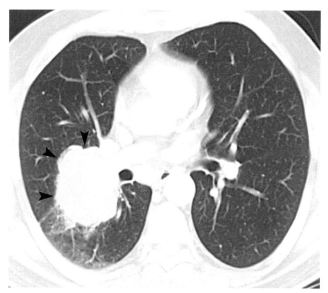

Fig. 6. Poorly differentiated adenocarcinoma in a 60-year-old man. CT shows a lobular mass in the right lower lobe with extension through the major fissure (*arrowheads*). The patient was treated definitively with concurrent chemoradiation

regional invasion is difficult to differentiate from abutment. MRI can be used to assess myocardial invasion and to evaluate superior sulcus tumors for involvement of the brachial plexus, regional vasculature, and adjacent spine and vertebra (Fig. 8). This is important since involvement of the brachial plexus roots or trunks superior to the T1 nerve root, invasion of the trachea or esophagus, and >50% invasion of a vertebral body are absolute contraindications to surgical resection [22, 23].

Tumor size, location, and extension are the fundamental T descriptors. The radiologist must have a thorough knowledge of the anatomic implications of the T descriptors in relation to surgery, radiotherapy, and chemotherapy.

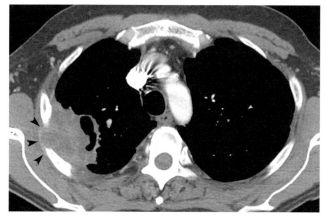

Fig. 7. Non-small-cell lung cancer in a 50-year-old man with chest-wall pain. CT shows a large cavitary mass in the right upper lobe with invasion of the chest wall (*arrowheads*). Note that chest wall invasion does not preclude surgery but usually changes the resection from a lobectomy to an en bloc resection of the lobe and chest wall

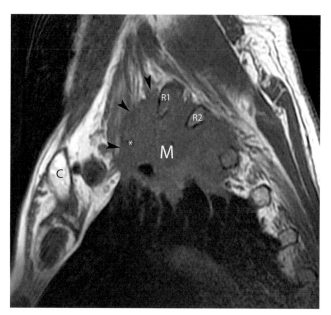

Fig. 8. Superior sulcus tumor in a 66-year-old man presenting with numbness of the upper arm extending to the elbow. Sagittal T1-weighted magnetic resonance image shows a mass (*M*) in the left upper lobe. The mass extends above the first rib and involves the C7 and C8 nerve roots of the brachial plexus (*arrowheads*). There is also extension of the mass into the soft tissues of the thorax posteriorly into the T1/2 and T2/3 intevertebral foramina. The mass encases the subclavian artery (*). Note that involvement of the brachial plexus roots superior to the T1 nerve root is an absolute contraindication to surgical resection. *C* clavicle, *R1* first rib, *R2* second rib

CT and MRI play fundamental roles in T descriptor determination. PET/CT is an additional tool in specific situations.

N Descriptor

The N descriptor, which specifies the presence and location of nodal metastatic disease, has a significant effect on management (Fig. 5). N descriptors are designated according to lymph node maps in which the nodal stations are numbered based on relationships to anatomic structures [24, 25]. For the 7th TNM edition, a standardized nodal map with seven node zones, created by unifying the Mountain/Dressler-ATS (MD-ATS) node map and the Japanese Naruke map, is used. The International Association for the Study of Lung Cancer (IASLC) nodal map designates the oncologic midline of the superior mediastinum to correspond with the left lateral border of the trachea, such that all nodes anterior to the trachea are grouped with right paratracheal nodes (Fig. 9). Surgical resection and the potential use of adjuvant therapy depend on the N descriptor, such that its accurate determination is important. Ipsilateral peribronchial, or hilar (N1) nodes are usually resectable while mediastinal nodes have a major influence on resectability. Specifically, ipsilateral mediastinal (including subcarinal) nodal metastasis (N2) can be resectable (usually after induction

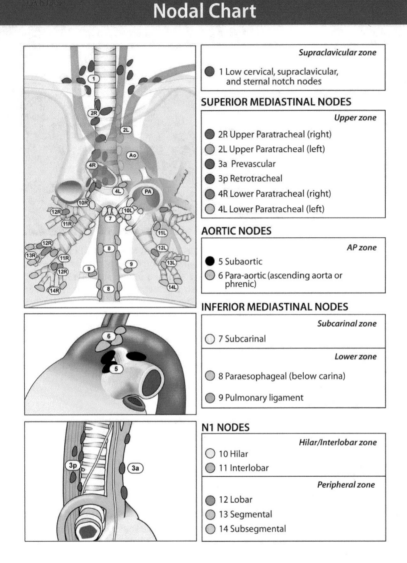

Fig. 9. Positions and descriptions of malignant nodes. Reprinted with courtesy permission of the International Association for the Study of Lung Cancer. Copyright 2009 IASLC and 2008 Aletta Ann Frazier

chemotherapy), while contralateral mediastinal and scalene or supraclavicular disease (N3) is not. To potentially improve patient management, data are currently being collected based on grouping nodal stations together in six zones within the current N1 and N2 patient subsets for further evaluation [26].

Role of Imaging in N Descriptor Determination

In the imaging evaluation of nodal metastasis, size is the only diagnostic criterion, with nodes >10 mm in their short-axis diameter considered abnormal. Chest radiographs are neither sensitive nor specific in evaluating nodal metastases. CT and MRI are better in this regard but their accuracy in detecting metastases to hilar and mediastinal nodes is not optimal because enlarged nodes can be hyperplastic and small nodes can contain metastases. A meta-analysis of CT accuracy for nodal staging in 3438 patients showed a sensitivity of 57%, a specificity of 82%, a positive predictive value of 56%, and a negative predictive value of 83% [27]. MRI has a reported sensitivity of 90.1%, a specificity of 93.1%, and an accuracy of 92.2% on a per patient basis in detecting nodal metastasis [28, 29]. FDG-PET and FDG-PET/CT have improved the sensitivity and specificity for detecting mediastinal nodal metastasis compared with CT alone (Fig. 10). A meta-analysis showed an overall sensitivity of 83% and specificity of 92% for

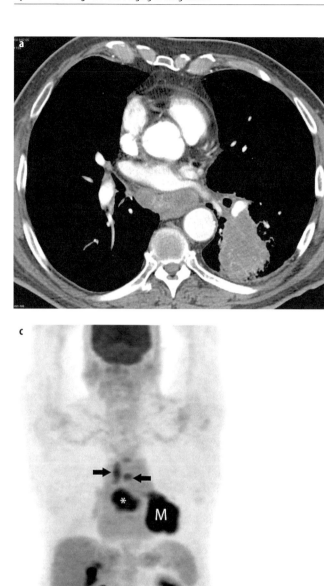

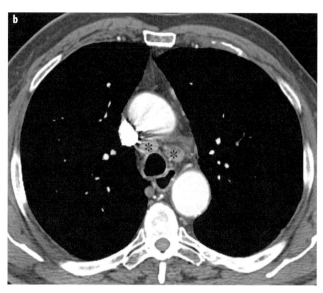

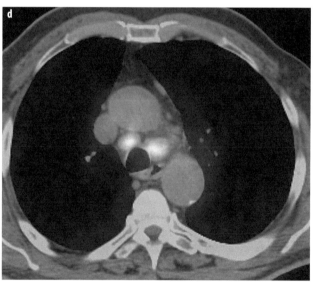

Fig. 10 a-d. Nodal metastasis in a 78-year-old man with non-small-cell lung cancer. **a, b** CT shows a large mass in the left lower lobe, enlarged subcarinal/azygo-esophageal (short-axis diameter >1 cm) nodes, and left and right lower paratracheal lymph nodes (* in **b**). **c** Whole-body PET maximum intensity projection image shows increased FDG uptake within the mass (*M*) and in the subcarinal/azygo-esophageal nodes (* in **c**) and paratracheal nodes (*arrows* in **c**). **d** FDG-PET/CT shows increased FDG uptake in the paratracheal nodes bilaterally. Mediastinoscopy confirmed nodal metastasis. Because N3 (contralateral mediastinal) nodal metastasis is nonresectable, the patient was treated palliatively

FDG-PET in detecting mediastinal nodal metastases compared with 59% and 78% on CT [30]. de Langen et al. showed that nodal sampling may not be necessary for nodes measuring 10–15-mm on CT, as long as they are negative on FDG-PET. However, mediastinal lymph nodes ≥16 mm, even if negative on FDG-PET, have a 21% post-test probability of metastatic involvement, necessitating preoperative pathologic staging [31]. Current recommendations for FDG-PET imaging are that it should be performed in patients with no CT findings of nodal metastatic disease to corroborate CT findings when there are no distant metastasis (M0), or to redirect nodal sampling by identifying an otherwise undetected site of metastasis.

The location of nodal metastasis is of major importance in determining management. Ipsilateral hilar (N1) nodes are resectable, ipsilateral mediastinal or subcarinal adenopathy (N2) may be resectable (usually after induction chemotherapy); contralateral mediastinal adenopathy and scalene or supraclavicular adenopathy (N3) are unresectable.

M Descriptor

Patients with NSCLC commonly have metastases to the lung, adrenals, liver, brain, bones, and extrathoracic lymph nodes at presentation. The M1 descriptor describes these metastases and is divided into two subsets based on outcome data showing a modest but significant survival difference [32]. M1a includes nodule(s) in the contralateral lung, pleural effusion and nodule(s), and pericardial nodule(s) while M1b designates extrathoracic metastasis (Fig. 5) [32, 33].

Role of Imaging in M Descriptor Determination

Detecting metastases is important to determine whether the patient will be a candidate for surgical resection or will receive palliative radiation and chemotherapy. CT is useful in determining the absence or presence of intrathoracic metastatic disease, including contralateral lung nodule(s), pleural and pericardial nodule(s), and effusions. Although a nodule in the contralateral lung is potentially a metastasis (M1a), most (approximately 75%) additional pulmonary nodules on CT imaging in patients with potentially operable clinical stages I to IIIA lung cancer are benign [34, 35]. Furthermore, an additional nodule can be a synchronous second primary lung cancer (incidence approximately 1.5–2% of patients per year) [34]. Additionally, pleural thickening and nodularity on CT suggest metastatic pleural disease (M1a) but these abnormalities may not be present in association with a malignant effusion and can occur with benign effusions (Fig. 11). Whole-body MRI is being used for the detection of M1b disease. A study in 203 patients with NSCLC who underwent whole-body MRI with diffusion-weighted imaging (DWI) reported a sensitivity of 68%, a specificity of 92%, and an accuracy of 88% in detecting distant (M1b) metastatic disease. Accordingly, with an accuracy equivalent to that of FDG-PET/CT, MRI with DWI may offer an alternative imaging option for the assessment of M1b in patients with NSCLC [36]. However, FDG-PET and FDG-PET/CT are more commonly used in detecting M1b disease as a means to improve the accuracy of CT staging [21]. Nonetheless, the appropriate role of FDG-PET/CT in the staging of patients with early-stage NSCLC is debated because occult distant metastases (M1b) are rarely detected (<5%) [37]. The incidence of occult metastatic disease discovered with FDG-PET increases with higher T and N descriptors [38]. In more advanced NSCLC, FDG-PET was shown to detect extrathoracic metastatic disease in up to 24% of patients potentially eligible for curative resection [38, 39]. Generally, CT is the primary modality used to diagnose and characterize intra-abdominal lesions, and a confident diagnosis of benignity or malignancy is frequently possible. For instance, CT and MRI are useful in the evaluation of adrenal masses and a confident diagnosis of benignity can be made if an adrenal mass has an attenuation value <10 HU on non-contrast-enhanced CT (Fig. 12) [40]. Although the

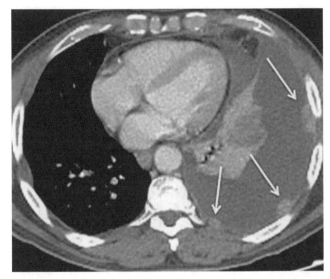

Fig. 11. Malignant pleural effusion in a 62-year-old man with non-small-cell lung cancer: Contrast computed tomography shows a large effusion and focal pleura thickening (*arrows*) due to metastases

finding of low attenuation is useful to characterize an adenoma, up to 30% of adenomas do not contain sufficient lipid to demonstrate low attenuation on CT imaging [41]. In these cases, delayed contrast-enhanced CT or MRI, using chemical shift analysis and dynamic gadolinium enhancement, has been shown to be of use in identifying lipid-poor adenomas [42-45]. FDG-PET/CT is also useful in detecting an adrenal metastasis and in distinguishing benign from malignant adrenal masses detected on CT [46]. A meta-analysis of 21 studies (1391 lesions), in which 5 specifically focused on patients with lung cancer, reported a combined sensitivity of 94% and a specificity of 82% of FDG-PET in detecting adrenal metastasis in patients with lung cancer [46]. FDG-PET/CT is now often used as the definitive imaging modality rather than MRI to evaluate an indeterminate adrenal mass, particularly when the adrenal mass is small (Fig. 13). Central nervous system metastases are common at presentation. Their detection rate in patients with CT and/or MRI and a negative clinical examination is low (0–10%) [47]. However, imaging of the brain may be indicated for the exclusion of brain metastases in patients with clinically resectable, locally advanced NSCLC with non-squamous histology. Furthermore, patients with clinical stage III or IV NSCLC should have routine imaging of the brain with MRI even if the clinical evaluation is negative for brain metastases [47]. FDG-PET/CT is more sensitive for osseous metastatic disease than bone scintigraphy with 99mtechnetium (Tc)-methylene diphosphonate (MDP). A meta-analysis reported an overall sensitivity and specificity of 92% and 98%, respectively, for osseous metastases on PET/CT, compared with a sensitivity of 86% and a specificity of 88% for 99mTc MDP bone scintigraphy. FDG PET/CT has to a large extent replaced the use of 99mTc MDP in patients with NSCLC (Fig. 14) [48-50].

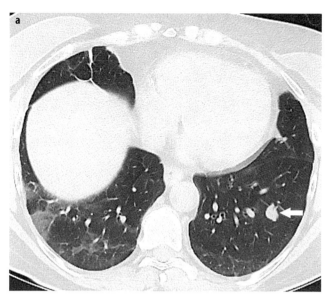
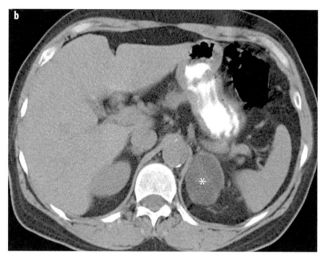

Fig. 12 a, b. Squamous cell carcinoma in a 61-year-old woman. **a, b** CT shows a 1.5-cm nodule in the left lower lobe (*arrow* in **a**) and a large, low-attenuation (<10 HU) left adrenal mass (* in **b**). Note that an attenuation value of <10 HU on non-contrast-enhanced CT is diagnostic of a benign etiology and no further evaluation is required

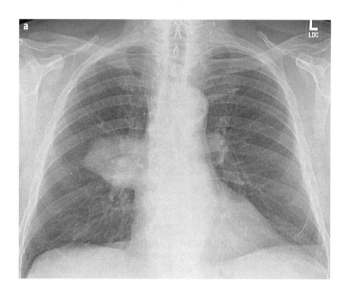
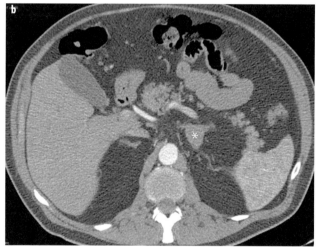

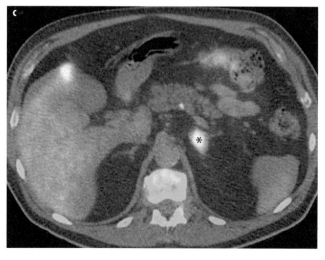

Fig. 13 a-c. Adrenal metastases in a 78-year-old man with non-small-cell lung cancer. **a** Chest radiograph shows a large mass in the right upper lobe. **b** CT shows a left adrenal mass (*). **c** FDG-PET/CT shows increased uptake by the adrenal metastasis (*)

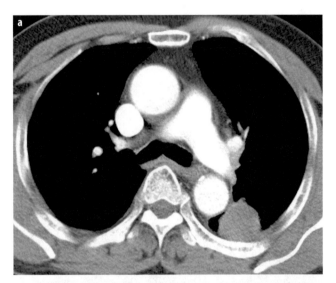

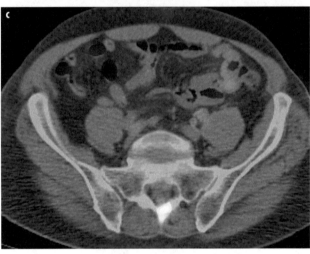

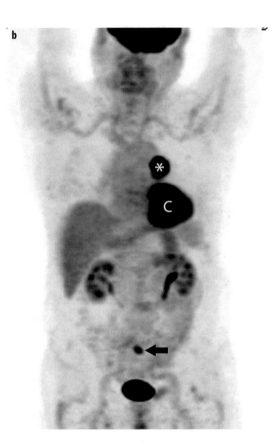

Fig. 14 a-c. Bone metastases in an 80-year-old man with non-small-cell lung cancer. **a** CT shows a mass in the left lower lobe. **b** Whole-body PET maximum intensity projection image shows increased FDG uptake within the mass (*) and focal increased uptake in the pelvis (*arrow*). **c** FDG-PET/CT reveals increased FDG uptake in the sacrum due to a metastasis. Note that FDG PET/CT is more accurate than CT in detecting occult metastasis. *C* cardiac uptake of FDG (physiologic)

The M1 descriptor is subclassified into M1a (additional nodules in the contralateral lung, malignant pleural effusions, pleural nodules) and M1b (distant metastases outside the lung and pleura). M disease precludes resection in most cases. CT is usually used to detect metastases. PET/CT is useful for detecting occult nodal and extrathoracic metastases and improves staging accuracy.

References

1. Ost DE, Yeung SC, Tanoue LT, Gould MK (2013) Clinical and organizational factors in the initial evaluation of patients with lung cancer: Diagnosis and management of lung cancer, 3rd Ed. American College of Chest Physicians evidence-based clinical practice guidelines. Chest 143(5 Suppl):e121S-141S.
2. Aberle DR, Berg CD, Black WC et al (2011) The National Lung Screening Trial: overview and study design. Radiology 258:243-253.
3. Detterbeck FC (2014) Overdiagnosis during lung cancer screening: is it an overemphasised, underappreciated, or tangential issue? Thorax 69:407-408.
4. Patz EF, Jr., Pinsky P, Gatsonis C et al (2014) Overdiagnosis in low-dose computed tomography screening for lung cancer. JAMA Intern Med 174:269-274.
5. Meza R, ten Haaf K, Kong CY et al (2014) Comparative analysis of 5 lung cancer natural history and screening models that reproduce outcomes of the NLST and PLCO trials. Cancer 120:1713-1724.
6. Hasegawa M, Sone S, Takashima S et al (2000) Growth rate of small lung cancers detected on mass CT screening. Br J Radiol 73:1252-1259.
7. Kakinuma R, Ohmatsu H, Kaneko M et al (2004) Progression of focal pure ground-glass opacity detected by low-dose helical computed tomography screening for lung cancer. J Comput Assist Tomogr 28:17-23.
8. Revel MP, Merlin A, Peyrard S et al (2006) Software volumetric evaluation of doubling times for differentiating benign versus malignant pulmonary nodules. AJR Am J Roentgenol 187:135-142.
9. Jennings SG, Winer-Muram HT, Tann M et al (2006) Distribution of stage I lung cancer growth rates determined with serial volumetric CT measurements. Radiology 241:554-563.
10. de Hoop B, Gietema H, van de Vorst S (2010) Pulmonary ground-glass nodules: increase in mass as an early indicator of growth. Radiology 255:199-206.
11. Henschke CI, Yankelevitz DF, Mirtcheva R et al (2002) CT screening for lung cancer: frequency and significance of part-solid and nonsolid nodules. AJR Am J Roentgenol 178:1053-1057.

12. Kishi K, Homma S, Kurosaki A et al (2004) Small lung tumors with the size of 1cm or less in diameter: clinical, radiological, and histopathological characteristics. Lung Cancer 44:43-51.

13. Godoy MC, Naidich DP (2009) Subsolid pulmonary nodules and the spectrum of peripheral adenocarcinomas of the lung: recommended interim guidelines for assessment and management. Radiology 253:606-622.

14. Austin JH, Garg K, Aberle D et al (2013) Radiologic implications of the 2011 classification of adenocarcinoma of the lung. Radiology 266:62-71.

15. Honda T, Kondo T, Murakami S et al (2013) Radiographic and pathological analysis of small lung adenocarcinoma using the new IASLC classification. Clin Radiol 68:e21-26.

16. Travis WD, Brambilla E, Noguchi M et al (2011) International association for the study of lung cancer/american thoracic society/european respiratory society international multidisciplinary classification of lung adenocarcinoma. J Thorac Oncol 6:244-285.

17. Hashimoto Y, Tsujikawa T, Kondo C et al (2006) Accuracy of PET for diagnosis of solid pulmonary lesions with 18F-FDG uptake below the standardized uptake value of 2.5. J Nucl Med 47:426-431.

18. Nomori H, Watanabe K, Ohtsuka T et al (2004) Evaluation of F-18 fluorodeoxyglucose (FDG) PET scanning for pulmonary nodules less than 3 cm in diameter, with special reference to the CT images. Lung Cancer 45:19-27.

19. MacMahon H, Austin JH, Gamsu G et al (2005) Guidelines for management of small pulmonary nodules detected on CT scans: a statement from the Fleischner Society. Radiology 237:395-400.

20. Naidich DP, Bankier AA, MacMahon H et al (2013) Recommendations for the management of subsolid pulmonary nodules detected at CT: a statement from the Fleischner Society. Radiology 266:304-317.

21. Silvestri GA, Gonzalez AV, Jantz MA et al (2013) Methods for staging non-small cell lung cancer: Diagnosis and management of lung cancer, 3rd ed: American College of Chest Physicians evidence-based clinical practice guidelines. Chest 143(5 Suppl):e211S-250S.

22. Bruzzi JF, Komaki R, Walsh GL et al (2008) Imaging of non-small cell lung cancer of the superior sulcus: part 1: anatomy, clinical manifestations, and management. Radiographics 28:551-560; quiz 620.

23. Bruzzi JF, Komaki R, Walsh GL et al (2008) Imaging of non-small cell lung cancer of the superior sulcus: part 2: initial staging and assessment of resectability and therapeutic response. Radiographics 28:561-572.

24. Mountain CF, Dresler CM (1997) Regional lymph node classification for lung cancer staging. Chest 111:1718-1723.

25. Naruke T, Suemasu K, Ishikawa S (1978) Lymph node mapping and curability at various levels of metastasis in resected lung cancer. J Thorac Cardiovasc Surg 76:832-839.

26. Rusch VW, Crowley J, Giroux DJ et al (2007) The IASLC Lung Cancer Staging Project: proposals for the revision of the N descriptors in the forthcoming seventh edition of the TNM classification for lung cancer. J Thorac Oncol 2:603-612.

27. Toloza EM, Harpole L, McCrory DC (2003) Noninvasive staging of non-small cell lung cancer: a review of the current evidence. Chest 123(1 Suppl):137S-146S.

28. Ohno Y, Hatabu H, Takenaka D et al (2004) Metastases in mediastinal and hilar lymph nodes in patients with non-small cell lung cancer: quantitative and qualitative assessment with STIR turbo spin-echo MR imaging. Radiology 231:872-879.

29. Ohno Y, Koyama H, Nogami M et al (2007) STIR turbo SE MR imaging vs. coregistered FDG-PET/CT: quantitative and qualitative assessment of N-stage in non-small-cell lung cancer patients. J Magn Reson Imaging 26:1071-1080.

30. Birim O, Kappetein AP, Stijnen T, Bogers AJ (2005) Meta-analysis of positron emission tomographic and computed tomographic imaging in detecting mediastinal lymph node metastases in nonsmall cell lung cancer. Ann Thorac Surg 79:375-382.

31. de Langen AJ, Raijmakers P, Riphagen I (2006) The size of mediastinal lymph nodes and its relation with metastatic involvement: a meta-analysis. Eur J Cardiothorac Surg 29:26-29.

32. Postmus PE, Brambilla E, Chansky K et al (2007) The IASLC Lung Cancer Staging Project: proposals for revision of the M descriptors in the forthcoming (seventh) edition of the TNM classification of lung cancer. J Thorac Oncol 2:686-693.

33. Rami-Porta R, Bolejack V, Goldstraw P (2011) The new tumor, node, and metastasis staging system. Semin Respir Crit Care Med. 32:44-51.

34. Detterbeck FC, Postmus PE, Tanoue LT (2013) The stage classification of lung cancer: Diagnosis and management of lung cancer, 3rd ed: American College of Chest Physicians evidence-based clinical practice guidelines. Chest 143(5 Suppl):e191S-210S.

35. Gould MK, Donington J, Lynch WR et al (2013) Evaluation of individuals with pulmonary nodules: when is it lung cancer? Diagnosis and management of lung cancer, 3rd ed: American College of Chest Physicians evidence-based clinical practice guidelines. Chest 143(5 Suppl):e93S-120S.

36. Ohno Y, Koyama H, Onishi Y et al (2008) Non-small cell lung cancer: whole-body MR examination for M-stage assessment—utility for whole-body diffusion-weighted imaging compared with integrated FDG PET/CT. Radiology 248:643-654.

37. Viney RC, Boyer MJ, King MT et al (2004) Randomized controlled trial of the role of positron emission tomography in the management of stage I and II non-small-cell lung cancer. J Clin Oncol 22:2357-2362.

38. MacManus MP, Hicks RJ, Matthews JP et al (2001) High rate of detection of unsuspected distant metastases by PET in apparent stage III non-small-cell lung cancer: implications for radical radiation therapy. Int J Radiat Oncol Biol Phys 50:287-293.

39. van Tinteren H, Hoekstra OS, Smit EF et al (2002) Effectiveness of positron emission tomography in the preoperative assessment of patients with suspected non-small-cell lung cancer: the PLUS multicentre randomised trial. Lancet 359:1388-1393.

40. Boland GW, Lee MJ, Gazelle GS et al (1998) Characterization of adrenal masses using unenhanced CT: an analysis of the CT literature. AJR AM J Roentgenol 171:201-204.

41. Pena CS, Boland GW, Hahn PF et al (2000) Characterization of indeterminate (lipid-poor) adrenal masses: use of washout characteristics at contrast-enhanced CT. Radiology 217:798-802.

42. Boland GW, Hahn PF, Pena C, Mueller PR (1997) Adrenal masses: characterization with delayed contrast-enhanced CT. Radiology 202:693-696.

43. Boland GW, Lee MJ (1995) Magnetic resonance imaging of the adrenal gland. Crit Rev Diagn Imaging 36:115-174.

44. Outwater EK, Siegelman ES, Huang AB, Birnbaum BA (1996) Adrenal masses: correlation between CT attenuation value and chemical shift ratio at MR imaging with in-phase and opposed-phase sequences. Radiology 200:749-752.

45. Schwartz LH, Ginsberg MS, Burt ME et al (1998) MRI as an alternative to CT-guided biopsy of adrenal masses in patients with lung cancer. Ann Thorac Surg 65:193-197.

46. Boland GW, Dwamena BA, Jagtiani Sangwaiya M et al (2011) Characterization of adrenal masses by using FDG PET: a systematic review and meta-analysis of diagnostic test performance. Radiology 259:117-126.

47. Kozower BD, Meyers BF, Reed CE (2008) Does positron emission tomography prevent nontherapeutic pulmonary resections for clinical stage IA lung cancer? Ann Thorac Surg 85:1166-1169; discussion 1169-1170.

48. Min JW, Um SW, Yim JJ et al (2009) The role of whole-body

FDG PET/CT, Tc 99m MDP bone scintigraphy, and serum al-
kaline phosphatase in detecting bone metastasis in patients with
newly diagnosed lung cancer. J Korean Med Sci 24:275-280.
49. Qu X, Huang X, Yan W et al (2012) A meta-analysis of
(1)(8)FDG-PET-CT, (1)(8)FDG-PET, MRI and bone scintigraphy for diagnosis of bone metastases in patients with lung cancer. Eur J Radiol 81:1007-1015.
50. Liu N, Ma L, Zhou W et al (2010) Bone metastasis in patients
with non-small cell lung cancer: the diagnostic role of F-18
FDG PET/CT. Eur J Radiol 74:231-235.

Computed Tomography Diagnosis and Management of Focal Lung Disease

Ioannis Vlahos[1], Gerald F. Abbott[2]

[1] Department of Radiology, St. George's Hospital and NHS Trust, St George's Medical School, University of London, UK
[2] Thoracic Imaging FND-202, Massachusetts General Hospital, Boston, MA, USA

Introduction

Focal pulmonary opacities can be broadly categorized as nodules, masses, or focal parenchymal airspace disease, but their diagnosis is often challenging. Computed tomography (CT), supplemented by thin section or high-resolution CT imaging, is better than chest radiography in the determination of the characteristics of these lesions.

Nodules are spherical well-defined opacities measuring <3 cm in diameter. In practice, ill-defined or irregular nodules are also included in the category of nodules, although more appropriately these should be considered as nodular opacities. The improved ability of CT to categorize nodules and masses is based on morphometric evaluation of their density and contour. However, CT densitometry is usually only a part of the evaluation of these abnormalities, as specific CT techniques to determine enhancement (nodule enhancement studies, dual-energy CT), follow-up imaging to verify evolution, positron emission tomography (PET)/CT to assess physiological activity and, ultimately, fine-needle aspiration or biopsy are also likely to play a role.

Features of Benign Solid Nodules

The principle application of CT in the evaluation of a solitary pulmonary nodule is in determining whether it has specific benign density characteristics, such as intralesional calcification or fat. The identification of either one is aided by the use of thin-section contiguous images (1–3 mm) through nodules of interest. These imaging techniques are preferably performed with a targeted reconstruction of the nodule itself (field of view: 10–12 cm). Although bulk fat may be evident by visual inspection alone, on CT fat will have an intensity of less than −30 to −40 Hounsfield units (HU) and often as low as −150 HU. Measurements should be performed using a suitably sized region of interest that encompasses an area that is still within the nodule on the slice above and the slice below the measured slice. This reduces the risk of

an erroneously low measurement due to partial volume average effects of the adjacent low-density lung parenchyma. Previously, pixel-mapping was used to identify voxels with HU <0 on thicker sections as it compensated for the partial volume average effects of more solid parts of the nodule. Today, in the era of isotropic data CT acquisition, this method is no longer advocated. There is no absolute HU measurement that confirms calcification, although measurements >200 are usually related to pixels occupied by calcific material. Visual comparison to other thoracic osseous structures is considered sufficient for determining the calcific nature of lesions.

Central, lamellated, or popcorn-type calcification is diagnostic of a benign lesion. The presence of central or lamellated calcification is usually indicative of granulomatous disease (Fig. 1). The presence of fat or popcorn

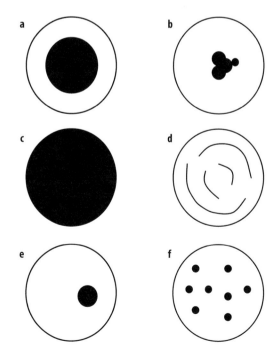

Fig. 1 a-f. Types of calcification. Benign: **a** central, **b** central multifocal, **c** uniform, **d** lamellar. Indeterminate: **e** eccentric, **f** stippled

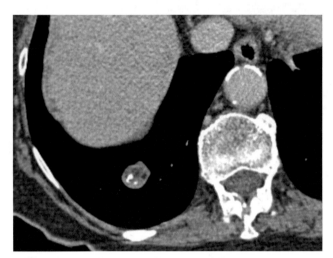

Fig. 2. Pulmonary hamartoma. Intralesional fat and popcorn calcification are seen

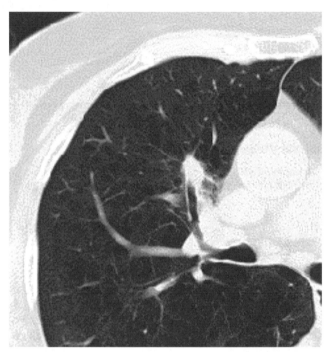

Fig. 3. CT bronchus sign in an adenocarcinoma of the lung

calcification is diagnostic of a pulmonary hamartoma (Fig. 2). It is important to determine the central location of a calcification on coronal or sagittal images, as the eccentric nature of calcification is often only noted in these planes. Eccentric calcification is most often benign, related to granulomatous disease; however, eccentric calcification occasionally reflects a small granuloma that has become engulfed within an enlarging adjacent neoplasm. Dystrophic or stippled calcifications are well-recognized to occur within carcinoid lesions, non-small cell carcinoma, and small cell-carcinoma; hence, they are not a helpful discriminator between benign and malignant nodules.

Other morphological features that are associated with benign lesions include a polygonal, elongated (length: width ratio >2), elliptical, linear, or plaque-like shape, particularly when related to the fissures or pleural surfaces. Indeed, not all such lesions are by definition strictly nodules, as some are best characterized as scars. Elliptoid nodules in the upper lobes are occasionally due to benign intrapulmonary lymph nodes. These findings are reported with variable incidence by pathologists and with variable incidence and confidence by radiologists. The confident accurate diagnosis of benign intrapulmonary lymph nodes requires an upper lobe location of an elongated nodule aligning lengthwise along typical lymphatic locations, such as the fissures or bronchi of the central axial interstitium.

Features of Malignant Solid Nodule

Specific features of malignancy are common in larger nodules but relatively uncommon in nodules smaller than 1 cm. Spiculation, microlobulation, pleural tags, satellite nodules, and the presence of a bronchus leading directly into a nodule ("CT bronchus sign") (Fig. 3) are associated with a high probability of neoplastic disease, although occasionally they are also seen in inflammatory or

infectious diseases, including mycobacterial disease. Cavitation is a feature that can be seen in neoplastic as well as benign infectious diseases (including bacterial, mycobacterial, and fungal diseases) and inflammatory diseases (e.g., vasculitides, Langerhans cell histiocytosis). The appearance of thicker-walled cavities on chest radiographs has historically been described as a feature favoring neoplasia [1]; however, this earlier radiographic interpretation has not been corroborated by CT evaluation of the wall thickness of nodules or masses [2].

CT Studies of Nodule Enhancement

Evaluation of the physiology of a solid lung nodule may be of assistance in determining whether the lesion is benign or malignant. Nodule enhancement studies consist of a non-contrast acquisition through the lesion at 120 kVp followed by repeated post-contrast acquisitions at 1, 2, 3, 4, and 5 min. Adapted protocols that evaluate initial nodule enhancement to extract perfusion metrics have also been developed. A multicenter study by Swensen et al. demonstrated that nodules that enhance <15 HU are highly likely to be benign [3]. Nodules that enhance more than 15 HU may be benign or malignant. Important caveats to this study are that the region of interest for evaluating nodule density before and after contrast should cover at least 70% of the lesion's surface area and that heterogeneous or cavitary lesions cannot be evaluated by nodule enhancement studies. Moreover, false-negative results are frequently obtained in mucin-rich lesions such as mucinous adenocarcinomas. The clinical value of

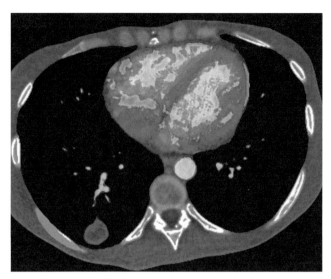

Fig. 4. Dual-energy CT demonstrating peripheral enhancement of a pulmonary metastasis

Table 1. Fleischner guidelines for incidentally detected solid nodules

Nodule size	Low risk	High risk
≤4 mm	No follow-up	12 months follow-up No change→Stop
>4–6 mm	12 months follow-up No change→Stop	6–12 months then 18–24 months follow-up No change→Stop
>6–8 mm	6–12 months then 18–24 months follow-up No change→Stop	3-6, 9–12 months, then 24 months follow-up No change→Stop
>8 mm	3, 9, 24 months follow-up, or CT/PET, or biopsy	

this imaging approach is in its very high negative predictive value (96%). However, in clinical practice only a small fraction of benign lesions exhibit low level enhancement; thus, even after this imaging approach the vast majority remain indeterminate. Therefore, PET/CT is gaining increasing favor as an alternative physiological assay of nodule activity, as it is more likely to alter the pre-test probability of malignancy or benignity.

The introduction of dual-energy CT, either by dual-source or rapid kVp switching, has permitted the accurate determination of contrast enhancement without the need for pre-contrast images [4]. This may be helpful in assessing the extent and pattern of lesion enhancement, perhaps as a surrogate marker of enhancement before and after treatment (Fig. 4). Yet, it is unclear whether this technological evolution can be used to distinguish benign from malignant disease. Certainly, the implementation of nodule enhancement is problematic in that in the original studies imaging was performed at 120 kVp. As such, appropriate thresholds for enhancement evaluation at kVp values ranging from 80 to 140 kVp have not been determined.

Indeterminate Solid Nodules

Unfortunately, the majority of nodules are indeterminate on CT imaging, as they do not demonstrate features that can be definitively considered as benign or malignant. In the Mayo screening series of more than 1,500 patients, over 3,300 indeterminate non-calcified nodules were identified, the vast majority of which were small (≤4 mm) and benign [5]. Even in established smokers, the risk of malignancy in nodules of this size is <1% [6]. The management of indeterminate nodules was previously a matter of debate. However, recent evidence-based guidelines from the Fleischner Society have greatly trans-

formed the management of these nodules [7]. It should be noted that the guidelines apply to the management of incidentally detected solid nodules in patients over the age of 35 who are not immune-suppressed. The guidelines vary according to whether patients are smokers (high risk) or non-smokers (low risk) but significantly eliminate the need for follow-up of small nodules in low-risk patients and greatly reduce the frequency of follow-up in other patients (Table 1). In addition, these guidelines do not apply to subsolid nodules, nor to patients with suspected neoplastic disease. In the former, a more infrequent follow-up may be appropriate (see below); in the latter, a more aggressive follow-up schedule or correlation with biopsy or PET may be indicated.

Role of Computer-Assisted Diagnosis for Solid Nodules

Computer-aided detection (CAD) improves the detection of pulmonary nodules, although its sensitivity varies depending on the characteristics of the lesion, including its size, density, and location. Sensitivity also depends on technical parameters, such as the thickness of the evaluated CT images. Moreover, there are vendor-specific issues related to CT algorithm optimization with the goal of obtaining high detection rates with an acceptable rate of false-positive detections. Most CAD systems also contain computer-aided diagnosis (CADx) features for the evaluation of pulmonary nodules. CADx systems may incorporate algorithms that can perform two- or three-dimensional analysis of the density of focal lung opacities as well as morphometry to determine the likelihood of malignancy, often expressed as a percentage probability of malignancy. But while this complex method of analysis performs better than human readers across multiple cases, it is difficult to reliably apply percentage probabilities to individual cases [8].

One of the most useful features of CADx is the ability to segment individual nodules, which permits a three-dimensional evaluation of the lesion's size and shape and can be coupled with follow-up examinations to determine volumetric growth. This approach is based on the observation that the doubling time of benign lesions is far

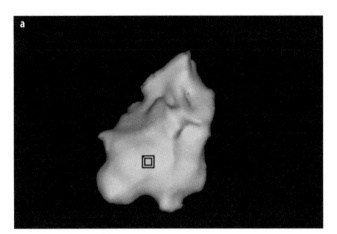
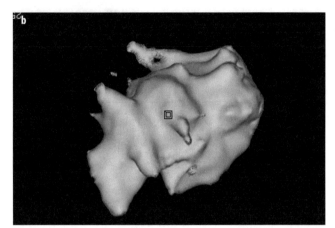

Fig. 5 a, b. Adenocarcinoma of the lung. Computer aided 3-D volumetric evaluation demonstrating asymmetric growth over an 11-month period. **a** Initial evaluation, **b** follow-up evaluation

longer than that of malignant lesions [9]. Volumetric evaluation of growth is also more reliable than reader-generated uni- or bidimensional size measurements [10]. Moreover, volumetric evaluation may be more sensitive to the detection of asymmetric growth, a feature that is limited to malignant lesions (Fig. 5). A commonly applied threshold for the volume doubling time of a solid lesion is 400 days, although several authors have advocated a threshold of 500 days [11-13]. This extended threshold is perhaps more prudent when the veracity of volumetric nodule evaluation is assessed. The accuracy and reproducibility of lung nodule segmentation have been confirmed in artificial and porcine models. However, the reproducibility of in vivo human nodule measurements can vary by up to 15%. This was demonstrated by evaluating the same nodule in different phases of inspiration or by using CT data based on different slice thicknesses or obtained with different software packages [13, 14]. Less significant changes may occur as a result of different reconstruction algorithms or radiation-dose variation. The presence or absence of intravenous contrast appears to play a largely inconsequential role. Nonetheless, by ensuring that a similar technique is employed on initial and follow-up examinations, lung nodule volumetry shows great promise and may further reduce the need for follow-up examinations.

Subsolid Nodules

Subsolid nodules include lesions that are pure ground glass in density as well as lesions that are partly solid and partly ground glass. Lesions with these characteristics, and especially those of the latter type, are associated with higher rates of malignancy than solid lesions (Fig. 6) [15]. Malignant sub-solid nodules lie along a spectrum of disease that extends from the suspected malignant precursor lesion of atypical adenomatous hyperplasia (AAH) to invasive adenocarcinoma. In 2011, a reclassification of pulmonary adenocarcinoma was introduced

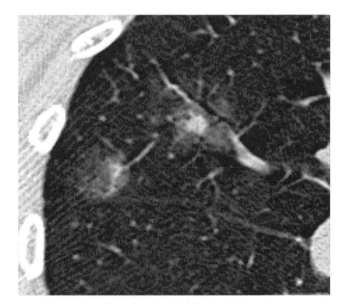

Fig. 6. Multifocal subsolid lesions. Mixed ground glass/solid-density lesions in a patient with multifocal adenocarcinoma

jointly by the International Association for the Study of Lung Cancer, the American Thoracic Society, and the European Respiratory Society [16]. This new classification was based on observations regarding heterogeneities in sub-solid neoplastic lesions that influenced their progression and clinical impact. For example, Aoki et al. [17] observed that AAH and lower-grade lesions of what was previously termed bronchioloalveolar cell carcinoma (BAC, Noguchi subtype A, B, C) were associated with lesions that were nearly exclusively ground glass in nature. Conversely, higher-grade lesions (Noguchi D, E, F) were associated with lesions that became progressively more reticular, demonstrated tractional bronchiolectasis, and, eventually, increasing solid components [17, 18].

The current 2011 classification replaces the heterogeneous lesion termed BAC with several different designations. Pre-invasive lesions, AAH, and adenocarcinoma in situ (AIS), are typically pure ground glass lesions <5 mm and 3 cm, respectively, in size. Minimally invasive adenocarcinoma (MIA) is typically a partly solid lesion with an invasive component measuring <5 mm. Larger subsolid lesions with more extensive solid invasive tumor are now termed lepidic predominant adenocarcinoma (LPA). Invasive multifocal mucinous adenocarcinoma replaces the entity of multicentric BAC.

Lesions that are exclusively ground glass or have minimal solid components were observed to progress with a very slow growth rate. In one study, a comparison of mean volume doubling times in lung cancer patients with solid, partly solid, or pure ground glass neoplastic lesions demonstrated a stepwise increase in the CT-calculated volume-doubling times (853 vs. 457 vs. 158 days) [19]. Therefore, for a subsolid lesion suspected to reflect a neoplasm in the adenocarcinoma spectrum, the demonstration of a 2-year stability may not be enough to ensure its benign nature. In these cases, an initial follow-up examination at 3 months may be performed to determine whether the lesion has persisted and is inflammatory. Follow-up may then be performed at longer intervals (1–2 years). In these irregular, ill-defined lesions, it can be difficult to measure incremental size; thus, evaluation should include comparison of comparable contiguous thin-section images and a determination of whether the ground glass or solid component geographically extends around more vessels or airways. In this setting, CAD may be of assistance. Although the technology is evolving to evaluate ground glass lesions, it remains less reliable than in solid lesions. It is also important to note that the natural evolution of these lesions also includes transient reduction in size that may occur when there is histological alveolar collapse.

The definitive determination that a subsolid lesion is malignant can be problematic. A progressive increment in the overall size or in the size of the solid component strongly favors malignancy. PET/CT imaging in these cases may be non-contributory because these lesions often have low SUVmax activity. Additionally, the evaluation of predominantly ground glass lesions by CT-guided fine-needle aspiration or biopsy should be considered with great caution, as the results are vulnerable to significant sampling-error effects and likely to vary significantly from the ultimate excision specimen. The extent of invasive adenocarcinoma in particular can be significantly underestimated by percutaneous needle sampling, even if directed to the more solid components.

There is no consensus on the optimal management of patients with single subsolid lesions. Patients with lesions characterized by a higher ground glass percentage composition are less likely to have nodal disease and have a better prognosis than patients with nodules having a greater solid component, in which invasive adenocarcinoma likely predominates [20, 21]. Expanding on the interim guideline published in 2009, the Fleischner Society's definitive guidelines, published in 2013, have helped to homogenize practice [22, 23]. They address

Table 2. Fleischner guidelines for subsolid nodules

Characteristics	Imaging/Management
Solitary pure ground glass nodule, ≤5 mm	No follow-up
Multiple pure ground glass nodule, ≤5 mm	2- and 4-year follow-up
Solitary pure ground glass nodule, >5 mm	3 months (then at 1, 2, and 3 years)
Multiple pure ground glass nodule, one >5 mm	3 months (then at 1, 2, 3 years)
Solitary part solid	3 months (then biopsy/resect) <5 mm solid (1, 2, 3 years?)
Multiple part solid	3 months (then biopsy/resect) Treat dominant lesion(s)

imaging strategies for single and multiple ground glass lesions and indicate potential clinical diagnostic and management pathways (Table 2), including more aggressive surgical management when a lesion exceeds 1 cm overall or when there is a significant increase in its solid component. Conversely, according to the recent guidelines, pure ground glass lesions less than 5 mm in size do not require follow-up as these almost always reflect benign entities or atypical adenomatous hyperplasia. The management of patients with multiple lesions of varying density is more complex, especially as radiologically it is not always possible to determine the extent of neoplasia in multiple ground glass opacities. Current treatment strategies may include resection of the initial lesions followed by localized resection of progressive or recurrent lesions, although there are no standardized long-term data to support this approach.

Focal Parenchymal Airspace Disease

A multitude of etiologies underlie the development of focal air-space opacities. The majority of these will be multifocal and infective in nature. A distinction of predisposing etiologies is impossible unless there are uncommon specific features, e.g., the ground-glass halo typical of invasive aspergillosis. The differential diagnosis may be narrowed by referring to a combination of radiological features, chronicity, progression, response to treatment, and the immune status of the patient.

The presence of cavitation in airspace disease can be helpful, although the differential can again be broad, incorporating staphylococcal or gram-negative bacterial infections, mycobacterial disease, or fungal infection. Rounded pneumonia is more common in children but it also occurs in adults, usually due to *S. pneumoniae* infection. Appearances are mass-like, without air-bronchograms resulting from disease propagation through the collateral air-drift mechanisms of the pores of Kohn and the canals of Lambert. Focal consolidative opacity that is chronic may be characterized by minor volume loss and tractional bronchiectasis; these features are more common in patients with chronic eosinophilic lung disease or organizing pneumonia. While organizing pneumonia may also present with a "reverse halo" appearance, central ground glass opacities with peripheral consolidation, this appearance is not specific for the disease. Progressive focal airspace disease may reflect neoplastic disease, including bronchoalveolar cell carcinoma, lymphoma, or, occasionally, mucinous metastases from gastrointestinal primary tumors. Calcification may be present in mycobacterial disease and in some cases of amyloidosis.

References

1. Woodring JH, Fried AM, Chuang VP (1980) Solitary cavities of the lung: diagnostic implications of cavity wall thickness. AJR Am J Roentgenol 135:1269-1271.
2. Honda O, Tsubamoto M, Inoue A et al (2007) Pulmonary cavitary nodules on computed tomography: differentiation of malignancy and benignancy. J Comput Assist Tomogr 31:943-949.
3. Swensen SJ, Viggiano RW, Midthun DE et al (2000) Lung nodule enhancement at CT: multicenter study. Radiology 214:73-80.
4. Chae EJ, Song JW, Seo JB et al (2008) Clinical utility of dual-energy CT in the evaluation of solitary pulmonary nodules: initial experience. Radiology 249:671-681.
5. Swensen SJ, Jett JR, Hartman TE et al (2005) CT screening for lung cancer: five-year prospective experience. Radiology 235:259-265.
6. Piyavisetpat N, Aquino SL, Hahn PF et al (2005) Small incidental pulmonary nodules: how useful is short-term interval CT follow-up? J Thorac Imaging 20:5-9.
7. MacMahon H, Austin JH, Gamsu G et al (2005) Guidelines for management of small pulmonary nodules detected on CT scans: a statement from the Fleischner Society. Radiology 237:395-400.
8. Li F, Aoyama M, Shiraishi J et al (2004) Radiologists' performance for differentiating benign from malignant lung nodules on high-resolution CT using computer-estimated likelihood of malignancy. AJR Am J Roentgenol 183:1209-1215.
9. Yankelevitz DF, Reeves AP, Kostis WJ et al (2000) Small pulmonary nodules: volumetrically determined growth rates based on CT evaluation. Radiology 217:251-256.
10. Jennings SG, Winer-Muram HT, Tarver RD, Farber MO (2004) Lung tumor growth: assessment with CT—comparison of diameter and cross-sectional area with volume measurements. Radiology 231:866-871.
11. Jennings SG, Winer-Muram HT, Tann M et al (2006) Distribution of stage I lung cancer growth rates determined with serial volumetric CT measurements. Radiology 241:554-563.
12. Revel MP, Merlin A, Peyrard S et al (2006) Software volumetric evaluation of doubling times for differentiating benign versus malignant pulmonary nodules. AJR Am J Roentgenol 187:135-142.
13. Honda O, Kawai M, Gyobu, T et al (2009) Reproducibility of temporal volume change in CT of lung cancer: comparison of computer software and manual assessment. Br J Radiol 82:742-747.
14. Bolte H, Riedel C, Muller-Hulsbeck S et al (2007) Precision of computer-aided volumetry of artificial small solid pulmonary nodules in ex vivo porcine lungs. Br J Radiol 80:414-421.
15. Henschke CI, Yankelevitz DF, Mirtcheva R et al (2002) CT screening for lung cancer: frequency and significance of part-solid and nonsolid nodules. AJR Am J Roentgenol 178:1053-1057.
16. Austin JHM, Garg K, Aberle D et al (2013) Radiologic implications of the 2011 classification of adenocarcinoma of the lung. Radiology 266:62-71.
17. Aoki T, Nakata H, Watanabe H et al (2000) Evolution of peripheral lung adenocarcinomas: CT findings correlated with histology and tumor doubling time. AJR Am J Roentgenol 174:763-768.
18. Noguchi M, Morikawa A, Kawasaki M et al (1995) Small adenocarcinoma of the lung. Histologic characteristics and prognosis. Cancer 75:2844-2852.
19. Hasegawa M, Sone S, Takashima S et al (2000) Growth rate of small lung cancers detected on mass CT screening. Br J Radiol 73:1252-1259.
20. Kodama K, Higashiyama M, Yokouchi H et al (2001) Prognostic value of ground-glass opacity found in small lung adenocarcinoma on high-resolution CT scanning. Lung Cancer 33:17-25.
21. Higashiyama M, Kodama K, Yokouchi H et al (1999) Prognostic value of bronchiolo-alveolar carcinoma component of small lung adenocarcinoma. Ann Thorac Surg 68:2069-2073.
22. Godoy MC, Naidich DP (2009) Subsolid pulmonary nodules and the spectrum of peripheral adenocarcinomas of the lung: recommended interim guidelines for assessment and management. Radiology 253:606-622.
23. Naidich DP, Bankier AA, MacMahon H et al (2013) Recommendations for the management of subsolid pulmonary lesions detected at CT: a statement from the Fleischner Society. Radiology 266:304-317.

Approach to Imaging of Mediastinal Conditions in the Adult

Sanjeev Bhalla[1], José Caceres[2]

[1] Mallinckrodt Institute of Radiology, Washington University, St. Louis, MO, USA
[2] Centro Medico Teknon, Barcelona, Spain

Introduction

The mediastinum is an anatomic space defined by the thoracic inlet superiorly and the diaphragm inferiorly. It extends from the sternum to the vertebral bodies. Yet, despite its landmarks, there are no structures that completely separate the mediastinum from the neck above or the retroperitoneum below. Thus, imaging of the mediastinum and generating a relevant different diagnosis rest on the principles of localization and characterization.

Once a process or mass can be localized to the mediastinum, it should be further localized within the mediastinum. Many of us use an approach first championed by Ben Felson. Using a lateral radiograph or sagittal computed tomography (CT) or magnetic resonance (MR) image, a line is drawn from the anterior tracheal wall to the posterior inferior vena cava. This line separates the anterior mediastinum from the middle mediastinum. A second line is drawn 1 cm posterior to the anterior margin of the vertebral body. This line separates the middle from the posterior mediastinum. No anatomic structures actually divide the mediastinal compartments but this approach can be useful in creating concise, meaningful differential diagnoses. Keep in mind that certain processes may involve more than one compartment and that a large mass may be hard to localize.

After localization, cross-sectional imaging (either CT or MR) should be performed for lesion characterization. Knowing whether a lesion has a significant vascular, fluid, or fat component can be very helpful in suggesting a more specific diagnosis. Positron emission tomography (PET-CT) is used mainly to evaluate lymph node metastases in lung cancer, but it can also be used in the evaluation of solid mediastinal masses.

This approach to localization and characterization will provide the interpreting radiologist with a solid foundation in mediastinal imaging.

Anterior Mediastinum

Most anterior mediastinal masses are thymic in origin. Even lymphomas and germ cell tumors tend to arise in cells within the thymus. A useful differential diagnosis should be based on patient age, as germ cell tumors are almost unheard of in individuals older than 45 years. Most anterior mediastinal massed tend to be lymphomas, germ cell tumors, or thymomas. Many texts will include thyroid goiter in the list of anterior mediastinal lesions. However, we have found that most goiters tend to extend into the middle mediastinum.

Observing fluid-attenuation or intensity can be very helpful in approaching anterior mediastinal masses. Pure cystic lesions are benign (usually thymic or pericardial cysts). As the amount of soft tissue within the lesion increases, one should consider the increased likelihood of a malignancy. Both lymphoma and cystic thymoma may have small areas of fluid, but these are far outweighed by the soft tissue elements. Germ cell tumors also follow this rule. The classic teaching is that the germ cell tumor have an attenuation like that of fat. Many teratomas do contain some fat elements, but almost all are cystic. As with the other lesions, if the soft tissue elements dominate, then a malignant germ cell tumor should be favored, such as seminoma. Interestingly, malignant germ cell tumors are quite rare in female patients.

Visualization of fat intensity or attenuation can also be very helpful (Fig. 1). In the anterior mediastinum, most fatty masses are benign. As described above, an anterior mediastinal mass with fat and fluid suggests a teratoma (benign germ cell tumor). If the mass is purely fat, it may be the very rare thymolipoma, but more likely it will be a fat pad or anterior hernia (Morgagni hernia). In our practices, patients with infarction of a pericardial fat pad or fat within the Morgagni hernia may present with chest pain. In the era of the frequent use of CT in the evaluation of potential pulmonary embolism or dissection, these areas of fat necrosis can simulate a neoplasm. Awareness of this potential pitfall will allow the patients to be treated appropriately.

Diseases of the Chest and Heart 2015-2018,
DOI: 10.1007/978-88-470-5752-4_3 © Springer-Verlag Italia 2015

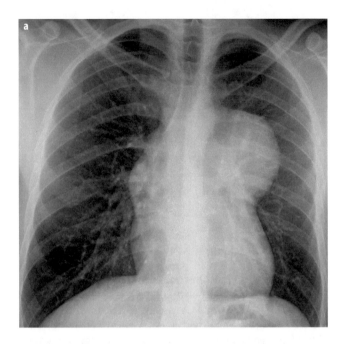

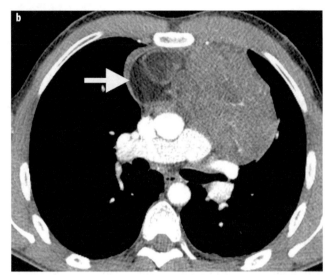

Fig. 1 a, b. Teratoma. Posteroanterior chest X-ray shows a left anterior mediastinal mass (**a**). Axial CT demonstrates a large soft-tissue mass with a fat component (**b**, *arrow*)

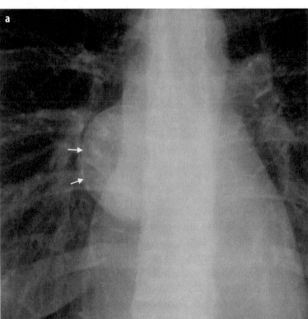

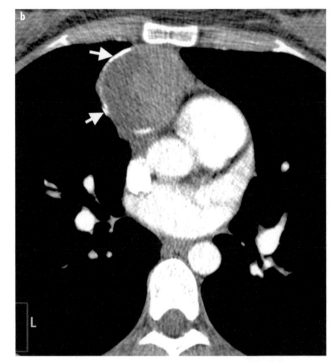

Fig. 2 a, b. Thymoma. Peripheral calcification is visible in the chest radiograph (**a**, *arrows*), confirmed with CT (**b**, *arrows*)

The incidence of calcification in thymomas varies from 10% to 40%. Circular peripheral calcification may occur in solid thymomas, simulating a cyst (Fig. 2). Teratomas contain calcium in about 35% of cases. Untreated lymphomas do not calcify and about 5% of them show calcifications after radiation therapy.

Vascular or hyperenhancing lesions may present within the anterior mediastinum. Occasionally, coronary or bypass aneurysms can simulate an anterior mediastinal mass. The key is to think about this potential, especially when a patient with median sternotomy wires presents for imaging.

Middle Mediastinum

Most middle mediastinal masses represent lymphadenopathy, foregut duplication cysts, vascular lesion, or esophageal processes. They usually present with right paratracheal widening on a frontal chest radiograph or, occasionally, the doughnut sign on a lateral examination. As with anterior mediastinal conditions, an assessment of attenuation or intensity can be helpful.

If the mass is fluid in character, the middle mediastinal mass most likely represents a foregut duplication cyst

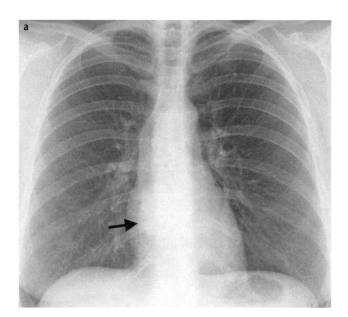 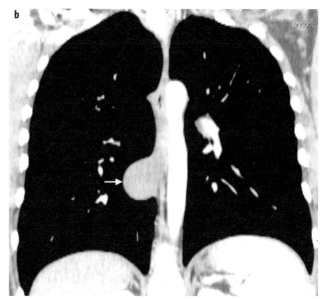

Fig. 3 a, b. Asymptomatic bronchogenic cyst. The cyst was discovered on the chest radiograph (**a**, *arrow*) and confirmed with CT (**b**, *arrow*). Note the high attenuation, similar to that of the soft tissue

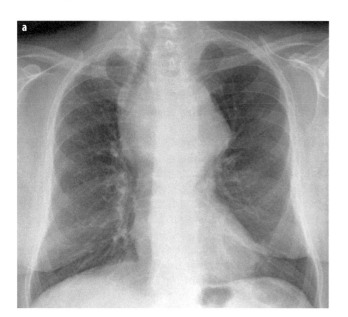 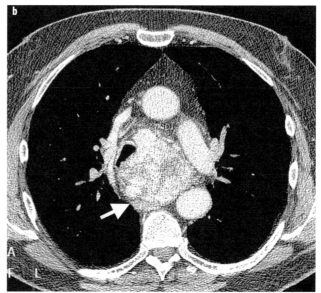

Fig. 4 a, b. Large endothoracic goiter. There is with marked tracheal displacement in the chest radiograph (**a**). Axial CT shows marked contrast enhancement of the thyroid tissue (**b**, *arrow*)

(either bronchogenic or esophageal). These cysts occasionally are higher in attenuation as a result of infection or hemorrhage (Fig. 3) and may even contain a fluid-calcium level from the milk of calcium. The risk of malignancy in these conditions tends to be low. As with anterior mediastinal lesions, the ratio of soft tissue to fluid needs to be considered. A foregut duplication cyst should have no soft tissue, enhancing element. If soft tissue is encountered, one must consider a potentially more significant process, usually low-attenuating lymphadenopathy. Such low-attenuating lymph nodes may be encountered in lung cancer, mucinous neoplasms, and mycobacterial disease.

Unlike the anterior mediastinum, fat in a middle mediastinal lesion cannot be considered benign. Although esophageal or tracheal lipomas and esophageal fibrovascular polyps contain fat, so may mediastinal liposarcomas. These rare lesions may insinuate through the mediastinum and often have a predilection for the middle mediastinum.

Hypervascular lesions in the middle mediastinum are most often hypervascular lymph nodes and intrathoracic extension of a goiter (Fig. 4). These hypervascular nodes (defined as higher in attenuation than skeletal muscle) may be seen with melanoma, plasmacytoma, Castleman's disease, Kaposi sarcoma, sarcomas, and thyroid and renal

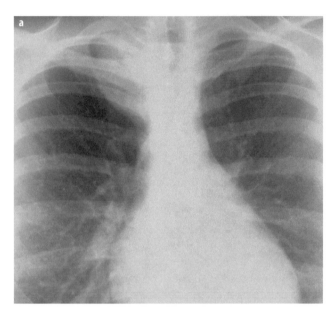 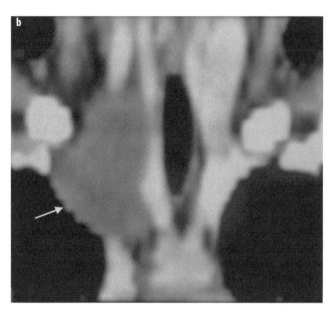

Fig. 5 a, b. Ganglioneuroma. The lesion, visible as a mass in the right apex (**a**), was confirmed with enhanced CT (**b**, *arrow*). Note the low CT density, which may create confusion with a cystic mass

cell cancers. When the high attenuating structure is tubular, a vessel must be considered. Aortic arch anomalies and azygos vein enlargement often present as a middle mediastinal mass on radiography.

Most mediastinal lymphadenopathy will present in the middle mediastinum. Occasionally, these nodes will be calcified. These calcified nodes are usually indicative of an old granulomatous process, such as healed tuberculosis or histoplasmosis or sarcoidosis, but care must be taken to remember that certain tumors also tend to present with calcified mediastinal lymph nodes, including ovarian serous adenocarcinomas, mucinous colon neoplasms, and osteosarcomas.

Another potential for a perceived middle mediastinal mass on radiography will be a dilated esophagus. Although a distal mass may also result in esophageal dilatation, it is usually only achalasia that results in esophageal widening that can be seen on a chest radiograph.

Posterior Mediastinum

A vast majority of posterior mediastinal masses will be neurogenic in origin. In adults, these tend to be benign nerve sheath tumors, usually schwannomas and neurofibromas. In children and younger adults, they tend to be sympathetic ganglion in origin, such as ganglioneuroblastoma, neuroblastoma, or ganglioneuroma. The key in separating the two groups is to assess the overall shape, comparing the z-axis to the xy-axis. Nerve sheath tumors tend to be spherical (equal in all 3 axes), while the ganglion lesions are longer in the z-axis and are more cylindrical. Osseous lesions represent the second most common group of posterior mediastinal disease. Although

metastases are often considered, one cannot forget about diskitis/osteomyelitis. This latter condition can present as insidious back pain and can easily be overlooked.

As with the other compartments, attenuation or intensity can be helpful. On CT, a potential pitfall is that myelin-rich neurogenic lesions may look cystic (Fig. 5). For this reason, with posterior mediastinal lesions we often rely on MR imaging. True posterior mediastinal cystic lesions are rare. Although neuroenteric cysts exist, they are often associated with vertebral anomalies and rarely encountered de novo in adults. Instead, a cystic lesion in the posterior mediastinum is much more likely to represent a lateral meningocele or post-traumatic nerve root avulsion.

Fatty lesions are unusual in the posterior mediastinum but when encountered may invoke extramedullary hematopoiesis. While rare, in patients with anemia, extramedullary hematopoiesis may develop in the posterior mediastinum. The etiology of this condition remains unknown. Some authors have postulated that it develops from extruded marrow while others have suggested that it develops from totipotent cells in the paravertebral space. When the patient is anemic, extramedullary hematopoiesis will present with bilateral masses that enhance similar to spleen without a connecting bridge. As the patient returns to normal hematocrit, the yellow marrow will take over. The net effect is bilateral posterior mediastinal fatty masses. In the elderly, Bochdalek hernias should be included in the differential diagnosis (Fig. 6).

Hypervascular lesions in the posterior mediastinum are less helpful than with the other compartments. Most often these are related to an aneurysmal aorta or enlarged collateral vessels as with aortic coarctation. As described above, extramedullary hematopoiesis may be seen with bilateral hypervascular paravertebral masses.

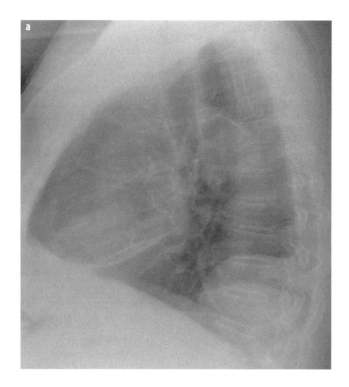 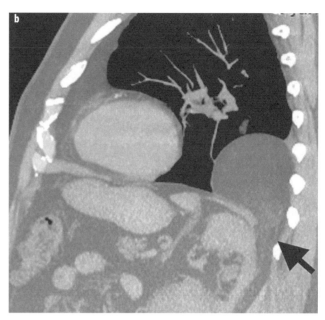

Fig. 6 a, b. Bochdalek hernia. Lateral chest radiograph shows a large posterior mediastinal mass (**a**). Sagittal CT demonstrates abdominal fat herniating through a posterior diaphragmatic defect (**b**, *arrow*)

Table 1. Mediastinal masses based on location and characteristics

Mediastinal compartment	Most common	Fluid	Fat	Hypervascular
Anterior	Thymoma Lymphoma Germ cell tumor	Thymic cyst Pericardial cyst Lymphoma	Teratoma Thymolipoma Fat pad Morgagni hernia	Heart Coronary arteries Ascending aorta
Middle	Lymphadenopathy Duplication cyst Vascular anomaly	Duplication cyst Lymphadenopathy	Lipoma Liposarcoma Fibrovascular polyp Hiatal hernia	Arch anomaly Azygos vein Lymph nodes Goiter
Posterior	Neurogenic Osseous metastases Diskitis	Neuroenteric cyst Lateral meningocoele Traumatic	Extramedullary hematopoiesis Bochdalek hernia	Aorta or collaterals
More than 1	Infection Hematoma Lung cancer	Lymphangioma	Liposarcoma Lipomatosis	Hemangioma

Conditions That Disregard the Compartment Model

Certain conditions tend to disregard the compartment model of the mediastinum. Even with these lesions, understanding the attenuation or intensity can be helpful. These include infection and hematoma, which will result in fat stranding and soft tissue attenuation throughout the mediastinum, often in more than one compartment.

Lymphangiomas and hemangiomas also tend to disregard the compartment model. The former tend to be fluid in their attenuation and insinuate throughout, while the latter will be higher in attenuation.

Of course, lung cancer may present with metastases to any compartment and, unfortunately, tends to metastasize to more than one region.

Conclusion

The mediastinum represents a space that may be impacted by a large number of lesions. Having an approach based on location and characterization will allow the radiologist the ability to create a useful, targeted differential diagnosis (Table 1).

Suggested Reading

Adam A, Hochholzer L (1981) Ganglioneuroblastoma of the posterior mediastinum: a clinicopathologic review of 80 cases. Cancer 47:373-381.

Baron RL, Sagel SS, Baglan RJ (1981) Thymic cysts following radiation therapy for Hodgkin disease. Radiology 141:593-597.

Chen JL, Weisbrod GL, Herman SJ (1988) Computed tomography and pathologic correlations of thymic lesions. J Thorac Imaging 3:61-65.

Cohen AJ, Thompson LN, Edwards FH et al (1991) Primary cysts and tumours of the mediastinum. Ann Thorac Surg 51:378-386.

Do YS, Im JG, Lee BH et al (1995) CT findings in malignant tumors of thymic epithelium. J Comput Assist Tomogr 19:192-197.

Erasmus JJ, McAdams HP, Donnelly LF, Spritzer CE (2000) MR imaging of mediastinal masses. Magn Reson Imaging Clin North Am 8:59-89.

Faul JL, Berry GJ, Colby TV et al (2000) Thoracic lymphangiomas, lymphangiectasis, lymphangiomatosis, and lymphatic dysplasia syndrome. Am J Respir Crit Care Med 161:1037-1046.

Gaerte SC, Meyer CA, Winer-Muram HT et al (2002) Fat-containing lesions of the chest. RadioGraphics 22:615-678.

Hoffman OA, Gillespie DJ, Aughenbaugh GL, Brown LR (1993) Primary mediastinal neoplasms (other than thymoma). Mayo Clin Proc 68:880-891.

Jeung M-Y, Gasser B, Gangi A et al (2002) Imaging of cystic masses of the mediastinum. RadioGraphics 22:S79-S93.

Jolles H, Henry DA, Roberson JP et al (1996) Mediastinitis following median sternotomy: CT findings. Radiology 201:463-466.

Knapp RH, Hurt RD, Payne WS et al (1985) Malignant germ cell tumors of the mediastinum. J Thorac Cardiovasc Surg 89:82-89.

Long JA Jr, Doppman JL, Nienhuis AW (1980) Computed tomographic studies of thoracic extramedullary hematopoiesis. J Comput Assist Tomogr 4:67-70.

Marano R, Liguori C, Savino G et al (2011) Cardiac silhouette findings and mediastinal lines and stripes radiograph and CT scan correlation. Chest 139:1186-1196.

McAdams HP, Rosado-de-Christenson M, Fishback NF, Templeton PA (1998) Castleman disease of the thorax: radiologic features with clinical and histopathologic correlation. Radiology 209:221-228.

Miles J, Pennybacker J, Sheldon P (1969) Intrathoracic meningocele. Its development and association with neurofibromatosis. J Neurol Neurosurg Psychiatry 32:99-110.

Miyake H, Shiga M, Takaki H et al (1996) Mediastinal lymphangiomas in adults: CT findings. J Thorac Imaging 11:83-85.

Moeller KH, Rosado-de-Christenson ML, Templeton PA (1997) Mediastinal mature teratoma: imaging features. AJR Am J Roentgenol 169:985-990.

Moran CA, Suster S (1997) Primary germ cell tumors of the mediastinum: I. Analysis of 322 cases with special emphasis on teratomatous lesions and a proposal for histopathologic classification and clinical staging. Cancer 80:681-690.

Nakata H, Nakayama C, Kimoto T et al (1982) Computed tomography of mediastinal bronchogenic cysts. J Comput Assist Tomogr 6:733-738.

Pombo F, Rodriguez E, Mato J et al (1992) Patterns of contrast enhancement of tuberculous lymph nodes demonstrated by computed tomography. Clin Radiol 46:13-17.

Rosado-de-Christenson ML, Galobardes J, Moran CA (1992) Thymoma: radiologic-pathologic correlation. RadioGraphics 12:151-168.

Rosado-de-Christenson ML, Pugatch RD, Moran CA, Galobardes J (1994) Thymolipoma: analysis of 27 cases. Radiology 193:121-126.

Rosado-de-Christenson ML, Templeton PA, Moran CA (1992) From the archives of the AFIP. Mediastinal germ cell tumors: radiologic and pathologic correlation. RadioGraphics 12:1013-1030.

Rossi SE, McAdams HP, Rosado-de-Christenson ML et al (2001) Fibrosing mediastinitis. RadioGraphics 21:737-757.

Shaffer K, Rosado-de-Christenson ML, Patz EF Jr et al (1994) Thoracic lymphangioma in adults: CT and MR imaging features. AJR Am J Roentgenol 162:283-289.

Spizarny DL, Rebner M, Gross BH (1987) CT evaluation of enhancing mediastinal masses. J Comput Assist Tomogr 11:990-993.

Strollo DC, Rosado-de-Christenson ML (1999) Tumors of the thymus. J Thorac Imaging 14:152-171.

Strollo DC, Rosado de Christenson ML, Jett JR (1997) Primary mediastinal tumors. Part 1: tumours of the anterior mediastinum. Chest 112:511-522.

Strollo DC, Rosado-de-Christenson ML, Jett JR (1997) Primary mediastinal tumors: part II. Tumours of the middle and posterior mediastinum. Chest 112:1344-1357.

Suwatanapongched T, Gierada DS (2006) CT of thoracic lymph nodes. Part II: diseases and pitfalls. Br J Radiol 79:999-1006.

Takahashi K, Al-Janabi NJ (2010) Computed tomography and magnetic resonance imaging of mediastinal tumors. J Magn Reson Imaging 32:1325-1339.

Whitten CR, Khan S, Munneke GJ, Grubnic S (2007) A diagnostic approach to mediastinal abnormalities. RadioGraphics 27:657-671.

Woodring JH, Loh FK, Kryscio RJ (1984) Mediastinal hemorrhage: an evaluation of radiographic manifestations. Radiology 151:15-21.

Zylak CJ, Eyler WR, Spizarny DL, Stone CH (2002) Developmental lung anomalies in the adult: radiologic-pathologic correlation. RadioGraphics 22:S25-S43.

Zylak CJ, Pallie W, Jackson R (1982) Correlative anatomy and computed tomography: a module on the mediastinum. RadioGraphics 2:555-592.

Current Approaches to Chronic and Acute Airway Diseases

Philippe A. Grenier[1], Jeffrey P. Kanne[2]

[1] University Pierre & Marie Curie, Hospital Pitié-Salpetrière, Paris, France
[2] University Of Wisconsin School Of Medicine and Public Health, Madison, WI, USA

Introduction

Volumetric multidetector computed tomography (MD-CT) using thin collimation during a single breath hold has become the ideal imaging technique for assessing airway diseases. Volumetric high-resolution data sets provide precise morphologic evaluation of both proximal and distal airways.

The different CT patterns of airways diseases and their main causes are reported in Tables 1–5. The different diseases affecting the airways that are presented in this chapter include neoplastic and non-neoplastic tracheobronchial diseases, bronchiectasis and small airway diseases, asthma, and chronic obstructive pulmonary disease (COPD).

Table 1. Luminal filling defect

- Benign tracheobronchial neoplasm
- Malignant primary tracheobronchial neoplasm
- Metastasis
- Mucus secretions
- Foreign body
- Broncholithiasis

Table 2. Multinodular appearance of the inner surface of the airway

- Granulomatosis with polyangiitis
- Tracheobronchial metastases (hematogeneous spread)
- Respiratory papillomatosis
- Adenoid cystic carcinoma (multicentric)
- Tracheobronchial amyloidosis
- Tracheobronchopathia osteochondroplastica

Table 3. Focal tracheobronchial narrowing

- Post-traumatic strictures
- Post-infectious stenoses (e.g. tuberculosis)
- Tracheobronchial neoplasms (primary and secondary malignant)
- Granulomatosis with polyangiitis
- Sarcoidosis
- Inflammatory bowel disease
- Extrinsic compression

Table 4. Diffuse tracheobronchial wall thickening

- Infectious tracheobronchitis (TB, aspergillosis)
- Relapsing polychondritis[a]
- Tracheobronchial amyloidosis
- Tracheobronchopathia osteochrondroplastica
- Tracheobronchitis associated with ulcerative colitis

[a] Calcific deposits

Table 5. Tracheobronchial dehiscence, fistulas, and diverticula

- Tracheal or bronchial rupture
- Bronchial dehiscence occurring after lung transplantation
- Tracheal diverticula (tracheocele)
- Accessory cardiac bronchus
- Multiple tracheobronchial diverticula (COPD)
- Nodobronchial and nodobronchoesophageal fistulas
- Tracheoesophageal fistulas
- Bronchopleural fistulas

CT Acquisition and Post-processing Techniques [1,2]

MDCT acquisition is performed through the entirety of the lungs at full suspended inspiration, using thin collimation (0.6–1.5 mm) without the administration of contrast material. Axial images are reconstructed with thin slice thickness (0.8–1.5 mm) and overlap (50% is ideal). Complementary MDCT acquisition at full continuous forced expiration using a reduced technique (120 Kv; 20–40 mA) is often recommended and is particularly useful for assessing tracheobronchial collapsibility and expiratory air trapping.

The images are best interpreted on a PACS workstation. Evaluation of the overlapped thin-section axial images in cine-mode allows the bronchial divisions to be easily followed, from the carina to the smallest peripheral bronchi visible on CT. Real-time manipulation of the data set allows the radiologist to select the optimal plane to better depict the distribution and extent of airway abnormalities. Furthermore, multiplanar reformations using minimum and maximum intensity projections can be

Diseases of the Chest and Heart 2015-2018,
DOI: 10.1007/978-88-470-5752-4_4 © Springer-Verlag Italia 2015

helpful to display airway abnormalities. Minimum intensity projections can highlight airway dilation, diverticula, and fistulas, as well as the extent of expiratory air trapping and emphysema. Maximum intensity projections accentuate foci of mucoid impaction and small centrilobular nodules and tree-in-bud opacities.

Volume-rendering techniques (CT bronchography) consist of segmentation of the lumen-wall interface of the airways. This technique has proven to be of particular interest in diagnosing mild changes in airway caliber and understanding complex tracheobronchial abnormalities. Virtual bronchoscopy provides an internal rendering of the tracheobronchial inner surface. It is used to detect mucosal nodularity indicative of granulomatous or tumoral lesions in proximal airways.

Tracheobronchial Tumors

MDCT plays a key role in depicting tumors of the tracheobronchial tree [3-5] and in assessing their extent within the lumen, airway wall, and surrounding structures before treatment planning. Airway lesions >5 mm are usually detected on CT because of the natural contrast between luminal air and soft-tissue attenuation of the lesions.

Primary Malignant Tumors

Compared to laryngeal or bronchial cancers, primary malignant tumors are rare in the trachea. The most frequent histological types are squamous cell carcinoma and adenoid cystic carcinoma, accounting for nearly 80% of all tracheal neoplasms.

Adenoid cystic carcinoma (sialadenoid tumor) is a low-grade malignancy that is not associated with cigarette smoking. It occurs in patients in their forties without any sex predilection. In the central airways, adenoid cystic carcinoma has a propensity to infiltrate the wall of the airways, with submucosal extension manifesting as a sessile, polypoid, annular, or diffuse infiltration. The inner surface is smooth and regular. Extraluminal growth, visible on CT scan, is a common feature.

Squamous cell carcinoma is the most common primary malignancy of the trachea and primarily occurs in older men with a history of cigarette smoking. On CT, the tumor appears as a polypoid intraluminal mass or as an eccentric irregular wall thickening with an irregular surface. The tumor has a tendency to spread to adjacent mediastinal lymph nodes and to directly invade the mediastinum.

Carcinoid tumor is a low-grade malignant neuroendocrine neoplasm representing 1–2% of primary lung tumors. It appears on CT scan as a well-circumscribed polypoid mass that protrudes into the airway lumen, usually located in a main or lobar bronchus. Segmental or lobar atelectasis and obstructive pneumonitis, as well as foci of calcification, are present in 30% of cases.

Marked homogeneous early contrast enhancement of an endobronchial nodule reflects the high vascularity of this tumor.

Mucoepidermoid carcinoma is a rare tumor that originates from the minor salivary glands lining the tracheobronchial tree. It occurs in young patients (<40 years-old) and mainly involves the segmental bronchi, resulting in airway obstruction. The typical CT appearance is a smooth, ovoid, or lobulated endobronchial mass with occasional punctuate calcifications and variable contrast enhancement.

Lymphoma of the trachea is rare and is usually related to mucosa-associated lymphoid tissue. The CT appearance is non-specific.

Secondary Tracheobronchial Malignancy

Direct invasion of the central airways by neoplasms of the thyroid, esophagus, lung, and larynx is much more common than hematogeneous metastases. CT demonstrates the primary neoplasm and its extension by contiguity within the main airways (endoluminal mass, destruction of cartilage, and tracheo-bronchial-esophageal fistula).

Many cancers have the potential to metastasize to the trachea and bronchi. Endotracheal or endobronchial metastases appear as endotracheal nodules or an eccentric thickening of the airway wall or as soft-tissue attenuation with contrast enhancement.

Benign Tracheobronchial Neoplasms

Benign tracheal neoplasms are rare, accounting for <2% of lung neoplasms. On CT, they present as endoluminal masses confined within the tracheobronchial lumen without evidence of involvement of surrounding structures. Benign neoplasms are typically sharply marginated, round, and <2 cm in diameter. Because they originate in the mucosa or submucosa, the overlying epithelium is usually intact, resulting in a smooth appearance of the tumor surface in the airway lumen.

Histology includes mainly hamartomas, lipomas, leiomyomas, fibromas, chondromas, and schwannomas. Endobronchial harmartomas account for 30% of intrathoracic hamartomas. The presence of fat with or without calcification is diagnostic.

Respiratory papillomatosis (laryngotracheobronchial papillomatosis) is a neoplastic disease caused by human papillomavirus infection transmitted from mother to child at birth or acquired from orogenital contact. Papillomas arise in the larynx and involve the trachea and proximal bronchi in up to 50% of cases. Involvement of the lungs is rare, occurring in <1% of patients, and manifests on imaging studies as multiple lung nodules and cavitary and cystic lesions in the parenchyma. Malignant transformation into squamous cell carcinoma is a rare but serious complication of respiratory papillomatosis.

Non-neoplastic Tracheobronchial Disorders [3, 6, 7]

Post-traumatic Stenoses

Post-traumatic strictures of the trachea are usually the result of ischemic injury from a cuffed endotracheal or tracheostomy tube or extrinsic neck trauma. These injuries initially heal by the formation of granulation tissue, with subsequent scarring characterized by dense mucosal and submucosal fibrosis associated with distortion of cartilage plates. The two principal sites of stenosis following intubation or tracheostomy tube are at the stoma or at the level of the endotracheal or tracheostomy tube balloon. CT with multiplanar reformations clearly depicts the severity and length of the stricture. Post-intubation stenosis extends for several centimeters and typically involves the trachea above the level of the thoracic inlet. Post-tracheostomy stenosis typically begins 1.0–1.5 cm distal to the inferior margin of the tracheostomy stoma and extends over 1.5–2.5 cm. These strictures typically have an hourglass configuration with a thickened tracheal wall. Less commonly, tracheal or bronchial stenosis may present as a thin membrane or granulation tissue protruding into the airway lumen. In select cases, the degree of stenosis may also be assessed by virtual bronchoscopy.

Infections

A number of infections, both acute but more often chronic, may affect the trachea and proximal bronchi, resulting in both focal and diffuse airway disease. Subsequent fibrosis can lead to localized airway narrowing. The most common causes of infectious tracheobronchitis are acute bacterial tracheitis in immunocompromised patients, tuberculosis, rhinoscleroma (*Klebsiella rhinoscleromatis*), and necrotizing invasive aspergillosis. CT clearly demonstrates the extent of irregular and circumferential tracheobronchial narrowing. In some patients an accompanying mediastinitis is evident, manifesting as infiltration of mediastinal fat. With active infection, the narrowed trachea and frequently one or more main bronchi have an irregularly thickened wall. In the fibrotic or healed phase, the airway is narrowed but the wall is smooth and of normal thickness. Occasionally, because of the presence of chronic fibrous or granulomatous hilitis/mediastinitis, tuberculosis of the trachea and/or proximal bronchi may mimic airway malignancy on CT.

Granulomatosis with Polyangiitis (Wegener Granulomatosis)

Involvement of the large airways is a common manifestation of granulomatosis with polyangiitis. Inflammatory lesions may be present with or without subglottic or bronchial stenosis, ulcerations, and pseudotumors. Radiologic manifestations include thickening of the subglottic and proximal trachea, with a smooth symmetric or asymmetric narrowing over variable length. Tracheal rings can become thickened and calcified. Cartilaginous erosions and ulcerations also may be seen. Stenosis may be present in any main, lobar, or segmental bronchus. Developing nodular or polypoid lesions can protrude into the airway lumen.

Relapsing Polychondritis

Relapsing polychondritis is a rare systemic autoimmune disease that affects cartilage at various sites, including the ears, nose, joints, and tracheobronchial tree. Histologically, the acute inflammatory infiltrate in both cartilage and perichondrial tissue induces progressive dissolution and fragmentation of the cartilage followed by fibrosis. Symmetric subglottic stenosis is the most frequent manifestation in the chest. As the disease progresses, the distal trachea and bronchi may be involved. CT scans show a smooth thickening of the airway wall associated with diffuse narrowing. In the early stages of the disease, the posterior wall of the trachea is spared but in advanced disease, circumferential wall thickening can occur. Trachcobronchomalacia can develop as a result of weakening of cartilage, resulting in considerable luminal collapse on expiration. Gross destruction of the cartilaginous rings with fibrosis may cause stenosis.

Amyloidosis

Amyloid deposition in the trachea and bronchi may occur in association with systemic amyloidosis or as an isolated process. The deposits can present as single, multifocal, or diffuse submucosal plaques or masses. The overlying mucosa is usually intact. Dystrophic calcification or ossification is frequently present. CT scans show focal or, more commonly, diffuse thickening of the airway wall and narrowing of the lumen. Calcification may be present. Narrowing of the proximal bronchi can lead to distal atelectasis, bronchiectasis, or both, with or without obstructive pneumonia.

Tracheobronchopathia Osteochondroplastica

This rare disorder is characterized by the presence of multiple cartilaginous nodules and bony submucosal nodules on the luminal surface of the trachea and proximal airways. Tracheobronchopathia osteochondroplastica involves males more frequently than females, and most patients are older than 50 years. Histologically, the nodules contain heterotopic bone, cartilage, and calcified acellular protein matrix. The overlying bronchial mucosa is normal, and, because it contains no cartilage, the posterior wall of the trachea is spared. On CT, tracheal cartilages are thickened and show irregular calcifications. The nodules may protrude from the anterior and lateral walls into the lumen; they usually show foci of calcification. The majority of patients are asymptomatic, with only a small number developing obstructive signs and symptoms.

Saber-sheath Trachea

Saber-sheath trachea is characterized by narrowing of the transverse diameter and an increase in the sagittal diameter of the intrathoracic trachea. It is almost always associated with COPD. The pathogenesis is unclear but is likely related to the altered mechanics resulting from the intrathoracic pressure changes associated with COPD. On radiographs and CT, the internal transverse diameter of the trachea is decreased to half or less than the corresponding sagittal diameter. The narrowing usually affects the whole intrathoracic trachea, with an abrupt return to normal caliber at the thoracic inlet. The trachea most often shows a smooth inner margin but occasionally has a nodular contour. Calcification of the tracheal cartilage is common.

Tracheobronchomegaly (Mounier-Kuhn Syndrome)

Tracheobronchomegaly is characterized by the abnormal dilation of the trachea and main bronchi and a recurrent lower respiratory tract infection. The etiology is not fully understood, but many patients have congenitally atrophic smooth muscle and elastin fibers. Mounier-Kuhn syndrome is often associated with tracheal diverticulosis and bronchiectasis. The diagnosis is based on radiologic findings. The immediately subglottic trachea typically has a normal diameter, but the tracheal diameter expands toward the carina, often involving the central bronchi. Prolapse of the atrophic mucosa between cartilage rings gives the trachea a characteristically corrugated appearance. The corrugations may become exaggerated to form sacculations or diverticula. On CT, a tracheal diameter of >3 cm (measured 2 cm above the aortic arch) and a diameter for the right and left bronchi of 2.4 cm and 2.3 cm, respectively, are diagnosing criteria. Additional findings include tracheal scalloping or diverticula (especially along the posterior membranous tracheal wall).

Tracheobronchomalacia

Tracheobronchomalacia [8, 9] is characterized by weakened tracheal cartilages and occurs in association with a number of disorders, including tracheobronchomegaly, COPD, diffuse tracheal inflammation such as relapsing polychondritis, as well as following trauma.

Dynamic expiratory multislice CT may offer a feasible alternative to bronchoscopy in patients with suspected tracheobronchomalacia. It may show complete collapse or collapse of >80% of the airway lumen. Involvement of the central tracheobronchial tree may be diffuse or focal. On expiration, the airway may have an oval or crescent shape. The crescent form is due to bowing of the posterior membranous trachea. The increased compliance reflects the loss of integrity of the wall's structural components and is particularly associated with damaged or destroyed cartilages. The coronal di-

ameter of the trachea becomes significantly larger than the sagittal one, producing a lunate configuration to the trachea.

Broncholithiasis

This rare condition is characterized by erosion into or distortion of a bronchus from an adjacent calcified lymph node. The underlying abnormality is usually granulomatous lymphadenitis caused by *Mycobacterium tuberculosis* or fungi such as *Histoplasma capsulatum*. A few cases associated with silicosis have been reported. Calcified material in the bronchial lumen or bronchial distortion results in airway obstruction, leading to collapse, obstructive pneumonitis, mucoid impaction, or bronchiectasis. Symptoms include cough, hemoptysis, and recurrent episodes of fever and purulent sputum production. Occasionally, patients will expectorate calcific fragments (lithoptysis). Broncholithiasis is recognized on CT by the presence of a calcified endobronchial or peribronchial lymph node, associated with bronchopulmonary complications related to obstruction in the absence of an associated soft-tissue mass.

Tracheobronchial Fistula and Dehiscence [2, 3]

Multidetector MDCT with thin collimation is the most accurate technique to identify peripheral bronchopleural fistulas, which are most commonly caused by necrotizing pneumonia or trauma. Nodobronchial and nodobronchoesophageal fistulas are characterized by the presence of gas in cavitated hilar or mediastinal lymph nodes adjacent to the airways and are usually the result of tuberculosis. Occasionally, congenital tracheal diverticula and tracheobronchoesophageal fistulas, especially the H-type, may not present until adulthood.

Malignant neoplasms, particularly esophageal, are the most common cause of tracheoesophageal fistula in adults. Infection and trauma are the most frequent nonmalignant causes.

MDCT has a high degree of sensitivity and specificity for depicting bronchial dehiscence occurring after lung transplantation. Bronchial dehiscence is seen as a bronchial wall defect at the anastomosis, associated with extraluminal gas collections.

The cardiac bronchus is an uncommon airway anomaly characterized by a supernumerary bronchus arising from the inferomedial aspect of the mid bronchus intermedius. The cardiac bronchus typically is a blind-ending pouch but occasionally supplies a very small number of pulmonary lobules. Most cardiac bronchi are clinically silent and thus are incidentally detected on chest CT. However, they may serve as a reservoir for retained secretions, leading to chronic inflammation and hypervascularity and thus to recurrent episodes of infection or hemoptysis. Importantly, a cardiac bronchus should not be mistaken for a bronchial fistula or tear.

Bronchiectasis

Bronchiectasis [3, 10-12] is a chronic condition characterized by local, irreversible dilation of bronchi, usually associated with inflammation. Despite the decreased prevalence of bronchiectasis in developed countries, it remains an important cause of hemoptysis and chronic sputum production. Among the many causes of bronchiectasis, there are three main underlying mechanisms: bronchial obstruction, bronchial wall damage, and parenchymal fibrosis. With the first two mechanisms, the combination of mucus plugging and bacterial colonization lead to a vicious cycle of progressive airway-wall damage, as a result of cytokine and enzyme release by inflammatory cells in addition to toxin secretion by bacteria. With parenchymal fibrosis, dilation of bronchi, termed traction bronchiectasis, occurs by the maturation and retraction of fibrous tissue formed in the parenchyma adjacent to an airway.

Pathology

Pathologically, bronchiectasis is classified into three subtypes, reflecting the increasing severity of the disease: (1) cylindrical, characterized by relatively uniform airway dilation; (2) varicose, characterized by non-uniform and somewhat serpentine dilation; and (3) cystic. As bronchiectasis progresses, the lung parenchyma distal to the affected airway shows increasing collapse.

CT Findings

The CT findings of bronchial dilation include lack of tapering of the bronchial lumina (the cardinal sign of bronchiectasis), an internal diameter of the bronchi greater than that of the adjacent pulmonary artery ("signet ring sign"), bronchi visible within 1 cm of the costal pleura or abutting the mediastinal pleura, and mucus-filled dilated bronchi. With varicose bronchiectasis, the bronchial lumen assumes a beaded configuration. Cystic bronchiectasis appears as a string of cysts caused by irregular dilated bronchi along their lengths, or a cluster of cysts, caused by multiple dilated bronchi lying adjacent to each other. Clusters of cysts are most commonly seen in an atelectatic lobe. Fluid levels, caused by retained secretions, may be present in the dependent portion of the dilated bronchi. Accumulation of secretions within bronchiectatic airways is typically recognizable as lobulated V- or Y-shaped structures ("finger in glove sign"). CT may show a completely collapsed lobe containing bronchiectatic airways. Subtle degrees of volume loss may present in lobes in relatively early disease.

Associated CT findings of bronchiolitis are present in about 70% of patients with bronchiectasis. These abnormalities are very common in patients with severe bronchiectasis and can even precede the development of bronchiectasis. The obstructive defect on pulmonary testing in patients with bronchiectasis is the consequence of

Table 6. Specific causes of disseminated bronchiectasis

- Acute, chronic, or recurrent infections
- Genetic abnormalities
  - Cystic fibrosis
  - Dyskinetic (immotile) cilia syndrome
  - Young syndrome
  - Williams-Campbell syndrome
  - Mounier-Kuhn syndrome (tracheobronchomegaly)
  - Immunodeficiency syndromes
  - Yellow nail syndrome
  - α-1-antitrypsin deficiency
- Noninfectious inflammatory diseases
  - Allergic bronchopulmonary aspergillosis
  - Asthma
  - Systemic diseases (rheumatoid arthritis, Sjögren syndrome, systemic lupus erythematosus, inflammatory bowel disease)
  - Post-transplantation bronchiolitis obliterans

an obstructive involvement of the small airways (constrictive). The extent and severity of bronchiectasis and bronchial wall thickening correlate with airflow obstruction. In patients with bronchiectasis, bronchial wall thickening and the extent of decreased lung attenuation are the strongest determinants of airflow obstruction. Bronchial wall thickening on baseline CT correlates with functional deterioration over time.

MDCT with thin collimation is the optimal imaging test to assess the presence and extent of bronchiectasis. Several studies have shown that multiplanar reformations increase the detection rate of bronchiectasis, readers' confidence as to the distribution of bronchiectasis, and agreement among observers as to the diagnosis of bronchiectasis.

The reliability of CT for distinguishing among the causes of bronchiectasis is somewhat controversial. An underlying cause for bronchiectasis is found in fewer than half of the patients, and CT features alone do not usually allow a confident distinction between idiopathic bronchiectasis versus known causes of bronchiectasis. The various specific causes of disseminated bronchiectasis are listed in Table 6.

Small Airway Diseases

Although normal bronchioles are below the resolution of thin-section CT, they can become detectable when inflammation of the airway wall and an accompanying exudate develop. Some bronchiolar changes are too small to be visible directly but result in indirect signs on CT. Bronchiolar obstruction can manifest as mosaic attenuation on CT, with decreased attenuation and abnormally smaller vessels as a result of reflex vasoconstriction. Expiratory CT confirms the presence of air trapping. Four different CT patterns can express small airway pathology [3, 4, 13].

Small Centrilobular Nodular and Branching Linear Opacities ("tree-in-bud")

Tree-in-bud opacities are defined as small centrilobular nodular and branching linear opacities, usually V- or Y-shaped, reflecting abnormally dilated bronchioles with thickened walls and mucus or exudate filling the lumens. Associated peribronchiolar inflammation is often present, contributing to the CT appearance. Tree-in-bud opacities are characteristic of acute or chronic infectious bronchiolitis. They also occur in diffuse panbronchiolitis and aspiration.

Poorly Defined Centrilobular Nodules

Poorly defined centrilobular nodules reflect the presence of peribronchiolar inflammation in the absence of airway filling. When the distribution of nodules is diffuse and homogeneous, the pattern is suggestive of bronchiolar or vascular diseases. Bronchiolar diseases associated with poorly defined centrilobular nodules include respiratory bronchiolitis, bronchiolitis associated with hypersensitivity pneumonitis, and follicular bronchiolitis.

Decreased Lung Attenuation and Mosaic Perfusion

Areas of decreased lung attenuation associated with decreased vessel caliber on CT reflect bronchiolar obstruction and associated reflex vasoconstriction. In acute bronchiolar obstruction, decreased perfusion represents a physiologic reflex of hypoxic vasoconstriction whereas irreversible vascular remodeling occurs with chronic bronchiolar obstruction. Areas of decreased lung attenuation related to hypoperfusion can be patchy or widespread. They are poorly defined or sharply demarcated, or have a geographical outline, but in all cases represent a collection of affected pulmonary lobules. Redistribution of blood flow to the normally ventilated areas causes localized increased attenuation. The patchwork of abnormal areas of low attenuation and normal lung or less diseased areas results in mosaic attenuation on CT, also termed mosaic perfusion. Expiratory CT accentuates the pattern of mosaic attenuation where areas of air trapping remain low in attenuation whereas normal lung increases in attenuation. Usually, the regional heterogeneity of lung attenuation is apparent on full inspiration on thin-section CT. However, with more extensive air trapping, the lack of regional homogeneity of lung attenuation can be challenging to detect on inspiratory scans; as a result, mosaic attenuation becomes visible only on expiratory scans. In patients with particularly severe and widespread involvement of the small airways, the patchy distribution of hypoattenuation and a mosaic pattern is lost. Inspiratory scans show an apparent uniformity of decreased attenuation in the lungs, and scans obtained at end expiration may appear normal. In these patients, the most striking features are the paucity of pulmonary vessels and the lack of a change in the cross-sectional area of lung between inspiration and expiration.

Mosaic attenuation is seen in patients who have constrictive bronchiolitis, bronchiolitis associated with hypersensitivity pneumonitis, asthma, and COPD.

Constrictive bronchiolitis, characterized by submucosal circumferential fibrosis along the central axis of ter-

Table 7. Causes of and association with obliterative (constrictive) bronchiolitis

- Post-infection
  - Childhood viral infection (adenovirus, respiratory syncytial virus, influenza, parainfluenza)
  - Adulthood and childhood (*Mycoplasma pneumoniae, Pneumocystis jirovecii* in AIDS patients, endobronchial spread of tuberculosis, bacterial bronchiolar infection)
- Post-inhalation (toxic fumes and gases)
- Diffuse aspiration bronchiolitis (chronic occult aspiration in the elderly, patients with dysphagia)
- Connective tissue disorders (rheumatoid arthritis, Sjögren syndrome)
- Allograft recipients (bone-marrow transplant, heart-lung, or lung transplant)
- Drugs (penicillamine, lomustine)
- Ulcerative colitis
- Other conditions
  - Bronchiectasis
  - Cystic fibrosis
  - Hypersensitivity pneumonitis
  - Diffuse idiopathic pulmonary neuroendocrine cell hyperplasia (DIPNECH)
  - Excessive *Sauropus androgynus* (katuk, sweet leaf, or star gooseberry) ingestion
- Idiopathic

minal bronchioles, has a variety of causes and, rarely, is idiopathic (Table 7). Bronchial wall thickening and bronchiectasis, both central and peripheral, are also commonly present.

Mosaic attenuation may also be seen in patients with chronic thromboembolic disease; however, in this condition, frank dilation of the proximal pulmonary arteries within the hyperattenuated areas and extensive areas of hypoattenuation and hypoperfusion are almost always present.

Expiratory Air Trapping

Lobular areas of air trapping may be readily apparent on expiratory CT but are occult on inspiratory CT. Foci of lobular air trapping are usually well demarcated, reflecting the geometry of individual or joined lobules. Lobular areas of air trapping may be present on expiratory CT scans of normal individuals, especially in the medial and posterior basal segments and apical portions of the superior segments of the lower lobes. However, when lobular air trapping occurs in the non-dependent portions of the lung or the overall extent is equal to or greater than one segment, the air trapping should be considered as abnormal. Expiratory air trapping occurs in smokers and in patients with asthma, constrictive bronchiolitis, and bronchiolitis associated with hypersensitivity pneumonitis and sarcoidosis.

Asthma

Asthma [3, 14-16] is a chronic inflammatory condition resulting from airway hyper-responsiveness to several stimuli. It is characterized by episodes of wheezing, coughing, and dyspnea due to airflow obstruction that resolves spontaneously or following treatment with bronchodilators. Over time, airway remodeling (fibrosis, smooth muscle hypertrophy and hyperplasia, and neovascularity) leads to persistent airflow obstruction.

The main clinical indication for imaging patients with asthma is to identify diseases that can mimic asthma clinically, particularly hypersensitive pneumonitis, constrictive bronchiolitis, and tracheal or carinal obstruction by neoplastic or non-neoplastic tracheal disorders. CT scans of patients with asthma can be normal or show bronchial abnormalities. Mucoid impaction and linear bands, reflecting subsegmental or segmental atelectasis, are reversible on follow-up. Bronchial wall thickening is commonly present and correlates with clinical severity and the duration of asthma and the degree of airflow obstruction. It also correlates with pathologic measures of remodeling from bronchial biopsies. Bronchiectasis may also be present; its extent is associated with an increased severity of asthma.

In patients with persistent moderate asthma, mosaic attenuation reflects remodeling in the small airways. The extent of expiratory air trapping does not change after inhalation of salbutamol. By contrast, in patients with mild or moderate uncontrolled asthma, therapy with inhaled corticosteroids reduces the degree of air trapping on CT, suggesting that CT can be used as a surrogate marker for assessing disease control.

Airway Disease in COPD

COPD consists of a group of diseases characterized by slow and progressive airway obstruction as a result of an exaggerated inflammatory response, typically from cigarette smoke [15, 17]. Progressive disease ultimately leads to the destruction of lung parenchyma (emphysema) and a permanent reduction in the number and caliber of the small airways (obstructive bronchiolitis). Both emphysema, because of the loss of alveolar attachments and decreased elastic recoil, and airway wall remodeling, with peribronchiolar fibrosis, are responsible for airflow limitation. The two types of lesions can coexist in the same patient, and small airway disease may precede the appearance of emphysema [18]. This explains why individuals with the same degree of functional impairment may have CT scans showing different morphologic appearances. For example, one patient with extensive emphysema on CT can have the same degree of airflow obstruction as another patient with little or no emphysema, suggesting small airway remodeling. These morphologic differences suggest differences in pathophysiology and the genomic profile. CT can help define the different phenotypes of COPD, allowing for better stratification of patients in clinical trials and, ultimately, for a more personalized treatment. Airway disease phenotypes of COPD include abnormalities of the small and large airways. Poorly defined

centrilobular nodules primarily in the upper lobes reflect inflammatory changes in and around the bronchioles (respiratory bronchiolitis), which can be reversible after smoking cessation and steroids. Mosaic attenuation and expiratory air trapping reflect obstructive bronchiolitis and remodeling of the small airways.

Large airway disease is also commonly present in COPD patients [19, 20]. Saber-sheath trachea occurs specifically in COPD, particularly males. Bronchial wall thickening and irregularities, although nonspecific, are frequently present. A quantitative assessment of bronchial wall thickening on CT scans can provide an estimate of airway remodeling in the absence of extensive emphysema. Bronchial wall thickness is one of the strongest determinants of FEV1 in patients with COPD. Moderate tubular bronchiectasis can occur, particularly in the lower lobes, following injury to cartilage. Bronchiectasis is often associated with more severe COPD exacerbations, lower airway bacterial colonization, and increased sputum inflammatory markers [21, 22]. However, the presence of bilateral varicose and cystic bronchiectasis in patients with panlobular emphysema should raise the diagnosis of α-1-antitrypsin deficiency. Cartilage deficiency in COPD may also induce abnormal collapse of the airway lumen at expiration, contributing to airflow limitation. Tracheomalacia can also develop.

References

1. Beigelman-Aubry C, Brillet PY, Grenier PA (2009) MDCT of the airways: technique and normal results. Radiol Clin North Am 47:185-201.
2. Grenier PA, Beigelman-Aubry C, Fetita C et al (2002) New frontiers in CT imaging of airway disease. Eur Radiol 12:1022-1044.
3. Naidich DP, Webb WR, Grenier PA et al (2005) Imaging of the airways. Lippincott Williams & Wilkins, Philadelphia, PA.
4. Hansell DM, Armstrong P, Lynch DA et al (2005) Imaging of diseases of the chest, 4th Ed. Elsevier Mosby, Philadelphia, PA.
5. Ferretti GR, Bithigoffer C, Righini CA et al (2009) Imaging of tumors of the trachea and central bronchi. Radiol Clin North Am 47:227-241.
6. Kang EY (2011) Large airway diseases. J Thorac Imaging 26:249-262.
7. Grenier PA, Beigelman-Aubry C, Brillet PY (2009) Nonneoplastic tracheal and bronchial stenoses. Radiol Clin North Am 47:243-260.
8. Lee EY, Litmanovich D, Boiselle PM (2009). Multidetector CT evaluation of tracheobronchomalacia. Radiol Clin North Am 47:261-269.
9. Ridge CA, O'Donnell CR, Lee EY et al (2011) Tracheobronchomalacia: current concepts and controversies. J Thorac Imaging 26:278-289.
10. Javidan-Nejad C, Bhalla S (2009) Bronchiectasis. Radiol Clin North Am 47:289-306.
11. O'Donnell AE (2008) Bronchiectasis. Chest 134:815-823.
12. Feldman C (2011). Bronchiectasis: new approaches to diagnosis and management. Clin Chest Med 32:535-546.
13. Pipavath SN, Stern EJ (2009) Imaging of Small Airway Disease (SAD). Radiol Clin North Am 47:307-316.
14. Boiselle P, Lynch D (2008) CT of the airways Humana Press, Totowa, NJ, USA.

36

15. Kauczor HU, Wielpütz MO, Owsijewitsch M et al (2011) Computed tomographic imaging of the airways in COPD and asthma. J Thorac Imaging 26:290-300.
16. Aysola RS, Hoffman EA, Gierada D et al (2008) Airway remodeling measured by multidetector CT is increased in severe asthma and correlates with pathology. Chest 134:1183-1191.
17. Ley-Zaporozhan J, Kauczor HU (2009) Imaging of airways: chronic obstructive pulmonary disease. Radiol Clin North Am 47:331-342.
18. McDonough JE, Yuan R, Suzuki M et al (2011) Small-airway obstruction and emphysema in chronic obstructive pulmonary disease. N Engl J Med 365:1567-1575.
19. Brillet PY, Fetita CI, Saragaglia A et al (2008) Investigation of airways using MDCT for visual and quantitative assessment in COPD patients. Int J Chronic Obstruct Pulm Dis 3:97-107.
20. Sverzellati N, Ingegnoli A, Calabrò E et al (2010) Bronchial diverticula in smokers on thin-section CT. Eur Radiol 20:88-94.
21. O'Brien C, Guest PJ, Hill SL, Stockley RA (2000) Physiological and radiological characterisation of patients diagnosed with chronic obstructive pulmonary disease in primary care. Thorax 55:635-642.
22. Martínez-García MÁ, Soler-Cataluña JJ, Donat Sanz Y et al (2011) Factors associated with bronchiectasis in patients with COPD. Chest 140:1130-1137.

Investigating a Child with a "Cough": A Pragmatic Approach

Maria do Rosario Matos[1], George A. Taylor[2], Catherine M. Owens[3]

[1] Radiology Department of Hospital Dona Estefânia, Centro Hospitalar de Lisboa Central, Lisbon, Portugal
[2] Harvard Medical School and Boston Children's Hospital, Boston, MA, USA
[3] Great Ormond Street Hospital for Children, London, UK

Introduction

Cough in children has a wide range of causes, is frequently misdiagnosed and consequently inappropriately treated [1].

A vast bibliography describing the assessment and management of cough is available, and guidelines have recently been proposed [1, 2]. This review discusses the role of imaging in the assessment of cough, in the investigation of a specific diagnosis. We emphasize important clues related to the patient's clinical condition that should be considered when selecting the most appropriate examination, as part of an organized investigation plan.

The pattern of respiratory illness in children is different from that in adults. The airways in children are less mature, as are the respiratory muscles, chest wall structure, sleep-related features, and respiratory reflexes. Viruses associated with common cold in adults can cause serious respiratory illnesses, such as bronchiolitis and croup, in previously well young children [3]. Also, the common "big three" causes of chronic cough in adults (cough variant asthma, postnasal drip and gastroesophageal reflux) [4] do not necessarily apply to the pediatric age. Other considerations for the etiology of cough include inhalation of a foreign body, airway lesions, environmental toxicants, respiratory infections, and otogenic causes [2, 5] (Table 1). Tumors are common in adults but are extremely rare in children, although this possibility must not be forgotten in a child with a specific chronic cough [6]. Medical history is often limited to parental perception, which may overestimate or misinterpret important situations of cough, like foreign-body aspiration.

Definitions

Cough is defined as a forced expulsive maneuver against a closed glottis and is associated with a characteristic sound [1].

Acute cough is defined as a recent onset of cough lasting <3 weeks; *chronic cough* is one that lasts >8 weeks [1, 7].

Prolonged acute cough resolves over a 3- to 8-week period. An example is *Pertussis* cough, which may need an additional period of time to elapse before further investigations are performed.

Recurrent cough refers to repeated (>2/year) cough episodes not related to head colds, each lasting >7–14 days [8, 9]. It can be difficult to distinguish from persistent chronic cough. Most simple infective causes of cough resolve in 3-4 weeks. Children with chronic cough may require further investigations.

Based on the suggested etiology, cough can be categorized as "normal" or "expected" cough, specific cough, and non-specific cough (Fig. 1). "Normal" children cough 11 times a day on average, although some children experience more than 30 episodes a day, as shown in recent studies [10, 11]. Frequency and severity increase during upper respiratory tract infection, which occurs in more frequently in the pediatric age group than in adults [1, 2].

Table 1. Influence of age on the causes of cough

Infancy	Early childhood	Late childhood
Gastroesophageal reflux	Post-viral airway hyper-responsiveness	Asthma
Infection	Asthma	Post-nasal drip
Congenital malformation	Passive smoking	Smoking
Congenital heart disease	Gastroesophageal reflux	Pulmonary tuberculosis
Passive smoking	Foreign body	Bronchiectasis
Environmental pollution	Bronchiectasis	Psychogenic cough
Asthma		

Diseases of the Chest and Heart 2015-2018,
DOI: 10.1007/978-88-470-5752-4_5 © Springer-Verlag Italia 2015

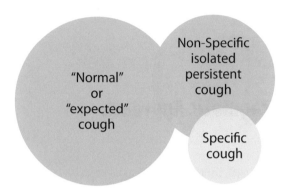

Fig. 1. Venn diagram of different types of cough

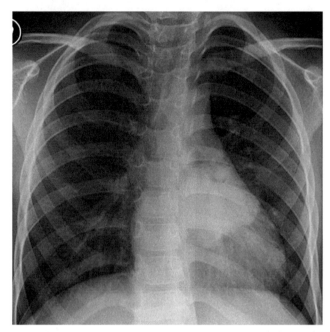

Fig. 2. Chest X-ray showing nodular consolidation behind the heart

When there are symptoms and signs that point to a certain diagnosis, thus demanding further investigation, cough is defined as specific.

Non-specific cough describes cases in which cough – usually dry – is the only symptom (isolated cough) and the child is otherwise well. Most cases are thought to be post-viral and related to increased cough receptor sensitivity [12, 13] and less likely to asthma or gastroesophageal reflux [1].

Acute Cough

Acute cough is most commonly caused by viral respiratory tract infections [14], which may or may not be associated with acute bronchitis. Other causes include seasonal allergic rhinitis, hay fever, an inhaled foreign body, and the first presentation of a chronic disorder.

According to British Thoracic Society guidelines [1], if acute cough is due to an uncomplicated upper respiratory tract infection (absence of fever, tachypnea, and chest signs), no further investigation is needed. If an inhaled foreign body is suspected as the cause, then an urgent rigid bronchoscopy should be performed. A chest radiograph is considered when lower respiratory signs are present (Fig. 2), when there are hemoptysis, or the suggestion of a chronic respiratory disorder or when a cough is relentlessly progressive beyond 2–3 weeks.

Chronic Cough

There may be an overlap between recurrent and chronic cough, which is why for investigation purposes these categories, along with prolonged acute cough, are not separated. Most children with chronic cough have recurrent viral bronchitis or post viral syndromes (subacute cough).

Causes of chronic cough may be classified in two groups [15]: (1) chronic isolated (no wheezing) non-specific cough in an otherwise healthy child and (2) a chronic cough in which the child has a serious underlying lung condition (Table 2).

Evaluation

Specific cough requiring further investigation is suggested by specific pointers identified in the history and clinical examination of the patient. Historical information includes time of onset, quality of cough, triggering and alleviating factors, and presence of hemoptysis (Table 3).

Table 2. Influence of pre-existing disease on the causes of cough

Chronic cough in an otherwise healthy child	Chronic cough with a significant underlying cause
Recurrent viral bronchitis	Cystic fibrosis
Post-infectious cough	Immune deficiencies
Pertussis-like illness	Primary ciliary dyskinesia
Cough variant asthma	Protracted bacterial bronchitis
Allergic rhinitis, post-nasal drip and sinusitis	Recurrent pulmonary aspiration
Psychogenic cough	Tracheoesophageal fistula, gastroesophageal reflux, hiatal hernia
Habit ("tic" like)	Retained inhaled foreign body
Bizarre honking cough	Tuberculosis
Gastroesophageal reflux	Anatomical disorder (airway or lung)
	Interstitial lung disease

Table 3. Influence of the time of onset on the causes of cough

Time of onset	Neonatal, infancy and childhood
Nature	Dry or productive
Quality	Brassy, croupy, honking, paroxysmal, staccato
Timing	Persistent, intermittent, nocturnal, on awaking
Triggering factors	Cold air, exercise, feeding, seasonal, starts with a head cold
Alleviating factors	Bronchodilators, antibiotics
Associated symptoms	Wheezing, shortness of breath

Clinical examination pointers include digital clubbing and asymmetrical auscultatory signs.

Two situations are commonly indicative of significant disease. The first is neonatal onset of the cough, suggesting: (a) a congenital defect leading to feeding problems and pulmonary aspiration, (b) cystic fibrosis, (c) primary ciliary dyskinesia, (d) an anatomical airways abnormality, for example a cyst compressing the airway or tracheomalacia, or (e) a chronic viral pneumonia (e.g., cytomegalovirus or *Chlamydia*) acquired in utero or during the perinatal period [1, 2].

The second situation is persistent productive (moist or wet) cough, which requires investigation for the presence of bronchiectasis or any specific suppurative lung condition [1, 2].

Investigation

A chest radiograph is indicated for most children with chronic cough, unless there is also a minor identified disorder, such as asthma or allergic rhinitis (Table 4). Spirometry should be always attempted in children capable of performing the maneuvers (generally those over the age of 5 years) [1, 2].

In children with a specific cough, further investigations may be warranted (Figs. 3, 4), except when asthma is the main cause [1, 2]. The next sections discuss the various etiologies of chronic cough.

Chronic Sinusitis

Sinusitis is a very common condition in children. Chronic sinusitis (lasting >3 months) involves symptoms that include nasal obstruction, nasal discharge, halitosis, and headache [16]. Although some authors report a high incidence of incidental sinus opacification in children [17], those data may be biased by different interpretations of mucosal thickening and by the true health condition of the population included in such studies [18]. Tatli et al. [18] found a 52% prevalence of moderate to severe opacification of the paranasal sinus on computed tomography (CT) in children with chronic cough, with 90% involvement of the maxillary sinuses.

Radiographs are used as a screening method for pathological conditions involving the sinuses but CT remains the imaging modality of choice for the evaluation of acute and chronic sinus inflammatory processes [19]. The association between adenoidal hypertrophy and rhinosinusitis with upper airway inflammation is increasingly recognized, with one study [20] stating that magnetic resonance imaging (MRI) can document changes in adenoid size associated with the resolution of rhinosinusitis (Fig. 5). Further studies are necessary to define the role of MRI in adenoidal hypertrophy.

Table 4. Imaging in a child with cough

Indication for chest X-ray	Features	Likely common diagnose
Uncertainty about the diagnosis of pneumonia	Fever and rapid breathing Chest signs Persisting high fever Unusual course in bronchiolitis Cough and fever persisting beyond 4–5 days	Pneumonia
Possibility of an inhaled foreign body	Choking episode may not have been witnessed Sudden onset Asymmetrical wheeze Hyperinflation	Inhaled foreign body X-ray may be normal Needs bronchoscopy
Suggestion of a chronic respiratory disorder	Failure to thrive Finger clubbing Overinflation Chest deformity	See Fig. 3
Unusual clinical course	Relentlessly progressive beyond 2–3 weeks Recurrent fever	Pneumonia Enlarging intrathoracic lesion Tuberculosis Inhaled foreign body Lobar collapse
Hemoptysis		Acute pneumonia Chronic lung disorder (e.g., cystic fibrosis) Inhaled foreign body Tuberculosis Pulmonary hemosiderosis Tumor

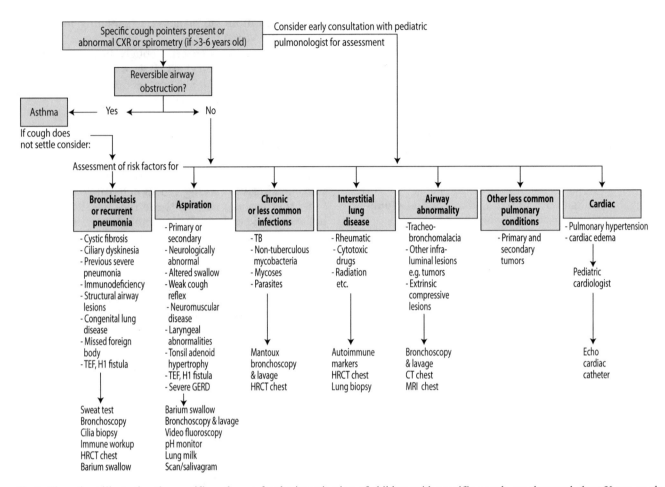

Fig. 3. Flow chart illustrating the specific pathways for the investigation of children with specific cough, an abnormal chest X-ray, or abnormal spirometry. TEF, tracheoesophageal fistula; GERD, gastroesophageal reflux disease; HRCT, high-resolution computed tomography, MRI, magnetic resonance imaging

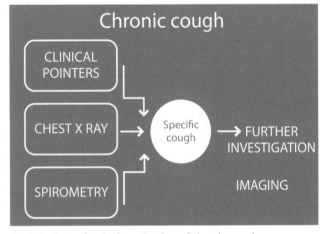

Fig. 4. Pathway for the investigation of chronic cough

Congenital Airway Disorders

Anatomical abnormalities of the airways may be the cause of chronic cough. Tracheobroncomalacia often causes a brassy, barking, or "seal-like" cough, with a neonatal onset.

Tracheoesophageal fistula (TEF) or laryngeal clefts cause cough due to aspiration, especially during meals. Following surgery for TEF or esophageal atresia, children usually have tracheomalacia and cough.

A seal-like barking cough occurs in children with any cause of airway compression or stenosis. In the study of Gormley et al. [21], 75% of children with tracheomalacia secondary to congenital vascular anomalies had persistent chronic cough at presentation. However, those authors did not take into account asymptomatic children. Mediastinal masses, such as bronchogenic cysts, need also to be considered in children presenting with the related symptoms (Fig. 6).

The barium esophagogram is the main imaging modality for identifying TEF. However, some infants with associated medical problems and on life support systems are poor candidates, in which case CT is an accurate diagnostic alternative [22]. The diagnostic utility of the new generations of multislice CT scans, performed appropriately with air insufflation into the trachea or esophagus during image acquisition, permits the rapid, safe, and accurate diagnosis of H-type TEF [23].

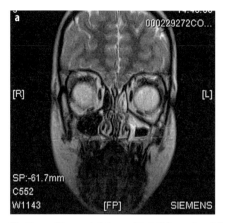
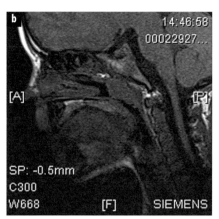
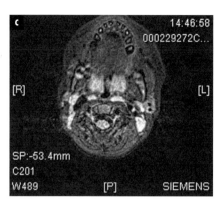

Fig. 5 a-c. Coronal (**a**), sagittal (**b**), and axial (**c**) T2-weighted spin echo magnetic resonance images illustrate paranasal sinus mucosal thickening and adenoidal hypertrophy in a child with chronic cough related to rhinosinusitis

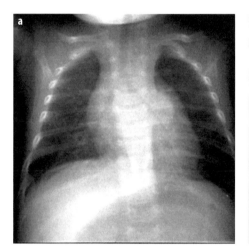
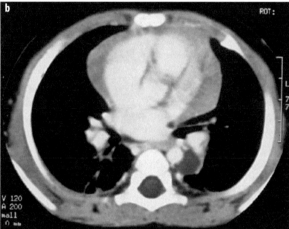

Fig 6. a, b. Chest X-ray (**a**) and axial contrast-enhanced computed tomography (CT) (**b**) in a child with cough due to a mediastinal bronchogenic cyst adjacent to the descending aorta

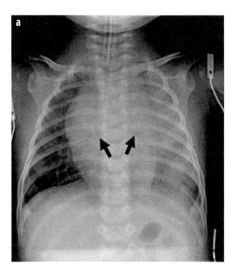
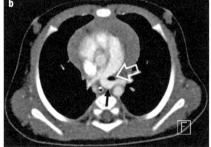
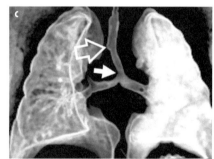

Fig. 7 a-c. Chest X-ray and axial contrast enhanced CT scan with volume rendered tomography (VRT) in a child with cough and stridor related to a pulmonary artery sling. **a** Chest X-ray shows splaying of the trachea (*arrows*), with an obtuse carinal angle. **b** Axial CT shows the narrow trachea (*open arrow*) with the abnormal LPA passing behind the trachea, in a sling like fashion. **c** The VRT image shows long segment tracheal stenosis with a rudimentary R apical tracheal bud (*open arrow*), with an obtuse carinal angle and narrowing of the origins of the R and L main bronchi (stovepipe trachea) (*white arrow*)

Barium swallow and echocardiography can demonstrate the presence of a vascular ring. Bronchoscopy in this context has to be defined prospectively [15]. Both CT and MRI are noninvasive imaging modalities that may help in the planning of surgery [24]. With the development of high-speed, high-resolution CT scanning, general anesthesia is usually unnecessary. According to Turner et al. [25], the first examination should be a barium swallow, followed by a high-resolution chest CT scan in the study of vascular rings (Fig. 7).

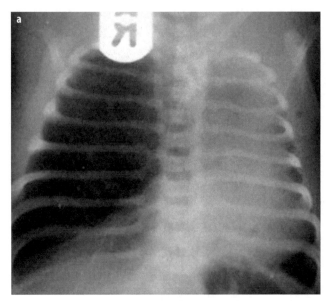
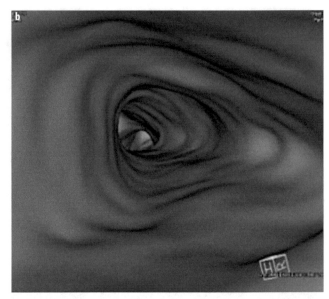

Fig. 8 a, b. An expiratory chest X-ray (**a**) and virtual bronchoscopy (**b**) show gross over-inflation, due to air trapping in a child with obstructive overinflation and ball valve effect in the right main bronchus due to an inhaled foreign body. This imaging approach increases the diagnostic accuracy for inhaled FB, whose findings include atelectasis, areas of unilateral or bilateral hyperinflation, or nonspecific opacification

Foreign-Body Aspiration

Cough may be an important symptom in acute foreign-material inhalation. Foreign-body aspiration (FBA) is much more frequent in boys than in girls and is more common in those under 4 years of age [15]. Although the presentation is usually acute [26], the problem may go unrecognized for prolonged periods of time if the diagnosis is missed initially [27]. In that case, the natural history may include hemoptysis, cough producing casts in the airways, associated wheezing, and associated recurrent pneumonia and infiltrates [1].

An expiratory chest X-ray increases the diagnostic accuracy in patients with FBA [7]. Findings include atelectasis, areas of unilateral or bilateral hyperinflation, or nonspecific opacification [28] (Fig. 8). However, a normal chest X-ray does not exclude the possibility of FBA. If the history is unclear and there are no localized physical or X-ray findings, flexible bronchoscopy should be performed to locate the inhaled object and rigid bronchoscopy to remove it [7, 29].

Virtual bronchoscopy associated with MCDT is a noninvasive modality for the identification of endobronchial lesions. Helical CT scanning with virtual bronchoscopy may be performed in selected cases of suspected FBA. When the chest radiograph is normal and the clinical diagnosis suggests an aspirated foreign body, helical CT and virtual bronchoscopy can be considered as a means to avoid rigid bronchoscopy if the clinical suspicion is low [30, 31].

Bronchiectasis

Bronchiectasis is defined as abnormal dilatation of thick-walled airways. Regardless of the etiology, symptoms

resulting from bronchiectasis are chronic cough and sputum production, although some patients may have a nonproductive cough [32].

Patients without an obvious cause of bronchiectasis should be diagnostically evaluated for an underlying disorder because the results may lead to treatment that can potentially slow or halt progression of the disease [32]. Cystic fibrosis (CF) occurs in 1 per 2,000–3,000 live births and is probably the most common identifiable cause of bronchiectasis in the United States and Europe [32]. CF-related cough may have a neonatal onset and can be productive or paroxysmal. It may be associated with hemoptysis, ill health, recurrent pneumonia, or pulmonary infiltrates [1]. Non-CF causes of bronchiectasis include post-infectious disease, primary ciliary dyskinesia, immunodeficiency states, retained airway foreign body, connective tissue disorders, chronic aspiration and allergic bronchopulmonary aspergillosis [33].

In patients with clinically suspected bronchiectasis without a characteristic chest radiograph, a CT scan can confirm the diagnosis. Criteria include an increased bronchial/adjacent pulmonary artery ratio, non-tapering bronchial walls, bronchi visualized at lung periphery, thickened bronchial walls, mucous plugging and focal air-trapping related to small airway disease [33, 34]. CT is also of great value in cases of superadded infection, such as allergic bronchopulmonary aspergillosis and nontuberculous mycobacterial infection [33] (Fig. 9).

Because CF may be diagnosed early in life due to nonpulmonary findings (e.g., meconium ileus, malabsorption, and failure to thrive due to pancreatic insufficiency), CT is used for the diagnosis of its complications rather than the primary diagnosis. However, in non-CF causes of bronchiectasis, CT plays a role in the primary diagno-

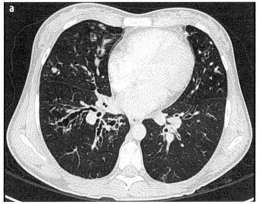
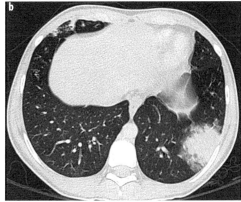

Fig. 9 a, b. CT is of value in patients with cystic fibrosis with superadded infection, such as allergic bronchopulmonary aspergillosis (**a**) and non-tuberculous mycobacterial infection (**b**)

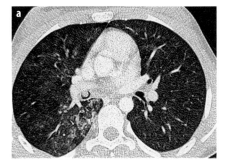
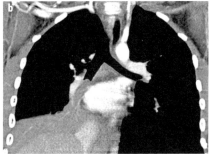
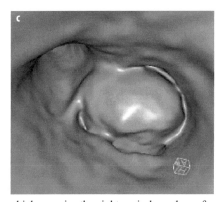

Fig. 10 a-c. Axial (**a**) and (**b**) sagittal CT scans and (**c**) virtual bronchoscopy show an endobronchial mass in the right main bronchus of a child with cough and hemoptysis related to endobronchial *Mycobacterium tuberculosis* infection.

sis and detection of complications (if chest X-ray is insufficient) as well as prior to lung surgery [33].

Tuberculosis

Chronic or less common infections that may lead to chronic cough are tuberculosis (TB) and non-tuberculous mycobacteria, fungal, and parasitic infections. TB should be considered in any child with a persistent productive cough, particularly if there are systemic features such as fever, weight loss, or general malaise. Specific pointers towards this diagnosis in cough investigation are hemoptysis, associated with severe ill health, recurrent pneumonia, or pulmonary infiltrates [1]. Since most TB infections are transmitted by inhalation, primary lesions occur in the lungs in over 95% of infected children [34].

Although chest radiography remains the first-line imaging technique in the evaluation of pulmonary TB in children, in selected cases CT can provide important information in the diagnosis and management of the disease. CT typically shows low-attenuation lymph nodes with rim enhancement and, eventually, calcification. These findings in HIV-positive patients are considered sufficient to warrant instituting empirical anti-TB therapy [35]. Parenchymal lesions include nodules of bron-

chogenic spread, miliary nodules, and segmental or lobar consolidation, which may evolve to caseating necrosis. CT also defines the extent of disease and its complications [36] (Fig. 10).

Considerations on Pediatric CT Radiation Burden

The utility of CT scans in the pediatric age needs to be balanced with radiation effects. Children are considerably more sensitive to radiation than adults and have a longer life expectancy, resulting in a higher lifetime cancer mortality risk [37].

CT settings in the diagnosis of chest disease can be reduced significantly while maintaining diagnostic image quality. Jogeesvaran and Owens [33] reported that the dose for a volumetric CT scan is between three and five times higher than for a non-contiguous high-resolution CT. Moreover, there is a strong argument that chronic diffuse diseases of the lung parenchyma are adequately imaged with non contiguous CT. The authors recommended a volumetric scan at the initial diagnostic stage of chronic lung disease to exclude co-existent or unsuspected tracheobronchial and vascular anomalies. For children suspected of having diffuse interstitial lung diseases at diagnosis and at follow-up of either airways or diffuse infiltrative lung disease, a limited, non-contiguous, conventional high-resolution CT should be the preferred exam.

Conclusion

In the management of illness in children, adult-based data should not be extrapolated: children are different from adults.

Most children with cough due to a simple upper respiratory tract infection will not need further investigations. Chest radiograph should be considered in the presence of: lower respiratory tract signs, relentlessly progressive cough, hemoptysis, or features of an undiagnosed chronic respiratory disorder.

Children with chronic cough require careful and systematic evaluation for the presence of specific diagnostic indicators and should undergo, as a minimum, a chest radiograph and spirometry.

In children with specific cough, further investigations may be warranted, except when asthma is the etiologic factor.

Children with chronic productive purulent cough should always be investigated, to document the presence or absence of bronchiectasis and to identify underlying and treatable causes such as CF and immune deficiency.

Chronic cough starting in the neonatal period usually indicates significant disease, especially if it starts in the first few days or weeks of life.

There are advantages of CT in children but the techniques and guidelines regarding the use of the different modalities in the pediatric population must be kept in mind, and the potential risks balanced accordingly.

References

1. Shields MD, Bush A, Everard ML et al (2008) Recommendations for the assessment and management of cough in children. Thorax 63:1-15.
2. Chang AB, Glomb WB (2006) Guidelines for evaluating chronic cough in pediatrics: ACCP evidence-based clinical practice guidelines. Chest 129: 260-283.
3. Couriel J (1998) Infection in children. In: Ellis ME (ed) Infectious diseases of the respiratory tract. Cambridge University Press, Cambridge, UK, pp 406-429.
4. D'Urzo A, Jugovic P (2002) Chronic cough. Three most common causes. Can Fam Physician 48:1311-1316.
5. Chang AB (2005) Cough: are children really different to adults? Cough 1:7.
6. Barr RL, McCrystal DJ, Perry CF, Chang AB (2005) A rare cause of specific cough in a child: the importance of following up children with chronic cough. Cough 1:8.
7. Massie J (2006) Cough in children: when does it matter? Paediatric respiratory reviews 7:9-14.
8. Sherrill DL, Guerra S, Minervini MC et al (2005) The relationship of rhinitis to recurrent cough and wheezing: a longitudinal study. Respir Med 99:1377-1385.
9. Chang AB, Phelan PD, Sawyer SM et al (1997) Airway hyperresponsiveness and cough receptor sensitivity in children with recurrent cough. Am J Respir Crit Care Med 155:1935-1939.
10. Munyard P, Bush A (1996) How much coughing is normal? Arch Dis Child 74:531-534.
11. Shann F (1996) How often do children cough? Lancet 348:699-700.
12. Chang AB, Phelan PD, Sawyer SM et al (1997) Airway hyperresponsiveness and cough-receptor sensitivity in children with recurrent cough. Am J Respir Crit Care Med 155:1935-1939.
13. Chang AB, Phelan PD, Sawyer SM et al (1997) Cough sensitivity in children with asthma, recurrent cough, and cystic fibrosis. Arch Dis Child 77:331-334.
14. Boujaoude ZC, Prat MR (2010) Clinical approach to acute cough. Lung 188(Suppl 1):4146.
15. Jongste JC, Shields MD (2003) Cough 2: Chronic cough in children. Thorax 58:998-1003.
16. Triulzi F, Zirpoli S (2007) Imaging techniques in the diagnosis and management of rhinosinusitis in children. Pediatr Allergy Immunol 18:46-49.
17. Glasier CM, Ascher DP, Williams KD (1986) Incidental paranasal sinus abnormalities on CT of children. Am J Neuroradiol 7:861-864.
18. Tatli M, Sanb I, Karaoglanogluc M (2001). Paranasal sinus computed tomographic findings of children with chronic cough. Int Journ Pediatr Otorhinolaryngol 60:213-217.
19. Mafee MF, Tran BH, Chapa AR (2006) Imaging of rhinosinusitis and its complications: plain film, CT, and MRI. Clin Rev Allergy Immunol 30:165-186.
20. Georgalas C, Thomas K, Owens C et al (2005) Medical treatment for rhinosinusitis associated with adenoidal hypertrophy in children: an evaluation of clinical response and changes on magnetic resonance imaging. Ann Otol Rhinol Laryngol 114:638-644.
21. Gormley PK, Colreavy MP, Patil N et al (1999) Congenital vascular anomalies and persistent respiratory symptoms in children. Int J Pediatr Otorhinolaryngol 51:23-31.
22. Johnson JF, Sueoka BL, Mulligan ME, Lugo EJ (1985) Tracheoesophageal fistula: diagnosis with CT. Pediatric Radiology 15:134-135.
23. Ou P, Seror E, Layouss W et al (2007) Definitive diagnosis and surgical planning of H-type tracheoesophageal fistula in a critically ill neonate: First experience using air distension of the esophagus during high-resolution computed tomography acquisition. Thorac Cardiovasc Surg 133:1116-1117.
24. Chun K, Colombani PM, Dudgeon DL et al (1992) Diagnosis and management of congenital vascular rings: a 22-year experience. Ann Thoraci Surg 53:597-602.
25. Turner A, Gavel G, Coutts J (2005) Vascular rings—presentation, investigation and outcome. Eur J Pediatr 164:266-270.
26. Mu L, He P, Sun D (1991) Inhalation of foreign bodies in Chinese children: a review of 400 cases. Laryngoscope 101:657-660.
27. Raman TS, Mathew S, Ravikumar, Garcha PS (1998) Atelectasis in children. Indian Pediatr 35:429-435.
28. Svedstrom E, Puhakka H, Kero P (1989) How accurate is chest radiography in the diagnosis of tracheobronchial foreign bodies in children? Pediatr Radiol 19:520-522.
29. Barben J, Berkowitz RG, Kemp A, Massie J (2000) Bronchial granuloma – where's the foreign body? Int J Pediatr Otorhinolaryngol 53:215-219.
30. Haliloglu M, Ciftci AO, Oto A et al (2003) CT virtual bronchoscopy in the evaluation of children with suspected foreign body aspiration. Eur J Radiol 48:188-192.
31. Sodhi KS, Saxena AK, Singh M et al (2008) CT virtual bronchoscopy: New non invasive tool in pediatric patients with foreign body aspiration. Indian Journal of Pediatrics 75:511-513.
32. Rosen MJ (2006) Chronic cough due to bronchiectasis: ACCP evidence-based clinical practice guidelines. Chest 129:122-131.
33. Jogeesvaran H, Owens CM (2010) Chronic diseases of lung parenchyma in children: the role. Pediatr Radiol 40:850-858.

34. Couriel J (2002) Assessment of the child with recurrent chest infections. Br Med Bull 61:115-132.
35. Pastores SM, Naidich DP, Aranda CR et al (1993) Intrathoracic adenopathy associated with pulmonary tuberculosis in patients with human immunodeficiency virus infection. Chest 103:1433-1437.
36. Kim W, Moon W, Kim IO et al (1997) Pulmonary tuberculosis in children: evaluation with CT. AJR Am J Roentgenol 68:1005-1009.
37. Brenner D, Elliston C, Hall E, Werdon B (2001) Estimated risks of radiation-induced fatal cancer from pediatric CT. AJR Am J Roentgenol 17:289-296.

Thoracic Manifestations of Pediatric Systemic Diseases

Edward Y. Lee[1], Alan S. Brody[2]

[1] Department of Radiology, Boston Children's Hospital and Harvard Medical School, Boston, MA, USA
[2] Department of Radiology and Pediatrics, Cincinnati Children's Hospital and the University of Cincinnati College of Medicine, Cincinnati, OH, USA

Introduction

There are a wide variety of systemic diseases that have a component of thoracic manifestations in pediatric patients. Although the imaging findings of these systemic diseases may be varied and non-specific, an understanding of their characteristic manifestations in the chest may allow the radiologist to suggest a diagnosis in often complex cases. Systemic diseases that have either a primary or a secondary component of thoracic manifestations in pediatric patients include collagen vascular diseases, immunodeficiencies, lysosomal storage disease, systemic granulomatous disorders, vasculitis, and miscellaneous conditions such as cystic fibrosis, sickle cell disease, Langerhans cell histiocytosis, and tuberous sclerosis. It is important to recognize that systemic diseases may have secondary effects that affect the chest. Abnormal host defenses result in increased infectious complications. Abnormal esophageal motility may result in aspiration. Fluid overload due to treatment may result in pulmonary edema. In many cases, these nonspecific findings are more common than the changes that are characteristic of a specific disease. The overarching goal of this chapter is to review the typical clinical presentation as well as the characteristic thoracic and extrathoracic imaging manifestations of important systemic diseases in the pediatric population.

Spectrum of Thoracic Manifestations of Pediatric Systemic Diseases

Collagen Vascular Diseases

The collagen vascular diseases are a subgroup of autoimmune connective tissue disorders, all of which have underlying inflammation or fragility of the connective tissues. The four most commonly encountered collagen vascular diseases in the pediatric population are juvenile idiopathic arthritis (JIA, previously referred to as juvenile rheumatoid arthritis), juvenile systemic sclerosis, juvenile dermatomyositis, and systemic lupus erythematosus (SLE) [1]. Of these collagen vascular diseases, JIA most commonly affects children whereas SLE is more often seen in adults than in children. In JIA particularly, findings on chest computed tomography (CT) are more common than clinically significant disease.

In general, collagen vascular diseases affect the lung less frequently in children than in adults. However, pediatric patients with this diverse group of collagen vascular diseases may have various lung abnormalities, including nonspecific interstitial pneumonitis (NSIP), pulmonary lymphoid hyperplasia, organizing pneumonia, hemorrhage, bronchiolitis, and bronchiectasis [2]. Ultimately pulmonary fibrosis and subsequent pulmonary hypertension, which can be a complication of pulmonary involvement by collagen vascular diseases, may develop (Fig. 1). On imaging studies such as chest radiograph and CT, these abnormalities can be suggestive of pulmonary nodules, diffuse ground glass opacities, and diffuse alveolar parenchymal opacities. Pleural effusion and pericardial effusion are also frequently present in pediatric patients with underlying collagen vascular diseases [1, 3, 4].

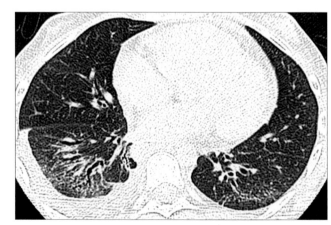

Fig. 1. A 13-year-old girl with juvenile idiopathic arthritis. Axial lung window computer tomography (CT) shows bronchiectasis in the posterior lower lobes. Right pleural effusion is also seen

Diseases of the Chest and Heart 2015-2018,
DOI: 10.1007/978-88-470-5752-4_6 © Springer-Verlag Italia 2015

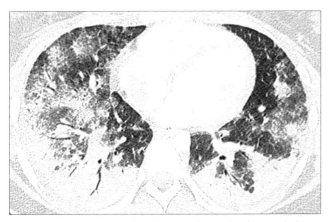

Fig. 2. A 15-year-old girl with a known diagnosis of systemic lupus erythematosus who presented with shortness of breath, desaturation, and decreased hematocrit. Axial lung window CT shows multifocal airspace opacifications compatible with pulmonary hemorrhage. A subsequently performed bronchoalveolar lavage confirmed the diagnosis

Some specific lung abnormalities are associated with a specific collagen vascular disease. For example, lipoid pneumonia, caused by deposition of cholesterol granulomas in the interstitium and alveoli, is associated with JIA, which may be related to an underlying macrophage activation syndrome that is often present in JIA [5]. Alveolar hemorrhage, which is more common in children than in adults, may present in pediatric patients with SLE and decreased hematocrit level (Fig. 2). The early and accurate diagnosis of alveolar hemorrhage in SLE patients is essential because it can be potentially treated successfully with steroids and cytotoxic agents. Furthermore, "shrinking lung syndrome," which describes a progressive decrease in lung volumes and is sometimes seen in patients with SLE, can be detected on imaging studies when there is a progressive elevation of the diaphragm despite attempted full inspiration [6]. Although the underlying etiology of "shrinking lung syndrome" is not known, a combination of pleural restriction due to recurrent pleural inflammation and pulmonary fibrosis, and weakness of the diaphragm and chest wall musculature may be responsible.

Immunodeficiencies

Defects in one or more of the essential components of the immune system can result in an increased risk of developing thoracic abnormalities in pediatric patients [3]. When assessing the chest of children with an immunodeficiency, the radiologist's role includes: (1) detecting characteristic imaging features of a specific immunodeficiency, (2) evaluating infections, and (3) detecting malignancies that can occur as a complication of certain immunodeficiencies. Because of the large number of immunodeficiencies, only the disorders that are the most common or have the most characteristic thoracic manifestations are discussed in the following.

Predominantly Antibody Deficiencies

The predominantly antibody deficiencies are characterized by a decreased ability to produce immunoglobulins from B-cells. The predominantly antibody deficiencies predispose affected patients to recurrent respiratory tract infection with encapsulated bacteria such as *Streptococcus* and *Haemophilus influenzae*. Recurrent infections from these organisms can lead to permanent lung damage such as irreversible bronchiectasis. The four most commonly encountered predominantly antibody deficiencies are IgA deficiency, X-linked agammaglobulinemia, common variable immunodeficiency disorder (CVID), and hyper-IgM syndrome.

In children with IgA deficiency, which is the most common primary immunodeficiency syndrome, pyogenic sinopulmonary infections are the most frequent finding [7]. X-linked agammaglobulinemia most often results from a mutation in the X-linked gene encoding Bruton tyrosine kinase (Fig. 3). Following recurrent pulmonary infections from *Streptococcus, H. influenzae,* and *Mycoplasma,* bronchiectasis in the lower lobes is often seen. Diminutive adenoid tissue on the lateral airway radiograph can be helpful clue for diagnosing X-linked agammaglobulinemia in affected children. CVID is described as "variable" because of the different clinical courses of different patients, rather than to changing manifestations over time in a single patient. CVID is caused by the failed terminal differentiation of B-cells to plasma cells, resulting in hypogammaglobulinemia. Approximately 75% of affected patients develop a lung disease characterized by bronchiectasis, bronchial wall thickening, and endobronchial mucus plugging closely resembling cystic fibrosis [8] (Fig. 4). Splenomegaly is seen in approximately 25% of patients with CVID [7]. Affected patients also have an increased risk for developing

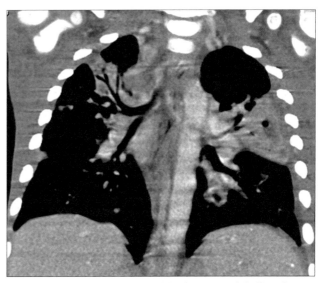

Fig. 3. A 3-year-old boy with X-linked agammaglobulinemia. Enhanced coronal reformatted CT shows multi-focal pneumonia from *Streptococcus* infection

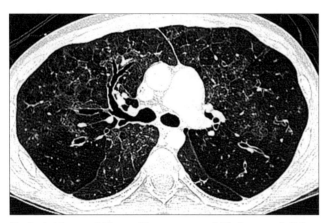

Fig. 4. A 16-year-old boy with common variable immunodeficiency disorder. Axial lung window CT shows bronchial wall thickening and bronchiectasis closely resembling cystic fibrosis

autoimmune cytopenia, lymphoproliferative disease, lymphoma, and gastric cancer. In addition, patients with CVID may develop granulomatous lymphocytic-interstitial lung disease (GLILD). On imaging studies, GLILD is characterized by a non-caseating granulomatous and lymphoproliferative histologic pattern often seen as pulmonary nodules, consolidation, and ground-glass or reticular opacities [9] (Fig. 5). Children affected with hyper-IgM syndrome may present with recurrent respiratory and gastrointestinal tract infections by encapsulated bacteria, viruses, fungi, and parasites [10]. An increased risk of developing *Pneumocystis jirovecii* pneumonia (PCP) and hepatocellular carcinoma has been also reported in patients with hyper-IgM syndrome.

Combined T-cell and B-cell Immunodeficiencies

Pediatric patients with combined T-cell and B-cell immunodeficiencies are at increased risk of developing

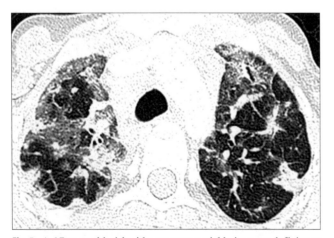

Fig. 5. A 17-year old girl with common variable immunodeficiency disorder. Axial lung window CT shows nodules as well as ground-glass and subtle reticular opacities in both lungs, compatible with granulomatous lymphocytic-interstitial lung disease (GLILD)

infections from the same pathogens that afflict those with antibody deficiencies. In addition, opportunistic infections from *Mycobacteria,* viruses, *Pneumocystis,* and other fungi can occur [11]. The two most common combined T-cell and B-cell immunodeficiencies are severe combined immunodeficiency (SCID) and combined immunodeficiency (CID).

In patients with SCID, the most severe form of the primary immunodeficiencies, recurrent, persistent, or opportunistic respiratory infections along with thrush, dermatitis, chronic diarrhea, or failure to thrive begin in early infancy. Without hematopoietic stem cell transplantation, gene therapy or enzyme replacement therapy, the disease is almost always fatal in the first two years of life [12]. In patients with CID, particularly with signal transducer and activator of transcription 5B (STAT5b) deficiency, the chronic lung disease in the form of lymphocytic interstitial pneumonitis can result in death from respiratory failure [13].

Well-Defined Syndromes Associated with Immunodeficiency

The five most common well-defined syndromes associated with immunodeficiency in the pediatric population are: (1) DiGeorge syndrome, (2) Wiscott-Aldrich syndrome, (3) hyper-IgE syndrome, (4) dyskeratosis congenita, and (5) ataxia-telangiectasia.

DiGeorge syndrome, also known as a velocardiofacial syndrome, is characterized by developmental malformation of the third and fourth pharyngeal pouches. This leads to distinctive facial features (hypertelorism, saddle nose, short philtrum, low-set ears, cleft palate), conotruncal malformations (including tetralogy of Fallot, interrupted aortic arch, or truncus arteriosus), thymic hypoplasia, and parathyroid hypoplasia [14]. Typical thoracic imaging findings that may be present in pediatric patients with DiGeorge syndrome are a narrowed mediastinum related to a small thymus, an abnormal cardiac silhouette related to a conotruncal malformation, and recurrent pulmonary infections. Large-airway abnormality, such as tracheobronchomalacia, and osseous anomalies involving the ribs or vertebrae may be also present. In Wiscott-Aldrich syndrome, pulmonary infections with encapsulated *Streptococcus pneumoniae* and *Pneumocystis* are often seen [15]. In patients with hyper-IgE syndrome, recurrent pneumonia, lymphadenopathy, post-infectious pneumatoceles, and bronchiectasis are typically features on imaging studies. In addition, some patients have osseous findings, including osteoporosis, fractures, and scoliosis [16]. Children with dyskeratosis congenita, which is a progressive multisystemic disorder, characteristically present with rapidly progressing pulmonary fibrosis after hematopoietic stem cell transplantation [17] (Fig. 6). Ataxia-telangiectasia is due to underlying autosomal recessive mutations in the *ATM* gene, which encodes a DNA damage response protein. Affected pediatric patients are highly susceptible to DNA damage from ionizing radiation and the subsequent

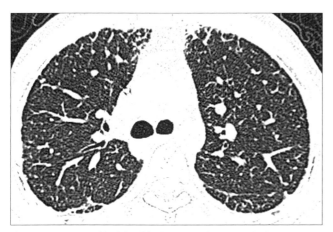

Fig. 6. A 15-year-old girl with dyskeratosis congenital status post hematopoietic stem cell transplantation. Axial lung window CT shows fibrotic lung changes in the peripheral portion of the lungs

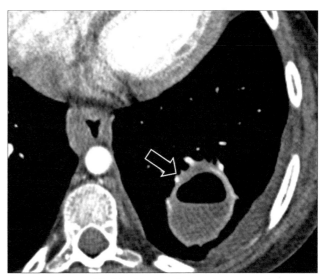

Fig. 8. A 14-year-old girl with chronic granulomatous disease. Enhanced axial CT shows a large lung abscess (*arrow*) from *S. aureus* infection. Also note the esophageal thickening due to chronic infective esophagitis

development of cancer, including lymphoma, leukemia, and leiomyosarcoma. Thus, in these patients, every effort should be made to limit imaging using ionizing radiation. Characteristic thoracic imaging findings include a small thymus, recurrent pneumonia (from *S. aureus, H. influenzae,* and *S. pneumoniae)*, bronchiectasis, and lymphadenopathy [18] (Fig. 7). In addition, a chronic interstitial lung disease unique to ataxia-telangiectasia (AT-ILD) may occur. On imaging studies it is characterized by pulmonary fibrosis presenting as interstitial and pleural thickening.

Congenital Defects of Phagocyte Number and/or Function

The most commonly encountered immunodeficiency syndrome related to congenital defects of phagocytes in children is chronic granulomatous disease (CGD). Affected children typically present with granuloma and ab-

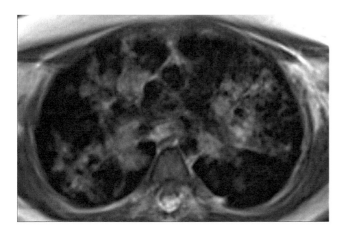

Fig. 7. An 11-year-old girl with ataxia-telangiectasis who underwent MRI of the lungs due to increased susceptibility to DNA damage from ionizing radiation associated with CT. Axial MRI shows multiple nodular and airspace opacities from histoplasmosis infection. The patient also later developed lymphoma (not shown)

scess formation from catalase-positive *S. aureus,* fungi, or atypical mycobacteria (Fig. 8). Although CGD can affect any organs, the lungs are the most common location of infection [19]. Depending on the infectious organism and disease chronicity, nodules, ground-glass opacities, consolidation, septal thickening, and cysts can be seen in the early phase. Later, recurrent and long-standing lung infections can lead to permanent damage, such as pulmonary fibrosis, honey-combing, and pulmonary hypertension. Extrapulmonary thoracic manifestations include suppurative lymphadenopathy, pleuritis, empyema, and rib or vertebral osteomyelitis.

Acquired Immunodeficiency

The two most commonly encountered acquired immunodeficiencies in the pediatric population are human immunodeficiency syndrome (HIV) and neutropenia due to chemotherapy for cancer or allogeneic hematopoietic stem cell transplantation. The lungs are the organ most commonly affected by infections in children with acquired immunodeficiency.

Many bacterial and viral infections have diverse nonspecific radiographic appearances in children with HIV. Pulmonary infection with PCP has more characteristic imaging findings; these include bilateral diffuse or patchy ground-glass or reticulonodular opacities with perihilar to peripheral progression [20]. In addition, pulmonary cysts, which can rupture and result in pneumothorax or pneumomediastinum, may also present on imaging studies in children with HIV. Lymphocytic interstitial pneumonitis (LIP) is a form of pulmonary lymphoid hyperplasia classically present in HIV-infected children older than 2 years of age. The imaging appearance of LIP includes nodules in a subpleural, septal centrilobular, or

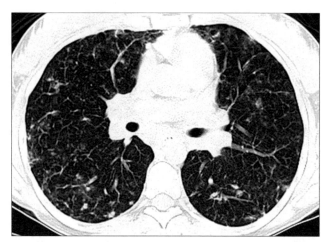

Fig. 9. An 18-year-old girl with lymphocytic interstitial pneumonitis. Axial lung window CT shows numerous small nodules and ground-glass opacities in both lungs

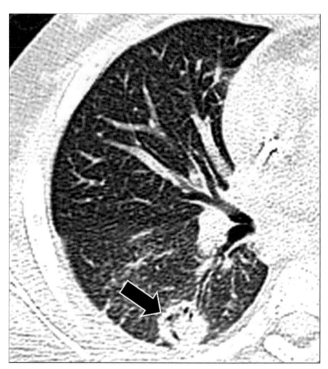

Fig. 11. A 10-year-old girl with aspergillus infection. Axial lung window CT shows a circumferential area of lucency ("air-crescent sign") within a nodular opacity (*arrow*) due to an underlying fungal ball

peribronchial distribution, and ground-glass opacities with or without lymphadenopathy [21] (Fig. 9). Other intrathoracic processes, such as thymic cysts and non-Hodgkin lymphoma, may occur in children with HIV infections.

In patients with acquired neutropenia, the characteristic imaging findings of the "halo sign" and the "air-crescent sign" can help radiologists make an early and accurate diagnosis. The "halo sign" consists of a ground-glass halo of alveolar hemorrhage around a nodular or consolidative focus of infarcting lung from fungal vascular invasion and thrombosis; it strongly suggests invasive fungal disease (Fig. 10). An "air-crescent" sign presents as a crescent-shaped or circumferential area of radiolucency within a parenchymal consolidation or nodular opacity, and strongly suggests an underlying fungal ball (Fig. 11). It important to recognize that children with acquired immunodefi-

ciency, particularly following allogeneic hematopoietic stem-cell transplantation, are susceptible not only to opportunistic pulmonary infections, but also to noninfectious pulmonary disorders including pulmonary edema, alveolar hemorrhage, drug reaction, bronchiolitis obliterans, graft-versus-host disease, and lymphoproliferative disease.

Lysosomal Storage Diseases

Lysosomal storage diseases (LSDs) result from the absence or dysfunction of a lysosomal enzyme, with subsequent accumulation of the lipid, glycol-protein, or mucopolysaccharide substrate. The three most commonly encountered LSDs in the pediatric population are Gaucher disease, Niemann-Pick disease, and mucopolysaccharidosis.

Gaucher disease, the most common LSD, is due to a congenital defect involving β-glucocerebrosidase. It results in the accumulation of glucocerebroside-laden macrophages in various organ systems, particularly the liver (hepatomegaly), spleen (splenomegaly and splenic infarcts), and bone marrow (osteonecrosis, endosteal scalloping, and Erlenmyer-flask deformities). Lung involvement is rare (~2%) but, when present, small nodules, ground-glass opacities, and septal thickening can be seen [22]. Niemann-Pick disease is due to the deficiency of sphingomyelinase, which results in the accumulation of "foamy" macrophages. Lung involvement as seen on imaging studies is characterized by diffuse interstitial

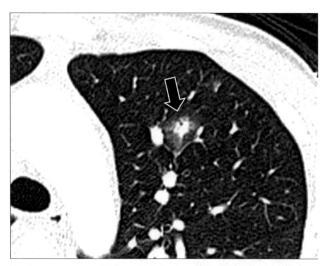

Fig. 10. A 14-year-old boy with leukemia. Axial lung window CT shows a round nodular opacity (*arrow*) surrounded by ground-glass opacity ("halo sign") from invasive aspergillus infection

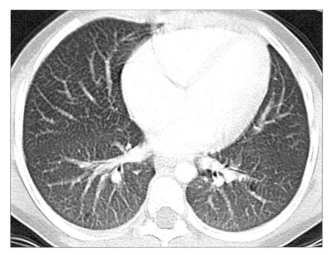

Fig. 12. A 5-year-old girl with Niemann-Pick disease. Axial lung window CT shows diffuse septal thickening in both lungs

thickening due to lipid-laden macrophages infiltrating the pulmonary interstitium [23] (Fig. 12). A "crazy-paving" appearance, which refers to the appearance of ground-glass opacities with superimposed interlobular septal thickening and intralobular reticular thickening, can be seen on the CT scans of patients affected with the type C2 form. The mucopolysaccharidoses (MPS) result from the accumulation of glycosaminoglycans in multi-organ systems. Affected children typically present with upper- and lower-airway obstruction, restrictive pulmonary disease, and respiratory tract infections. Large-airway involvement in MPS reflects excessive gly-cosaminoglycan deposition in the airway walls, which may result in tracheobronchomalacia, airway-wall deformity, and airway luminal narrowing. Underlying concomitant skeletal dysplasia limiting chest wall motion and hepatosplenomegaly limiting diaphragmatic motion can cause extrinsic restrictive lung disease in affected children [24].

Systemic Granulomatous Disorders

Two important systemic granulomatous disorders in pediatric patients are sarcoidosis and Crohn's disease [1, 3, 25]. Sarcoidosis is characterized by the presence of multiple small and well-circumscribed granulomas without necrosis that are typically located along lymphatic pathways [25]. It is a systemic disease process of unknown etiology with multisystem involvement. Pulmonary involvement of sarcoidosis is traditionally classified into four different stages of disease progression: (1) isolated lymphadenopathy, (2) lymphadenopathy with pulmonary disease, 3) isolated pulmonary disease, and 4) pulmonary fibrosis [1, 25]. The imaging findings of sarcoidosis mainly depend on the state of disease progression. In patients with stages 1–3 pulmonary sarcoidosis, small peribronchial nodules (<3 mm) and interstitial thickening intermixed with the areas of

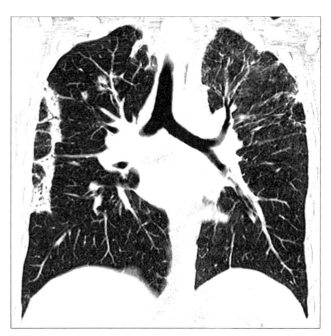

Fig. 13. A 16-year-old girl with Crohn's disease who presented with progressively worsening shortness of breath. Axial lung window CT shows bronchiectatic areas associated with ground glass and consolidative opacities

ground-glass opacities and consolidation are often seen [1, 25]. In patients with stage 4 disease, pulmonary fibrosis characterized by underlying architectural distortion, septal thickening, traction bronchiectasis, and honeycombing are the predominant findings [1, 3, 25]. Although much less frequent than intestinal manifestations, abnormalities involving the lung parenchyma (eosinophilic pneumonia, organizing pneumonia, granulomatous pneumonitis, interstitial pneumonitis), the small airways (bronchiolitis obliterans), and the large central airways (chronic bronchitis and bronchiectasis) may be seen in pediatric patients with Crohn's disease [26] (Fig. 13).

Vasculitis

Vasculitis is an inflammatory disease of the blood vessel walls. According to the size of the vessel affected, vasculitis can be classified as: 1) large-vessel disease, e.g., Takayasu's arteritis, temporal arteritis, and polymyalgia rheumatic; 2) medium-size vessel disease, e.g., Kawasaki disease, polyarthritis nodosa, Buerger's disease, and cutaneous vasculitis; and 3) small-vessel disease, e.g., granulomatosis with polyangiitis, Henoch-Schonlein purpura, Behcet's syndrome, and Churg-Strauss syndrome [1, 3]. Among them, granulomatosis with polyangiitis, formerly known as Wegener granulomatosis, is the most common pediatric necrotizing systemic vasculitis with thoracic manifestations and is thus the only one discussed in this review [1, 3].

Granulomatosis with polyangiitis is a rare systemic disorder that primarily affects the upper and lower respi-

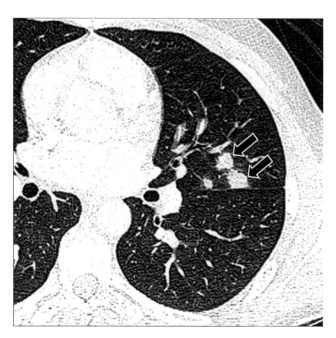

Fig. 14. A 14-year-old boy with granulomatosis with polyangiitis (Wagner granulomatosis). Axial lung window CT shows pulmonary nodules (*arrows*)

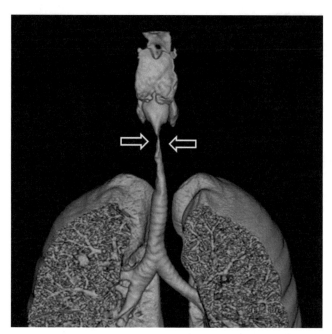

Fig. 16. A 13-year-old boy with granulomatosis with polyangiitis who presented with neck pain and shortness of breath. Frontal 3D volume-rendered image of the large airway shows a marked narrowing (*arrows*) of the subglottic airway

ratory tract and the kidney. Typical thoracic manifestations include multiple pulmonary nodules usually ranging in size from 2 mm to several centimeters in diameter [1, 3] (Fig. 14). Associated cavitation is seen in larger pulmonary nodules (>2 cm). Consolidation due to underlying pulmonary hemorrhage and/or ischemic necrosis may also be present (Fig. 15). In addition, there may be large-airway involvement, such as tracheobronchial wall thickening, tracheobronchial stenosis, or bronchiectasis [3] (Fig. 16).

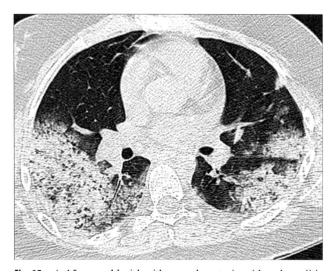

Fig. 15. A 15-year-old girl with granulomatosis with polyangiitis who presented with dyspnea and a decreased hematocrit. Axial lung window CT shows multifocal airspace consolidations in both lungs, compatible with pulmonary hemorrhage

Miscellaneous Disorders

Cystic Fibrosis

Cystic fibrosis (CF), the most common cause of pulmonary insufficiency in childhood, is caused by a mutation in the gene encoding the cystic fibrosis transmembrane regulator (CFTR) [1, 3]. CF typically affects children of European heritage, with an estimated incidence of 1:2,500 live births. Affected individuals commonly present with failure to thrive, meconium ileus syndrome, malabsorption syndrome, or chronic respiratory infection. The diagnosis is currently most often made during newborn screening. An abnormal sweat test or genetic test can provide a definite diagnosis.

In children with early stage of CF, the thoracic manifestations include mild to moderate air trapping (hyperinflation) due to an underlying obstruction of the small airways by abnormally viscid mucus and/or bronchial wall thickening. Upper lobe predominant bronchiectasis, peribronchial wall thickening, centrilobular nodular and tree-in-bud opacities, and mucus plugging with air-trapping are usually present in children with later or advanced CF [1, 3] (Fig. 17a). Because of the chronic and recurrent superimposed lung infection, concomitant reactive hilar and mediastinal lymphadenopathy as well as enlarged bronchial arteries are also often present (Fig. 17b). Although many patients with CF are evaluated by chest radiograph, it is not sensitive enough to detect the early or subtle lung changes. Currently, high-resolution CT is the most sensitive diagnostic imaging modality for assessing the morphologic changes of CF lung disease.

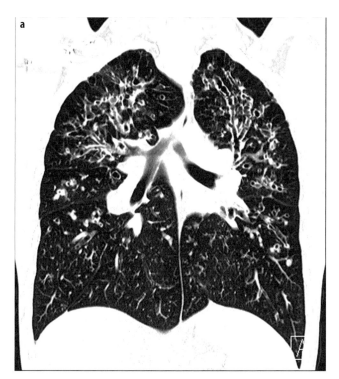
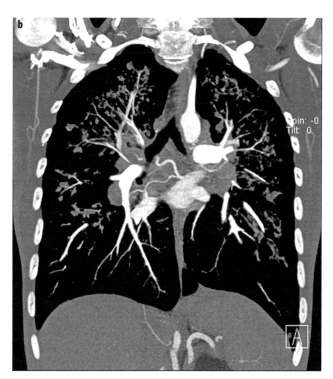

Fig. 17 a, b. A 15-year-old girl with cystic fibrosis. **a** Coronal lung window CT shows extensive upper-lobe-predominant bronchiectatic changes consistent with lung changes due to cystic fibrosis. **b** Coronal soft-tissue window CT shows extensive mucus plugging and enlarged bronchial arteries from chronic infection

A previously published study showed that CT is more sensitive than chest radiographs for detecting CF-related lung abnormalities, and that the CT score correlates well with the forced vital capacity (FVC), one-second forced expiratory volume (FEV1) ratio on a pulmonary function test [27]. A major consideration in the imaging of CF patients is the higher risk posed by ionizing radiation exposure. Therefore, in CF patients, MRI with advanced techniques including fast imaging sequences, high-resolution sequences, and hyperpolarized gas is being actively investigated for evaluating CF lung disease [28]. In addition to pulmonary disease, pancreatic disease is another primary abnormality in CF patients.

Although lung infections are treated with antibiotics, lung transplantation may be required for survival in pediatric patients with advanced CF. A broad range of therapies, including mucolytics and inhaled antibiotics, have improved both the life expectancy and the quality of life in CF patients. New medications targeting the specific defect in CFTR have recently become available, and gene therapy continues to be investigated as a potential treatment.

Sickle Cell Disease

Sickle cell disease is due to an abnormality in the oxygen-carrying hemoglobin molecule of red blood cells, such that the cells have a propensity for to assume an abnormal, sickle-like shape. Overproduction of abnormal

hemoglobin can result in anemia and bone marrow infarction. Eventually, sickle cell disease leads to various acute and chronic complications in multi-organ systems.

Two main chest complications of sickle cell disease are acute chest syndrome (ACS) and pneumonia [1, 3]. The former refers to the clinical situation in which patients with sickle cell disease develop a new opacity on chest radiographs accompanied by chest pain, fever, and respiratory syndrome [29] (Fig. 18). Possible underlying etiologies for ACS include infection, pulmonary infarction, and fat embolism from vaso-occlusive crises involving the bone marrow. A lack of interval resolution of the pulmonary opacities on the follow-up study should raise the possibility of a superimposed infectious process such as pneumonia. The two most common cardiovascular imaging findings in pediatric patients with sickle cell disease are cardiomegaly and pulmonary vascular plethora related to chronic anemia. Abnormal osseous changes due to underlying bone infarction are also frequently present. In the spine, recurrent bone infarction causes indentation of the upper and lower vertebral endplates (H-shaped vertebral bodies). Humeral head sclerosis or fragmentation related to bone infarction can be observed on chest radiographs. Hand-foot syndrome, which is characterized by a painful swelling of the hands and feet, may occur in young infants and children. Pediatric patients with hand-foot syndrome may also have soft-tissue swelling and periosteal new bone formation (Fig. 19). In addition, the spleen, the function of which is to clear red blood cells,

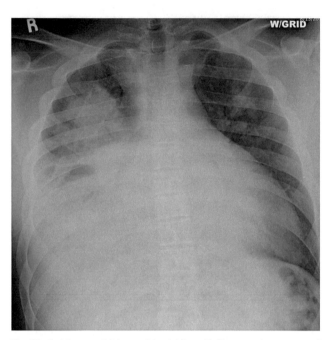

Fig. 18. A 17-year-old boy with sickle cell disease who presented with chest pain, fever, and respiratory distress. Frontal chest radiograph shows new airspace opacities in the right lung and cardiomegaly, compatible with acute chest syndrome

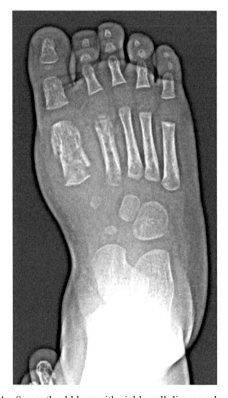

Fig. 19. An 8-month-old boy with sickle cell disease who presented with pain and swelling involving the right foot. Frontal radiograph of the right foot shows lytic bony changes associated with sclerotic new bone formation involving the first and second metatarsals. Soft-tissue swelling overlying the first metatarsal is also seen. The constellation of imaging findings is compatible with hand-foot syndrome in a sickle cell disease patient

is almost always infarcted before the end of childhood in affected patients. The functional asplenia can lead to an increased susceptibility to infections caused by bacteria with polysaccharide capsules.

Langerhans Cell Histiocytosis

Langerhans cell histiocytosis (LCH) is characterized by a clonal proliferation and the subsequent infiltration of tissues by Langerhans cells originating from the bone marrow [3]. In the past, LCH was classified into eosinophilic granuloma, Letterer-Siwe disease, and Hand-Schuller-Christian disease. The current classification divides affected patients into two groups: single-organ system involvement and multisystem involvement. The latter is more frequently seen in pediatric patients younger than 2 years old. Pulmonary involvement by LCH can be seen in pediatric patients with either single-organ system (primary pulmonary LCH) or multisystem disease. A recent study of 420 pediatric patients with multisystem LCH reported that pulmonary involvement was present at diagnosis in 24% of affected patients [30]. Pediatric patients with pulmonary LCH typically present with nonspecific symptoms such as cough, dyspnea, tachypnea, and chest pain.

Pulmonary manifestations of LCH can be categorized into two stages: early and advanced [1, 3]. Randomly distributed reticular nodular opacities with or without cysts are usually seen in patients with early-stage pulmonary involvement by LCH. Cysts in affected patients can sometimes rupture and result in spontaneous pneumothorax (Fig. 20). In patients with advanced or long-standing disease, both pulmonary fibrosis characterized by areas of architectural distortion and cysts are present. LCH involvement of other organ systems includes thymus (calcification, cyst formation, and enlargement), liver (hepatomegaly), and spleen (splenomegaly). Recognition of the characteristic pulmonary manifestation of LCH in conjunction with other organ system involvement can be helpful in reaching an early diagnosis.

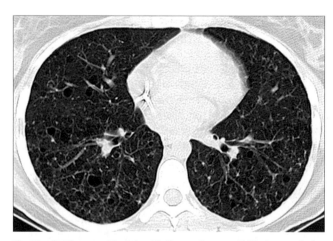

Fig. 20. A 17-year-old girl with Langerhans cell histiocytosis involving the lungs. Axial lung window CT shows randomly distributed reticulonodular opacities and cysts in both lungs

Tuberous Sclerosis

Tuberous sclerosis (TS) is a multisystem genetic disease that results from a mutation of either of two genes, TSC1 and TSC2, which code for hamartin and tuberin, respectively. These two proteins act as tumor growth suppressors regulating cell proliferation and differentiation. Affected patients typically present with the classic clinical triad of mental retardation, seizures, and adenoma sebaceum.

Two characteristic pulmonary manifestations of TS are lymphangioleiomyomatosis (LAM) and multifocal micronodular pneumocyte hyperplasia (MMPH) [1, 3]. Dyspnea or acute respiratory distress related to spontaneous pneumothorax is the usual clinical presentation in a TS patient with lung involvement from LAM. On imaging studies, multiple small cysts with thin or imperceptible walls that are evenly distributed throughout the lungs are seen in affected children with early-stage LAM (Fig. 21). These cysts are located within adjacent normal lung parenchyma and usually do not coalesce. Concomitant spontaneous pneumothorax or chylous effusions may also present. Patients with late-stage LAM with extensive cystic lung involvement eventually require lung transplantation for survival. In TS patients with MMPH, multiple, well-defined pulmonary nodules that may resemble metastases can be seen on imaging studies. These represent proliferations of enlarged type II pneumocytes that form ill-defined papillae and fill the alveolar spaces. Because the imaging findings of these pulmonary nodules are non-specific, lung biopsy with pathological evaluation may be required for a definitive diagnosis.

In addition to lung abnormalities, pediatric patients with TS often present with characteristic findings indicating the involvement of other organ systems, such as giant cell astrocytoma, cortical tubers, sub-ependymal nodules of the brain (Fig. 22a), rhabdomyomas of the heart (Fig. 22b), and angiomyolipomas of the kidneys and liver (Fig. 22c). Recognition of the characteristic pulmonary manifestation of TS in conjunction with other organ system involvement can be helpful in reaching an early diagnosis.

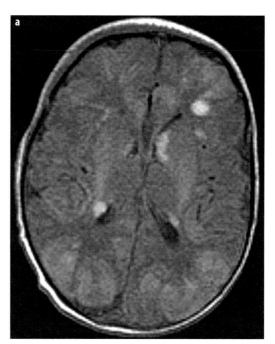
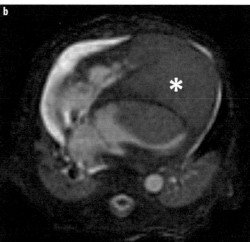
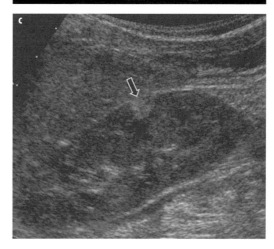

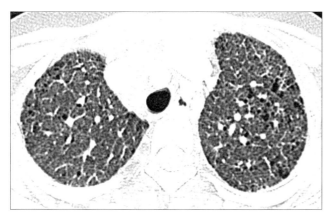

Fig. 21. A 15-year-old girl with tuberous sclerosis and lymphangioleiomyomatosis. Axial lung window CT shows multiple small thin-walled cysts distributed relatively evenly in both lungs

Fig. 22 a-c. A 5-day old boy with tuberous sclerosis. **a** Axial T1 FLAIR MRI shows cortical tubers. **b** Axial T2 MRI demonstrates a large cardiac rhabdomyoma (*asterisk*). **c** Longitudinal renal ultrasound shows echogenic renal lesion (*arrow*) consistent with renal angiomyolipoma

Conclusion

With clear knowledge of the characteristic thoracic imaging features of systemic diseases, the radiologist may be the first to suggest a particular diagnosis, which in turn can lead to early and optimal pediatric patient care.

References

1. Garcia-Pena P, Boixadera H, Barber I et al (2011) Thoracic findings of systemic diseases at high-resolution CT in children. Radiographics 31:465-482.
2. Dishop MK (2011) Diagnostic pathology of diffuse lung disease in children. Pediatr Allergy Immunol Pulmonol 23:69-85.
3. Lee EY, Cleveland RH, Langston C (2012) Interstitial lung disease in infants and children: new classification system with emphasis on clinical, imaging, and pathological correlation. In: Cleveland RH (Ed) Imaging in Pediatric Pulmonology, Springer.
4. Athreya BH, Doughty RA, Bookspan M et al (1980) Pulmonary manifestations of juvenile rheumatoid arthritis. A report of eight cases and review. Clin Chest Med 1:361-374.
5. Kimura Y, Weiss E, Haroldson KL et al (2013) Pulmonary hypertension and other potentially fatal pulmonary complications in systemic juvenile idiopathic arthritis. Arthritis Care Res (Hoboken) 65:745-752.
6. Ferguson PJ, Weinberger M (2006) Shrinking lung syndrome in a 14-year-old boy with systemic lupus erythematosus. Pediatr Pulmonol 41:194-197.
7. Cunningham-Rundles C (2012) The many faces of common variable immunodeficiency. Hematology Am Soc Hematol Educ Program 2012:301-305.
8. Touw CML, van de Ven AA, de Jong PA et al (2010) Detection of pulmonary complications in common variable immunodeficiency. Pediatr Allergy Immunol 21:793-805.
9. Park JH, Levinson AI (2010) Granulomatous-lymphocytic interstitial lung disease (GLILD) in common variable immunodeficiency (CVID). Clin Immunol 134:97-103.
10. Winkelstein JA, Marino MC, Ochs H et al (2003) The X-Linked hyper-IgM syndrome: clinical and immunological features of 79 patients. Medicine (Baltimore) 82:373-384.
11. Buckley RH (2004) Pulmonary complications of primary immunodeficiencies. Paediatr Respir Rev 5 (Suppl A):S225-233.
12. Griffith LM, Cowan MJ, Notarangelo LD et al (2009) Improving cellular therapy for primary immune deficiency diseases: recognition, diagnoses, and management. J Allergy Clin Immunol 123:1152.
13. Nadeau K, Hwa V, Rosenfeld RG (2011) STAT5b deficiency: an unsuspected cause of growth failure, immunodeficiency, and severe pulmonary disease. J Pediatr 158:701-708.
14. Demczuk S, Aurias A (1995) DiGeorge syndrome and related syndromes associated with 22q11.2 deletions. A review. Ann Genet 38:59-76.
15. Notarangelo LD, Miao CH, Ochs HD (2008) Wiskott-Aldrich syndrome. Curr Opin Hematol 15:30-36.
16. Chandesris MO, Melki I, Natividad A et al (2012) Autosomal dominant STAT3 deficiency and hyper-IgE syndrome: molecular, cellular, and clinical features from a French National Survey. Medicine 91:e1-e19.
17. Giri N, Rees L, Faro A et al (2011) Lung transplantation for pulmonary fibrosis in dyskeratosis congenital: case report and systematic literature review. BMC Blood Disorders 11:3. Doi: 10.1186/1471-2326-11-3.
18. Schroeder SA, Zielen S (2013) Infections of the respiratory system in patients with ataxia-telangiectasia. Pediatr Pulmonol doi:10.1002/ppul.22817.
19. Mahdaviani SA, Mohajerani SA, Rezaei N et al (2013) Pulmonary manifestations of chronic granulomatous disease. Expert Rev Clin Immunol 9:153-160.
20. George R, Andronikou S, Theron S et al (2009) Pulmonary infections in HIV-positive children. Pediatr Radiol 39:545-554.
21. Theron S, Andronikou S, George R et al (2009) Non-infective pulmonary disease in HIV-positive children. Pediatr Radiol 39:555-564.
22. Goitein O, Elstein D, Abrahamov A et al (2001) Lung involvement and enzyme replacement therapy in Gaucher's disease. QJM 94(8):407-415.
23. Nuillemot N, Troadec C, de Villemeur TB et al (2007) Lung disease in Niemann-Pick disease. Pediatr Pulmonol 42:1207-1214.
24. Berger KI, Fagondes SC, Giugliani R et al (2013) Respiratory and sleep disorders in mucopolysaccharidosis. J Inherit Metab Dis 36:201-210.
25. Milman N, Hoffman AL, Byg KE (1998) Sarcoidosis in children. Epidemiology in Danes, Clinical features, diagnosis, treatment and prognosis. Acta Paediatr 87:871-878.
26. Al-Binali AM, Scott B, Al-Garni A et al (2003) Granulomatous pulmonary disease in a child: an unusual presentation of Crohn's disease. Pediatr Pulmonol 36:76-80.
27. Bhalla M, Turcios N, Aponte V et al (1991) Cystic fibrosis: scoring system with thin-section CT. Radiology 179:783-788.
28. Gorkem SB, Coskun A, Yikilmaz A et al (2013) Evaluation of pediatric thoracic disorders: comparison of unenhanced fast-imaging-sequence 1.5T MRI and contrast-enhanced MDCT. AJR Am J Roentgenol 200:1352-1357.
29. Martin L, Buonomo C (1997) Acute chest syndrome of sickle cell disease: radiographic and clinical analysis of 70 cases. Pediatr Radiol 27:637-641.
30. Ronceray L, Potschger U, Janka G et al (2012) Pulmonary involvement in pediatric-onset multisystem Langerhans cell histiocytosis: effect on course and outcome. J Pediatr 161:129-133.

Modern Diagnosis in the Evaluation of Pulmonary Vascular Disease

Alexander A. Bankier[1], Christoph Engelke[2]

[1] Department of Radiology, Beth Israel Deaconess Medical Center, Harvard Medical School, Boston, MA, USA
[2] Department of Radiology, University of Goettingen, Goettingen, Germany

Introduction

Conventional chest radiography, computed tomography (CT), and, with restrictions, magnetic resonance imaging (MRI) are the three most commonly used imaging modalities for evaluating patients with suspected pulmonary vascular disease. Very recently, the clinical usefulness of fluorodeoxyglucose positron emission tomography (FDG-PET) and FDG-PET/CT in the diagnosis of large-vessel vasculitis also has been recognized. However, in daily general clinical routine, most patients with suspected pulmonary vascular disease will be evaluated by CT. Moreover, the utility of CT has been improved by technical developments such as dual-source and dual-energy scanners, which simultaneously generate morphological and functional information from a sole dataset. In patients with pulmonary vascular diseases, this approach is of major interest for three main reasons: (1) Pulmonary vascular disorders require a thorough morphological evaluation, not only of the vascular tree per se, but also of the surrounding lung parenchyma; (2) given that we have reached an upper limit in terms of morphologic image resolution, but can simultaneously obtain functional information, CT ideally combines high-end morphologic imaging with perfusion and ventilation imaging; and (3) it is becoming increasingly important to determine the cardiac consequences or causes of pulmonary vascular diseases, which requires all of the advantages that CT can provide. For these reasons, and because of the general importance of CT, it is the focus of this chapter. Other imaging modalities are not ignored; rather, they are discussed in case-based presentations and in their distinct clinical contexts.

Optimized Evaluation of Pulmonary Vessels on Chest CT Examinations

Temporal Resolution of Pulmonary CT Angiograms

Given the anatomical complexity of the lungs, a crucial prerequisite for optimal chest imaging is a high spatial resolution, not only to detect subtle morphologic abnormalities but also to adequately visualize the thoracic vessels on CT angiography (CTA) and to differentiate between normal and abnormal vascular dimensions. However, high spatial resolution is optimally employed when short overall examination times and high temporal resolution (i.e., short acquisition times of the individual axial image planes) are available simultaneously. This enables the analysis of high-resolution images with a minimum of motion artifacts. The development of multidetector-row CT (MDCT) has allowed radiologists to image the entire thorax with increasing spatial resolution in shorter time intervals. Consequently, more patients are able to maintain a breath-hold throughout the entire period of data acquisition, which results in a substantial decrease in the number and frequency of respiratory motion artifacts. Furthermore, shorter CT rotation times have enabled shorter acquisition times and thus contributed to the substantial reduction in artifacts caused by cardiac motion. In the past, cardiac motion artifacts not only reduced the quality of images obtained close to the heart but also caused pulsation artifacts at the anatomical level of the systemic and pulmonary vessels, thus mimicking endovascular abnormalities such as thrombi and neoplastic lesions. To image patients with the highest temporal resolution and shortest examination time possible requires the shortest rotation time and the highest pitch, defined as the table feed per rotation divided by the nominal beam width at the isocenter of the scanner. For example, on a 64-slice MDCT using a single X-ray source, rotation times range from 0.30 and 0.40 s, resulting in a temporal resolution per image not better than half the rotation time, and with pitch values usually not exceeding 1.5 [1]. The introduction of dual-source 64-slice MDCT has improved the technical requirements for CT. When both available tubes are operated at the same kilovoltage, the temporal resolution of each image is 1/4 of the rotation time, each of the two detectors contributing 90° of data in parallel-ray geometry to each image plane [2]. Moreover, the second measurement system of dual-source CT (DSCT) allows for a higher pitch mode than available with a single-

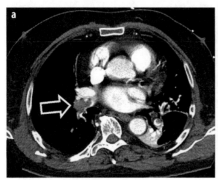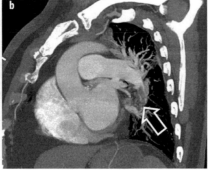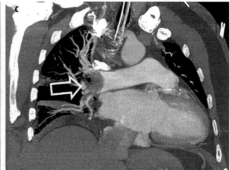

Fig. 1 a-c. Acute pulmonary embolism. Transverse contrast-enhanced CT section (**a**) allows the diagnosis of a large intraluminal clot (*arrow*). Multiplanar reconstructions in the sagittal (**b**) and coronal (**c**) planes show the true sagittal and coronal extent of the clot (*arrows*)

source CT, but without image distortion inside the field of view of the second detector. Tacelli et al. showed that this scanning mode yields CTA examinations of excellent quality for thoracic applications in routine clinical practice, including in patients in pulmonary vascular diseases such as acute pulmonary embolism (PE) (Fig. 1) [3].

Improved Morphological Evaluation of the Peripheral Pulmonary Vasculature

With the introduction of MDCT, CTA is now recognized as the reference standard for diagnosing acute PE [4]. A main advantage of MDCT over single-slice CT is the ability to scan the entire volume of the thorax with submillimetric collimation in a very short period of time, most often under the duration of a single breath-hold. This is particularly useful when evaluating dyspneic patients. These technological advances have improved both evaluations of the peripheral pulmonary arteries and the accuracy of CT in the workup of acute PE. Simultaneously, MDCT allows radiologists to scan patients at a low kilovoltage, with reductions in the dose of contrast material and the overall radiation dose. This is of particular importance in young female patients who may be exposed to substantial levels of radiation to breast tissue. In the context of acute PE, the latter concern is clinically relevant given the lower prevalence of acute PE, which has dropped from 33% on angiographic studies to <20% on CT/MDCT scans. To date, several studies have investigated the clinical benefits of low-kilovoltage techniques, i.e., 80–100 kV(p) vs. 120–140 kV(p), the parameters at which CTA is typically performed. However, for obvious ethical reasons, these studies were based on the comparative analysis of different populations scanned with single-source CT [5-8]. The limitations of these comparisons include the lack of systematic adjustment for individual patient morphology, cardiac hemodynamics, and potential underlying respiratory disease. With the introduction of DSCT, the two tubes can be set at different kilovoltages. In addition to the opportunity to evaluate lung perfusion, there are benefits for standard CTA as this scanning mode has been shown

to improve the visualization of small pulmonary arteries at 80 kV(p) [9].

Perfusion Imaging with Dual-Energy CT

Lung perfusion with dual-energy CT does not reflect blood flow analysis per se, as it provides a measurement at only one time point; rather, it yields an iodine map of the lung microcirculation at a particular time point. Numerous parameters are known to influence the distribution of iodine within pulmonary capillaries; some are technique-related whereas others are due to the anatomical and/or physiological circumstances under which the data were acquired. Dual-energy CTA is performed using a scanning protocol similar to the one used in clinical practice. The acquisitions proceed from the top to the bottom of the chest, with an injection protocol similar to that of standard CTA obtained with a single energy on a 64-slice scanner. Two categories of images can be reconstructed: Diagnostic scans correspond to contiguous 1-mm-thick transverse CT scans generated from the raw spiral projection data of tube A and tube B (60% from the acquisition by tube A; 40% from the acquisition by tube B). Lung perfusion scans (i.e., images of the perfused blood volume of the lung parenchyma) are generated after determination of the iodine content of every voxel of the lung parenchyma on the separate 80- and 140-kVp images. The images can be rendered in gray-scale or color-coded. All images can be displayed as transverse scans, complemented as needed by corona land sagittal reformats. Even though a dual-energy acquisition does not correspond to true perfusion imaging, several applications of this pulmonary micro-CTA technique have been investigated [10].

Acute Pulmonary Embolism

Dual-energy CT can detect endoluminal clots on averaged images obtained with tubes A and B as reliably as can single-source CTA [11]. In a preliminary study, the detectability of perfusion defects beyond obstructive clots was validated. Perfusion defects in the adjacent lung parenchyma have the typical perfusion-territorial triangular shape well known from pulmonary angiographic, scintigraphic, and MRI perfusion studies. Dual-energy CTA can help predict perfusion defects without directly identifying peripheral endoluminal clots that may be located in subsegmental or more distal pulmonary arterial branches. It can also help differentiate lung infarction from less specific peripheral lung consolidation.

Chronic Pulmonary Embolism

Dual-energy CTA can depict perfusion defects distal to chronic clots (Fig. 2). Three vascular characteristics of chronic PE may manifest on dual-energy CT imaging. First, chronic PE causes a mosaic pattern of lung attenuation, characterized by areas of ground-glass attenuation, with enlarged vascular segments intermingled with areas of normal lung attenuation and smaller vascular segments. When present, these findings are suggestive of blood flow redistribution, but they are not consistently seen on conventional CT in patients with chronic PE. In these patients, dual-energy CT can detect ground-glass attenuation of vascular origin based on the high iodine content within the areas of ground-glass attenuation, thus enabling their distinction from ground-glass attenuation secondary to bronchial or alveolar diseases [12]. Second, chronic PE can cause calcifications within partially or completely occlusive chronic clots as well as within pulmonary artery walls, when chronic PE is complicated by longstanding or severe pulmonary hypertension. The calcifications are detectable using virtual non-contrast imaging, accessible by dual-energy CT imaging. Third, the images generated at 80 kV can improve visualization of the systemic collateral supply characteristic of chronic PE and originating from bronchial and non-bronchial systemic arteries.

Obstructive Airways Diseases

Abnormalities of pulmonary perfusion are a feature of numerous smoking-related respiratory diseases. Peinado et al. showed that endothelial dysfunction of the pulmonary arteries is present even in patients with mild chronic obstructive pulmonary disease (COPD) [13]. In these patients, as well as in smokers with normal lung function, some arteries show a thickened intima, suggesting that tobacco consumption plays an important role in the pathogenesis of pulmonary vascular pathologies in COPD. Several structural changes in the early stages of COPD have been described in experimental and animal models, including proliferation of smooth-muscle fibers within peribronchiolar arterioles and collagen and elastin deposition in the thickened intima of vessels [14, 15]. In preliminary studies, Hoffman et al. [16] showed an increased heterogeneity of the local mean transit times of contrast material within the pulmonary microvasculature of smokers with normal pulmonary function tests. In their dual-source, dual-energy CTA study of pulmonary lobar perfusion in COPD patients, Pansini et al. [17] found that nonsmokers had no alterations in lung structure and observed a uniform distribution of iodine content within the upper and lower lobes and between the right and left lungs. Perfusion scans showed significantly lower iodine content within the lung microcirculation of the upper lobes in emphysematous patients than in smokers without emphysema and a significantly lower perfusion in the upper than in the lower lung zones, consistent with the destruction of the lung parenchyma. These structural abnormalities have important implications given the epidemiologic and socioeconomic burden of COPD.

Restrictive Airways Diseases

The substantial importance of pulmonary hypertension on the clinical course and prognosis of patients with

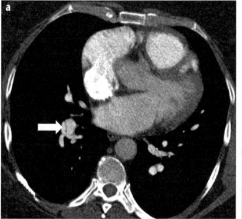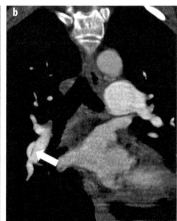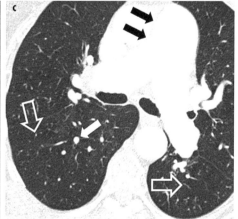

Fig. 2 a-c. Chronic thromboembolic disease. Transverse CT section (**a**) shows a web in the pulmonary artery of the right lower lobe (*arrow*), which is confirmed (*arrow*) by a coronal multiplanar reconstruction (**b**). Lung window (**c**) shows a dilated main pulmonary artery (*black arrows*), dilated peripheral pulmonary artery (*white arrow*), and parenchymal areas of hypoperfusion (*open arrows*)

fibrotic lung disease has been extensively recognized. However, the mere measurement of pulmonary artery diameters might not be a reliable parameter in the assessment of disease severity, due to the potentially confounding role of parenchymal traction on central and peripheral pulmonary vessels. Moreover, because of the age of the population in which these diseases usually occur, age-related changes have to be taken into account in morphometric-based clinical decision-making and disease classification. Overall, and despite promising initial scientific evidence, the roles of MDCT and DSCT in assessing patients with fibrotic lung diseases still need to be determined. The many ongoing pharmacological trials, notably in patients with usual interstitial pneumonits, may provide an ample study ground in this field.

Are There Indications for ECG-Gated CTA Examinations When Exploring Pulmonary Vascular Diseases?

Pulmonary Hypertension

Although a pulmonary trunk diameter ⩾33.2 mm has 95% sensitivity for the diagnosis of pulmonary hypertension (PHT), the specificity of this measurement is only 58%, which is insufficient for the accurate diagnosis of PHT, notably in patients with mild disease [18]. Moreover, no correlation has been found between the degree of PHT and pulmonary trunk diameter. Electrocardiograph (ECG)-gated MDCT acquisitions of the entire thorax enable the evaluation of novel functional parameters in addition to the standard morphology. In patients with PHT, right pulmonary artery distensibility was recently shown to be an accurate predictor of PHT on ECG-gated 64-slice MDCT scans of the chest [19]. In that study, its diagnostic value was superior to that of the single measurement of pulmonary trunk diameter.

Right Ventricular Function

Fast rotation speed and dedicated cardiac reconstruction algorithms designed to extend the conventional multislice acquisition data scheme have opened up new opportunities for cardiac and thoracic imaging applications. The first method for ECG-gated examinations of the entire thorax was introduced by Flohr et al., using 4-slice MD-CT technology [20]. This approach provided greater anatomical coverage than achieved with standard ECG-gated spiral scanning. When used with reconstruction approaches for cardiac applications, precise morphologic data at the level of the larger mediastinal vessels can be obtained. Despite this improvement, major progress in fast-scanning multislice CT technology came with the introduction of 16-slice MDCT, which allowed the integration of cardiac functional information. Three approaches were proposed: (1) investigating cardiac global function during a whole-chest multislice CT acquisition with a 16-×1.5-mm collimation to ensure an acceptable breath-hold duration [21], (2) a two-phase protocol to scan both the entire thorax and cardiac cavities with the highest spatial resolution [22], and (3) a dedicated cardiac MD-CT protocol to assess right ventricular function and myocardial mass [23]. In a comparison of ECG-gated 16-slice MDCT with equilibrium radionuclide ventriculography, these studies confirmed both the feasibility of the former in a population of hemodynamically stable patients and the accuracy of the CT-estimated right ventricular ejection fraction. The introduction of 64-slice scanners also offered further improvement in the integration of morphology and cardiac function. Salem et al. reported that right and left ventricular function was assessable in 93% of their study patients with various respiratory disorders; in the remaining patients, an imprecise segmentation of the right and left ventricular cavities was the limiting factor for precise calculation of end-systolic and end-diastolic ventricular volumes [24]. The positive results were achievable with dose length-product (DLP) values lower than those recommended for standard non-ECG-gated examinations. This was possible because of the concurrent use of two-dose modulation systems, in particular, the adjustment of the milliampere setting for patient size and anatomical shape and an ECG-controlled tube current.

Overall, there is increased evidence and awareness in the radiological community that new scanner technology has opened up new opportunities for imaging the cardiopulmonary system [25, 26]. The techniques have also received increased attention in the field of translational research [27].

Imaging of Pulmonary Vasculitis

Systemic primary vasculitides are idiopathic diseases that cause an inflammatory injury to the vessel walls. Pulmonary involvement is frequent, and chest-CT often in combination with PET/CT is the reference imaging technique in its assessment. Pulmonary vasculitis occurs in a wide variety of systemic and pulmonary vascular disorders. Most vasculitic entities affecting the lung induce overlapping disease patterns such as pneumonitis with or without capillaritis, diffuse alveolar damage, and acute pulmonary hemorrhage, or inflammatory obstruction of the central pulmonary arteries down to the small vessels, with chronic secondary pulmonary hypertension with or without interstitial lung disease. Therefore the clinical symptoms per se or the CT-morphology alone are often nonspecific.

Owing to their complimentary value in the imaging of central and peripheral vascular territories and their secondary parenchymal or interstitial abnormalities, CTA, high-resolution CT, and fusion imaging play key roles in the noninvasive workup of patients with suspected pulmonary vasculitis. They can indicate the need for further clinical tests, imaging, or invasive diagnostics and direct medical treatment during follow-up.

The Role of CT in the Differential Diagnosis of Pulmonary Vasculitis

In large-vessel vasculitis, CT is the method of choice, often in combination with PET, to discriminate macrospcopic vascular abnormalities presenting key pathological features, such as pulmonary arterial wall thickening with late enhancement, steno-occlusive or thrombo-obliterating disease with resulting oligemia, infarction in the dependent lung, or arterial aneurysms, as a facultative cause of massive pulmonary hemorrhage. CT is the modality of choice to demonstrate the effects of peripheral small-vessel pulmonary vasculitis on the central pulmonary arteries, such as secondary chronic pulmonary hypertension due to reduction of the total cross-sectional area with arteriolar remodeling or narrowing of the capillary bed in capillaritis.

Because CT-determined pathologies of the lung parenchyma, vessels, and airways are highly variable, diagnosis is a challenging interdisciplinary task. Clinical and laboratory data have to be included in close cooperation with the findings of the referring physician. However, many vasculitic disorders present characteristic CT features. CT-pathologic correlates of the peribronchovascular axial interstitium, pulmonary hemorrhage, types of inflammatory parenchymal infiltration, and secondary pathologies such as organizing pneumonia, should be considered with reference to the revised 2012 International Chapel Hill Consensus Conference on Pulmonary Vasculitis and the American College of Rheumatology [28].

Acknowledgment. We thank Prof. Martine Remy-Jardin, Lille, France, for her previous work in this field, which served as an inspiration and blueprint for this contribution.

References

1. Rogalla P, Kloeters C, Hein PA (2009) CT technology overview: 64-slice and beyond. Radiol Clin North Am 47: 1-11.
2. Petersilka M, Bruder H, Krauss B et al (2008) Technical principles of dual source CT. Eur J Radiol 68:362-368.
3. Tacelli N, Remy-Jardin M, Flohr T et al (2010) Dual-source chest CT angiography with high temporal resolution and high pitch modes: evaluation of image quality in 140 patients. Eur Radiol 20:1188-1196.
4. Remy-Jardin M, Pistolesi M, Goodman LR et al (2007) Management of suspected acute pulmonary embolism in the era of CT angiography: a statement from the Fleischner Society. Radiology 245:315-329.
5. Holmquist F, Nyman U (2006) Eighty-peak kilovoltage 16-channel multidetector computed tomography and reduced contrastmedium doses tailored to body weight to diagnose pulmonary embolism in azotaemic patients. Eur Radiol 16:1165-1176.
6. Sigal-Cinqualbre AB, Hennequin R, Abada H et al (2004) Low-kilovoltage multi-detector row chest CT in adults: feasibility and effect on image quality and iodine dose. Radiology 231:169-174.
7. Schueller-Weidekamm C, Schaefer-Prokop CM, Weber M et al (2006) CT angiography of pulmonary arteries to detect pulmonary embolism: improvement of vascular enhancement with low kilovoltage settings. Radiology 241:899-907.
8. Heyer CM, Mohr PS, Lemburg SP et al (2007) Image quality and radiation exposure at pulmonary CT angiography with 100- or 120-kVp protocol: prospective randomized study. Radiology 245:577-583.
9. Gorgos AB, Remy-Jardin M, Duhamel A et al (2009) Evaluation of peripheral pulmonary arteries at 80 kV and at 140 kV: dual-energy computed tomography assessment in 51 patients. J Comput Assist Tomogr 33:981-986.
10. Remy-Jardin M, Faivre JB, Pontana F et al (2010) Thoracic applications of dual energy. Radiol Clin North Amer 48:193-205.
11. Pontana F, Faivre JB, Remy-Jardin M et al (2008) Lung perfusion with dual-energy multidetector-row CT (MDCT): Feasibilityfor the evaluation of acute pulmonary embolism in 117 consecutive patients. Acad Radiol 15:1494-1504.
12. Pontana F, Remy-Jardin M, Duhamel A et al (2010) Lung perfusion with dual energy multidetector-row CT: can it help recognize ground glass opacities of vascular origin? Acad Radiol 17:587-594.
13. Peinado VI, Barberà JA, Ramirez J et al (1988) Endothelial dysfunction in pulmonary arteries of patients with mild COPD. Am J Physiol 274:L908-L913.
14. Yamato Y, Sun JP, Churg A et al (1997) Guinea pig pulmonary hypertension caused by cigarette smoke cannot be explained by capillary bed destruction. J Appl Physiol 82:1644-1653.
15. Santos S, Peinado VI, Ramirez J et al (2002) Characterization of pulmonary vascular remodelling in smokers and patients with mild COPD. Eur Respir J 19:632-638.
16. Hoffman EA, Simon BA, McLennan G (2006) A structural and functional assessment of the lung via multidetector-row computed tomography. Proc Am Thorac Soc 3:519-534.
17. Pansini V, Remy-Jardin M, Faivre JB et al (2009) Assessment of lobar pulmonary perfusion in COPD patients: preliminary experience with dual-energy CT angiography. Eur Radiol 19:2834-2843.
18. Edwards PD, Bull RK, Coulden R (1998) CT measurement of main pulmonary artery diameter. Br J Radiol 71:1018-1020.
19. Revel MP, Faivre JB, Remy-Jardin M et al (2009) Pulmonary hypertension: ECG-gated 64-section CT angiographic evaluation of new functional parameters as diagnostic criteria. Radiology 250:558-566.
20. Flohr T, Prokop M, Becker CR et al (2002) A retrospectively ECG-gated multislice spiral CT scan and reconstruction technique with suppression of heart pulsation artifacts for cardiothoracic imaging with extended volume coverage. Eur Radiol 12:1497-1503.
21. Coche E, Vlassenbroeck A, Roelants V et al (2005) Evaluation of biventricular ejection fraction with ECG-gated 16-slice CT: preliminary findings in acute pulmonary embolism in comparison with radionuclide ventriculography. Eur Radiol 15:1432-1440.
22. Delhaye D, Remy-Jardin M, Teisseire A et al (2006) Estimation of right ventricular ejection fraction by multidetector row-CT: comparison with equilibrium radionuclide ventriculography, Part I. AJR Am J Roentgenol 187:1597-1804.
23. Kim TH, Ryu YH, Hur J et al (2005) Evaluation of right ventricular volume and mass using retrospective ECG-gated cardiac multidetector computed tomography: comparison with first-pass radionuclide angiography. Eur Radiol 15:1987-1993.
24. Salem R, Remy-Jardin M, Delhaye D et al (2006) Integrated cardiothoracic imaging with ECG-gated 64-slice multidetector-row CT: Initial findings in 133 patients. Eur Radiol 16:1973-1981.
25. Lu GM, Zhao Y, Zhang LJ, Schoepf UJ (2012) Dual-energy CT of the lung. AJR Am J Roentgenol 199:S40-53.
26. Ko JP, Brandman S, Stember J, Naidich DP (2012) Dual-energy computed tomography: concepts, performance, and thoracic applications. J Thorac Imaging 27:7-22.

27. Badea CT, Guo X, Clark D et al (2012) Dual-energy micro-CT of the rodent lung. Am J Physiol Lung Cell Mol Physiol 302:1088-1097.

28. Jennette JC, Falk RJ, Bacon PA et al (2012) Revised International Chapel Hill Consensus Conference Nomenclature of Vasculitides. Arthritis & Rheumatism Vol. 65, No. 1, January 2013, 1.11.

Imaging of Pulmonary Infections

Philip Goodman[1], Helmut Prosch[2], Christian J. Herold[2]

[1] Duke University Medical Center, Durham, NC, USA
[2] Department of Radiology, Vienna General Hospital, Medical University of Vienna, Vienna, Austria

Introduction

Pulmonary infection is one of the most frequent causes of morbidity and mortality throughout the world. Many infections occur in individuals with concomitant intrapulmonary or extrathoracic diseases; however, they commonly develop in otherwise healthy people. In the non-immunocompromised population, pneumonia is the most prevalent community-acquired infection and the second most common nosocomial infectious disorder. In immunocompromised patients, in children, and in the elderly, pneumonia, as well as other pulmonary infections, may develop into a life-threatening condition.

In this chapter, the most important principles regarding the epidemiology, pathogenesis, classification, and clinical and radiographic diagnoses of pneumonias are reviewed. Our aim is to formulate an integrated approach to the diagnosis of pneumonia that combines clinical and radiologic information. As such, we focus on: (1) community-acquired pneumonia (CAP); (2) nosocomial pneumonia (NP); and (3) pneumonia in immunocompromised patients including those infected with the human immunodeficiency virus (HIV). The differentiation between CAP, NP, and other forms of pneumonia is of paramount importance because of the potentially different etiologies, clinical features, diagnostic approaches, radiologic patterns, and therapeutic strategies. Although the spectrum of causative organisms differs between these disorders, there is considerable overlap with regard to their radiologic features.

Community-Acquired Pneumonia

Pathogenesis

Pneumonias acquired in the community are the form of pneumonia most often seen in the offices of general practitioners, private radiologists, and, in a hospital setting, in the outpatient department or the emergency room. Most CAP patients are children (15–35 of 1,000 children per year) and the elderly (30–40 per 1,000 persons per year). The mode of transmission in CAP is usually person-to-person, via water or mucus droplets laden with viruses or bacteria. The most frequent pathogens are gram-positive bacteria, such as *Streptococcus pneumoniae* (*Pneumococcus*) and *Staphylococcus aureus,* and gram-negative bacteria, such as *Haemophilus influenzae* and atypical bacteria, including *Mycoplasma pneumoniae, Chlamydia pneumoniae,* and *Legionella pneumophila.* Viral forms commonly include those caused by respiratory viruses, such as influenza viruses, human metapneumovirus, respiratory syncytial virus (RSV), rhinovirus, parainfluenza viruses, adenoviruses, and corona viruses. According to the literature, the spectrum of organisms varies according to patient-related, temporal, geographic, and diagnostic factors.

In CAP, the patient's health and socioeconomic status may provide clues as to the spectrum of causative organisms. Healthy people are most likely to contract mycoplasma pneumonia or a mild form of pneumococcal pneumonia. Debilitated patients, alcoholics, and the chronically ill more often present with severe pneumococcal pneumonia or infections caused by *H. influenzae, S. aureus,* or gram-negative bacilli. *L. pneumophila* and *Chlamydia* infections are more common in patients with some form of mild immunologic compromise. Patients with poor oral hygiene and occasional loss of consciousness (epilepsy, alcoholism) may suffer from anaerobic pulmonary infections. In these patients, *Mycobacterium tuberculosis* infections are more prevalent than in healthy individuals without risk factors. Recurrent pneumonia in outpatients usually indicates an underlying problem, such as congenital or acquired immunologic disorder; airway abnormalities, such as chronic bronchitis, bronchiectasis, and bronchogenic carcinoma; cardiac conditions (congestive heart failure); or systemic diseases, such as diabetes, chronic alcoholism, and intravenous drug abuse. Up to 10% of CAPs are aspiration pneumonias caused by the aspiration of colonized oropharyngeal or gastric contents. The

Diseases of the Chest and Heart 2015-2018,
DOI: 10.1007/978-88-470-5752-4_8 © Springer-Verlag Italia 2015

most frequently isolated pathogens in aspiration pneumonia are gram-negative bacteria. Aspiration pneumonia must be differentiated from aspiration pneumonitis, which is a chemical pneumonitis that results from the aspiration of noncolonized gastric contents (Mendelson's syndrome).

The definition of CAP has been challenged over the last few years, as it also includes pneumonia in patients from nursing homes, rehabilitation hospitals, and outpatient-based surgical centers who routinely receive invasive medical treatment. The bacteriology and outcome of these patients are more similar to those of NPs. Therefore, it has been proposed that pneumonia in outpatients hospitalized for more than 2 days over the previous 3 months or who reside in nursing homes or extended-care facilities should be categorized as health-care-associated pneumonia (HCAP).

Clinical Diagnosis

Patients suffering from CAP usually present with fever, cough, dyspnea, sputum production, and pleuritic chest pain, as well as laboratory signs, such as leukocytosis. Because the clinical symptoms are nonspecific, most people who have fever and cough do not have pneumonia; in fact, about 30% of patients, and especially the elderly, are afebrile at presentation. Imaging is one of the most important tools in the diagnosis of CAP. The radiographic identification of a new pulmonary infiltrate is, in the appropriate clinical setting, indicative of pneumonia. Conversely, a patient who has fever and cough but does not have radiologic proof of pneumonia cannot be considered to have pneumonia. In CAP, the causative organism is frequently not identified because noninvasive tests such as sputum cultures correctly identify the offending organism in only 50% of cases, and invasive procedures are rarely used in patients with pneumonia.

Radiographic Diagnosis

In patients with CAP, the primary role of the radiologist is to detect or to exclude pneumonia. A second task is to aid the clinician in determining the etiologic diagnosis. Categorization of the causative organism is sometimes possible by integrating clinical and laboratory information with radiographic pattern recognition (see the section "Radiographic Patterns"). A specific etiologic diagnosis, however, is difficult to establish, given the increasing spectrum of causative organisms and their overlapping radiographic features. In a prospective study of 359 adults with CAP, Fang and coauthors compared the radiographic, clinical, and laboratory features of patients with bacterial pneumonia (caused by *H. influenzae, S. pneumoniae, S. aureus,* and aerobic gram-negative bacilli) and those with atypical pneumonia (caused by *M. pneumoniae* and *Chlamydia* spp.). The authors found no features that could reliably differentiate these two groups. Another

group prospectively compared the clinical and radiologic features of CAP caused by *L. pneumophila* to those of patients with pneumococcal infections AUHA (Ahuja and Kanne, 2014). The authors concluded that *Legionella* infection may clinically as well as radiologically resemble a typical bacterial pneumonia.

The chest radiogram is the first-line tool in evaluating patients with suspected CAP. Computed tomography (CT) is reserved for assessing complications or for guiding further diagnostic procedures. It is definitely indicated in investigating patients with recurrent or persistent pulmonary opacifications.

Nosocomial Pneumonia

By definition, NPs develop in a hospital environment. The incidence of NP ranges from 0.5 to 5 cases per 100 admissions, but in the subgroup of ventilated patients in an intensive care setting it may reach 7–41%. Mortality rates reported for NPs range from 20% in multihospital studies to ≥50% in single referral centers and university hospitals.

Mortality is related to the causative agent. The prognosis associated with aerobic gram-negative pneumonias is considerably worse than that associated with gram-positive or viral agents.

Pathogenesis

NP develops from bacterial colonization of the oropharynx followed by the aspiration of oropharyngeal secretions and gastrointestinal contents into the lungs. The majority of NPs are caused by gram-negative bacilli, including *Pseudomonas aeruginosa, Klebsiella* spp., *Enterobacteriaceae* spp., *Escherichia coli, Serratia marcescens,* and *Proteus*, and to a lesser extent by gram-positive cocci, atypical bacteria such as *L. pneumophila,* and viruses such as RSV. Microbial contamination of inserted tubes, lines, and catheters is an important source of infection. Less commonly, NP is the result of bacteremia originating from right-sided endocarditis or septic pelvic thrombophlebitis. Risk factors are either patient-related (underlying illness, previous surgery, prolonged hospital care) or iatrogenic (intravascular catheters, tracheal tubes, indwelling catheters, respirator equipment). Sources of infections are hospital personnel and patients with active infections. The inappropriate use of broad-spectrum and prophylactic antibiotics is an additional and important factor leading to an increased susceptibility to NPs.

Clinical Diagnosis

Compared with CAP, it may be difficult for the clinician to diagnose pneumonia in a hospitalized patient. The classical findings for pneumonia, such as new fever, new pulmonary opacification on chest radiographs, cough, sputum production, and elevated leukocyte count may not be present in the hospitalized patient with NP. Moreover, even if these symptoms are present, they may not necessarily be caused by pneumonia. Microbiologic evaluation of the patient with suspected NP (sputum, bronchoalveolar lavage) may or may not be helpful because of the difficulties in differentiating contamination from true infection. In addition, pulmonary disease in a hospital environment may be caused by more than one agent. Therefore, identifying a pulmonary infection, the various methods used to obtain a specimen, and the value of isolating potential pathogens are matters of constant discussion in the clinical diagnosis of NP.

Radiographic Diagnosis

Because of the potential difficulties in the clinical diagnosis of pneumonia in the hospitalized patient, the radiologist has an important role in detecting and classifying suspected cases. However, the radiographic diagnosis of a pulmonary opacity in suspected NP is not as straightforward as it is in patients with CAP. The radiographic diagnosis of a pneumonia may be hampered by preexisting disorders or concomitant lung disease, such as fibrosing alveolitis, lupus pneumonitis, hemorrhage or contusion, acquired respiratory distress syndrome (ARDS), tumor, atelectasis, and embolic infarcts. These disorders may obscure or alter the otherwise characteristic radiographic appearance of a pulmonary opacification and thus render the etiologic approach using pattern recognition difficult.

The difficulties in diagnosing NP can be readily demonstrated by two examples. Winer-Muram et al. assessed the diagnostic accuracy of bedside chest radiography for pneumonia in ARDS patients. The overall diagnostic accuracy in these patients was only 42% because of false-negative and false-positive results originating from diffuse parenchymal areas of increased opacity that obscured the radiographic features of pneumonia. Wunderink et al. compared premortem chest radiographic findings with pulmonary autopsy studies in ventilated patients with NP. No radiographic sign had a diagnostic efficiency greater than 68%. The only radiographic sign that correlated with pneumonia, correctly predicting 60% of the cases, was the presence of an air bronchogram.

CT is used more often when an NP is suspected than in patients with CAP, as it can detect early morphologic signs of infection (for example, ground-glass densities). CT can also identify a pulmonary opacification in areas of preexistent disease, detect complications, and guide invasive diagnostic procedures, such as bronchoscopy or percutaneous biopsy.

Radiographic Patterns

In general terms, imaging patterns can be grouped into airspace consolidation (lobar pneumonia), bronchiolar disease (bronchopneumonia) and bilateral diffuse disease.

Most commonly, consolidation, confined to a segment or a lobe of one or both lungs, is caused by typical and atypical bacteria, whereas bronchopneumonia commonly relates to *Staphylococcus aureus*, *Haemophilus*, *Mycoplasma*, and tuberculous infection. Diffuse bilateral lung disease, frequently developing over time, can in most cases be attributed to viruses and fungi such as *Pneumocystis jirovecii*. Nodular disease may be attributed to septic emboli (small nodules), larger nodules can be caused by *Nocardia* and fungal disorders in immunocompromised hosts.

Again, these patterns are nonspecific, they overlap, may be mimicked by non-infectious lung disease and masked by pre- or coexisting lung conditions. Patterns can be identified both on chest radiography and CT but CT may help to identify complex or coexisting patterns and aid the novice in establishing a diagnosis.

Opportunistic Infections

Infectious agents that cause opportunistic pneumonia in humans include representatives from the classifications bacteria, virus, fungus, protozoa, and parasite. In the following, we review some of these pathogens and their appearance on chest film and CT. Usually, the chest radiograph will reveal the abnormality but, occasionally, the increased sensitivity of CT is necessary and even recommended to see the pneumonia. Whereas the findings on chest imaging may not be totally pathognomonic of the underlying etiology of infection, they may still be highly suggestive and will certainly lead to a reasonable differential diagnosis.

Human Immunodeficiency Syndrome

Since the first description of HIV/acquired immune deficiency syndrome (AIDS), pneumocystis pneumonia caused by *Pneumocystis jirovecii* (PJP) has been one of its most common complications. (Previously it was thought that *Pneumocystis carinii* was the cause of these infections, but this is not the case. The abbreviation PCP is still used in some circles to refer to pneumocystis pneumonia.) In recent years the incidence of PJP as a presenting abnormality in patients with AIDS has decreased. Nevertheless it still accounts for a considerable amount of diseases in patients not on highly active antiretroviral therapy (HAART) or prophylactic therapy and should be considered as a diagnosis when characteristic radiographic findings are noted. Patients with PJP typically present with increasing shortness of breath; the disease may run a gradual or fulminant course. Chest films classically reveal a bilateral fine to medium reticulonodular pattern, generally bilateral but occasionally focal or unilateral. If the patient remains untreated, the radiograph progressively becomes more opaque and bilateral homogeneous opacities may ultimately be seen. While upper lobe involvement is more frequent, any lobe may be involved. On CT imaging PJP presents as ground-glass opacification in the areas of involvement, typically perihilar in distribution. The chest film occasionally may worsen within a few days of intravenous trimethoprim-sulfamethoxazole treatment secondary to overhydration and the production of pulmonary edema, but this can be treated quite effectively with diuretics.

Otherwise, with treatment, the radiographic course is one of steady improvement, with complete resolution usually occurring by day 11. Pneumatoceles , as seen on chest films, develops in ≥10% of patients; the incidence is probably higher in patients evaluated by CT scanning. These air-filled cysts are frequently multiple, located in the upper lobes, measure 1–5 cm in diameter, and will resolve within 2 months. However, in 35% of patients, pneumatoceles may lead to pneumothorax, which can be extremely difficult to treat. Overall, pneumothorax develops in 5% of patients with PJP and AIDS. In about 10% of patients with PJP, the chest film may be normal. In some of these patients with normal radiographs, a CT scan will show the typical geographic, ground-glass opacities associated with pneumocystis pneumonia. Lymphadenopathy and pleural effusions are not part of the PJP picture.

Cytomegalovirus (CMV) may mimic the appearance of PJP on chest film, with diffuse bilateral fine to medium reticulonodular opacities. On CT, centrilobular nodules and ground-glass opacities are reported. In some patients with CMV, the presence of discreet nodules, sometimes several centimeters in size, may help distinguish between these two entities. Lymphocytic interstitial pneumonia may also mimic PJP with fine reticular opacities on chest radiographs, ground-glass opacities on CT scans, and air-filled cysts seen on both forms of imaging.

Disseminated fungal infections, such as histoplasmosis and coccidiomycosis, generally produce bilateral, fairly symmetric, coarse, nodular opacities on chest radiographs.

The nodules and occasionally reticular opacities are larger than those seen with PJP, which may aid in distinguishing between the two processes. Discreet larger nodule(s) or disseminated disease may be seen with other fungal infections such as aspergillosis and cryptococcosis. With angio-invasive fungal infections cavitation may occur secondary to ischemia, regardless of the CD-4 lymphocyte count.

The imaging appearance of tuberculosis (TB) depends on the patient's immune status. In patients with relatively normal CD-4 lymphocyte cell counts, TB will look much like it does in the general population. That is, with primary infection, patients will present with a homogeneous lobar opacity and ipsilateral hilar and/or mediastinal adenopathy. With post-primary infection, chest films will show apical and posterior upper-lobe and/or superior segment lower-lobe heterogeneous opacities with or without cavitation; on CT scans, imaging may also demonstrate centrilobular nodules and/or tree-in-bud opacities. In patients with low CD-4 cell counts and primary infection, homogeneous lobar opacities with adenopathy similar to immune competent hosts may be seen on chest films, but increased adenopathy may also be present. With post-primary disease, the organism disseminates more widely, creating a diffuse, coarse, nodular pattern on chest film similar to the pattern seen with fungal infections. Cavitation does not develop, as the body's immune response is weak, such that well-formed granulomas and necrosis are unusual. In patients with improving cell-mediated immunity secondary to HAART, more typical findings of cavitation might be seen. If the organism is sensitive to the appropriate therapy, then some resolution of the abnormal findings should be observed on chest film within 1 week.

Ordinary bacterial infections now occur with increased frequency and among some patients with HIV are the most common type of infection. This increasing percentage of bacterial infections may reflect the larger number of pulmonary infections in populations in whom antiretroviral and prophylactic therapy is available. Common organisms are S. pneumoniae, H. influenzae, S. aureus, and P. aeruginosa. In the immunocompromised, pneumonias caused by these bacteria usually appear as they do in normal hosts, i.e., as homogeneous, peripheral, lobar opacities. Parapneumonic effusions may be present. S. aureus, and P. aeruginosa pneumonias may present with cavitations. These should begin to resolve within days of instituting antibacterial therapy, with complete resolution of abnormalities usually occurring in about 2 weeks. Other bacterial etiologies, such as Rhodococcus equi and Nocardia asteroides, are less common and may present as nodules or masses with or without cavitation.

With the use of antiretroviral therapy, noninfectious etiologies of disease have become more prevalent, such as pulmonary hypertension and chronic obstructive pulmonary disease (COPD), including emphysema and chronic bronchitis. Also, the immune reconstitution inflammatory syndrome (IRIS), occurring in up to 30% of patients after the initiation of antiretroviral treatment, may cause confusing clinical and radiological findings. With improving immune status, patients are able to mount a greater inflammatory response to existing organisms, resulting in worsening clinical disease and increasing lung parenchymal abnormalities and lymphadenopathy. This usually develops in individuals with low CD-4 counts and high viral loads, typically about one month after starting therapy (but as early as within days and as late as after several months). It is more commonly seen in patients with partially treated tuberculosis or non-tuberculous mycobacterial infection. Worsening of other infections and the development of sarcoidosis have also been attributed to HAART and IRIS.

Two infection-related neoplasms, non-Hodgkin's lymphoma (NHL) and Kaposi's sarcoma, may also be seen in patients with AIDS and could cause confusion in generating a differential diagnosis. NHL will produce well-defined, discete, nodules on chest films. The nodules range in size from about 1 cm to several centimeters. Solitary or multiple nodules may be noted. Lymphadenopathy and pleural effusions are also observed. The nodules have a tendency to grow extremely rapidly.

Whereas the nodules with NHL are very well defined, those associated with Kaposi's sarcoma are not. This disease produces poorly marginated nodules that tend to coalesce and occur in the perihilar lung and lower lobes. On CT, the distribution is along bronchovascular pathways.

(Other diseases seen in HIV/AIDS patients which occur along the bronchovascular bundles include lymphocitic interstitial pneumonia (LIP), Castleman disease, and sarcoidosis). In almost all cases of Kaposi's sarcoma involving the lungs, cutaneous lesions are also common, as is pleural fluid.

Other Conditions of the Immune-Compromised

Increasing numbers of transplant procedures, both solid organ and hematopoietic stem cell, have led to new populations of immunosuppressed individuals. The underlying diseases (e.g. leukemia) or the widespread use of induced immunosuppression for treatment purposes may result in neutropenia or other causes of immune dysfunction. Steroids are also being used with increased frequency for a number of medical conditions. Thus, infectious and non-infectious complications in the setting of transplantation or steroid use have become a major problem. Prophylactic drug treatment for pneumocystis, CMV, and occasional fungi may reduce the number of infections in some, but not all of these patients.

Bacterial pneumonias caused by a variety of organisms (e.g., *Pseudomonas*, *Nocardia*, *Legionella*) have a typical appearance of peripheral homogeneous opacification with or without air-bronchograms. More than one lobe might be involved. In the case of *Legionella* the opacification may simulate a mass.

The appearances on chest film and CT scans of CMV will be similar to that seen in patients with HIV infection, as described above. Other viral pathogens are also seen in this setting, including RSV, parainfluenza virus, adenovirus, and influenza virus in lung transplant patients, and varicella zoster, which may be seen in patients with lymphoma and those undergoing steroid therapy.

These same organisms are responsible for infections in patients who develop graft versus host disease. Many of these viral pneumonias have a similar appearance, including ground-glass and consolidative opacities, centrilobular and tree-in-bud opacities, and a frequently bi-

lateral involvement. On chest film, varicella pneumonia usually produces bilateral symmetric acinar opacities (poorly marginated nodules 7–10 mm in diameter) that may coalesce as the disease worsens. CT shows similar-sized nodules and distribution as well as ground-glass opacities.

Among the fungal organisms seen with some regularity in this group of immunocompromised patients are PJP, *Cryptococcus*, and *Aspergillus*. Other emerging agents include *Pseudallescheria/Scedosporium species, Fusarium* spp., and *Mucorales* spp. The appearance of PJP is similar to that described for patients with HIV/AIDS. A recent report suggested that PJP in patients with HIV/AIDS as opposed to non-HIV/AIDS patients might have a higher incidence of pneumatoceles, but less extensive ground-glass opacities (Hardak et al., 2010).

Cryptococcus has numerous types of presentation on chest film. Perhaps most common is the appearance of well-defined nodules, usually solitary but sometimes multiple. If the nodules become masses, the margins may become indistinct. The nodules may cavitate. *Cryptococcus* may also manifest as a lobar pneumonia or diffuse heterogeneous reticulonodular opacities.

Aspergillus fumigatus is responsible for many lung infections. Up to 10% of pneumonias following allogeneic transplantation are due to *Aspergillus*. The pattern of abnormality seen on chest film depends on the patient's immune status. In the setting of immunosuppression (neutropenia), the typical appearance is that of invasive aspergillosis. In this form, the chest film initially demonstrates a poorly marginated area or areas of homogeneous opacity that may resemble ordinary bacterial pneumonia in appearance and distribution but is occasionally rounder and farther from the subpleural lung than common community infections. In some cases, the disease is peripheral and wedge-shaped secondary to infarction caused by the angio-invasive obstruction of pulmonary vessels. In time, the lesions become more discreet and rounder, thus resembling lung masses.

As patients are treated and immune status improves, there may be cavitation within the masses with the formation of an air crescent. Wall thickness of the cavity is generally moderate. The air crescent is created by the contained necrotic debris within the cavity. On CT, initially, the areas of homogeneous opacity may have air bronchograms, and commonly, additional regions of involvement are identified. A ground glass opacity that surrounds (frequently incompletely) a more opaque center of the lesion results in the "halo sign," in which the ground glass portion is an area of hemorrhage and the central area is necrotic lung. This sign was thought to be pathognomonic of invasive aspergillosis but it is also a feature of other infections, neoplasms, and inflammatory diseases. CT may also reveal bronchial wall thickening, peribronchial opacities, and small centrilobular nodules.

Take-Home Messages: Usefulness of Imaging Methods in Pulmonary Infections

Despite the increasing use of CT imaging for diagnosing chest disorders, plain film radiography remains the primary imaging modality for patients with suspected pneumonia. The presence of an appropriate lung opacity on a chest radiograph is considered the gold standard for diagnosing pneumonia. Extensive knowledge of the radiographic appearances of pulmonary infections, their complications, and their course is essential in aiding the referring clinician and, ultimately, the patient. CT imaging is useful in patients with CAP and NP when there is a non-resolving or complicated chest film and at times in immunocompromised patients with suspected pulmonary infections. CT can help differentiate infectious from noninfectious abnormalities. CT may detect empyema, cavitation, and lymphadenopathy when chest films cannot. CT should be performed in immunocompromised patients with a clinical suspicion of pneumonia when the chest film is normal. This is especially true when the early diagnosis of pneumonia is critical, as is the case with immunocompromised and severely ill patients.

To reiterate: No pattern of abnormality seen on chest films can be considered pathognomonic of a specific infection. However, the distribution and appearance of lung opacities, especially in conjunction with clinical information, should enable one to produce a useful, ordered list of most likely possibilities helpful to our clinical colleagues and, most importantly, to our patients.

Suggested Reading

Ahuja J, Kanne JP (2014) Thoracic infections in immunocompromised patients. Radiol Clinics of North Am 52:121-136.

Albaum MN, Hill LC, Murphy M (1996) Interobserver reliability of the chest radiograph in community-acquired pneumonia. Chest 110:343.

Aquino SL, Dunagan DP, Chiles C, Haponik EF (1998) Herpes simplex virus 1 pneumonia: patterns on CT scans and conventional chest radiographs. J Comput Assist Tomogr 22: 795-800.

Aviram G, Boiselle PM (2004) Imaging features of bacterial respiratory infections in AIDS. Curr Opin Pulm Med 10: 183-188.

Bartlett JG, Dowell SF, Mandell LA et al (2000) Practice guidelines for the management of community-acquired pneumonia in adults. Infectious Diseases Society of America. Clin Infect Dis 31:347-382.

Bartziokas K, Daenas C, Preau S et al (2010) Vibration Response Imaging: evaluation of rater agreement in healthy subjects and subjects with pneumonia. BMC Medical Imaging 10:6.

Basi SK, Marrie TJ, Huang JQ, Majumdar SR (2004) Patients admitted to hospital with suspected pneumonia and normal chest radiographs: epidemiology, microbiology, and outcomes. Am J Med 117:305.

Bierry G, Boileau J, Barnig C et al (2009) Thoracic manifestations of primary humoral immunodeficiency: a comprehensive review. Radiographics 29:1909-1920.

British Thoracic Society Standards of Care Committee (2001) BTS guidelines for the management of community acquired pneumonia in adults. Thorax Suppl 4: IV1-IV64.

Carmona EM, Limper AH (2010) Update on the diagnosis and treatment of Pneumocystis pneumonia. Ther Adv Respir Dis 5:41-59.

Choi MH, Jung JI, Chung WD et al (2014) Acute complications in patients with hematologic malignancies. RadioGraphics 34:1755-1768.

Chou S-H S, Prabhu SJ, Crothers K et al (2014) Thoracic diseases associated with HIV infection in the era of anti-retroviral therapy: clinical and imaging findings. RadioGraphics 34:895-911.

Conees DJ (1999) Endemic fungal pneumonia in immunocompromised patients. J Thorac Imaging 14:1-8.

Connolly JE Jr, McAdams HP, Erasmus JJ et al (1999) Opportunistic fungal pneumonia. J Thorac Imaging 14:51-62.

Coy DL, Ormazabal A, Godwin JD et al (2005) Imaging evaluation of pulmonary and abdominal complications following hematopoietic stem cell transplantation. RadioGraphics 25:305-318.

Crothers K, Huang L, Goutlet JL et al (2010) HIV infection and risk for incident pulmonary diseases in the combination anti-retroviral therapy era. Am J Respir Crit Care Med [Epub ahead of print].

Donnelly LF (1999) Maximizing the usefulness of imaging in children with community-acquired pneumonia. AJR Am J Roentgenol 172:505-512.

Ellis SM (2004) The spectrum of tuberculosis and non-tuberculous mycobacterial infection. Eur Radiol 14(Suppl 3):E34-E42.

Escuissato DL, Gasparetto EL, Marchiori E et al (2005) Pulmonary infections after bone marrow transplantation: high-resolution CT findings in 111 patients. AJR Am J Roentgenol 185:608-615.

Fang GD, Fine M, Orloff J et al (1990) New and emerging etiologies for community-acquired pneumonia with implications for therapy. A prospective multicenter study of 359 cases. Medicine (Baltimore) 69:307-316.

Franquet T, Gimenez A, Hidalgo A (2004) Imaging of opportunistic fungal infections in immunocompromised patients. Eur J Radiol 51:130-138.

French MA (2009) Immune reconstitution inflammatory syndrome: a reappraisal. Clin InfectDis 48:101-107.

Goodman P (2006) Radiographic assessment of HIV-related diseases. In: Peiperl L, Volberding P (eds) HIV InSite Knowledge Base. CD-ROM version.

Goodman PC (2007) Pulmonary infection in adults. In: Grainger RG, Allison DJ, Dixon AK (eds) Grainger & Allison's diagnostic radiology: a textbook of medical imaging, 5th Ed. Churchill Livingstone, London, New York, NY.

Hansell DM, Armstrong P, Lynch DA, McAdams HP (2005) The immunocompromised patient. In: Rozenshtein A (ed) Imaging of diseases of the chest, 4th Ed. Elsevier Mosby, Philadelphia, PA.

Hardak E, Brook O, Yigla M (2010) Radiological features of Pneumocystis jirovecii pneumonia in immunocompromised patients with and without AIDS. Lung 188:159-163.

Herold CJ, Sailer JG (2004) Community-acquired pneumonia and nosocomial pneumonia. Eur Radiol 14:E2-E20.

Heussel CP, Kauczor HU, Ullmann AJ (2004) Pneumonia in neutropenic patients. Eur Radiol 14:256-271.

Huang L, Cattamanchi A, Davis JL et al (2011) HIV-Associated pneumocystis pneumonia. Proc Am Thorac Soc 8:294-300.

Huang L, Crothers K (2009) HIV-associated opportunistic pneumonias. Respirology 14:474-485.

Ibrahim EH, Traey L, Hill C (2002) The occurrence of ventilator-associated pneumonia in a community hospital: risk factors and clinical outcomes. Radiology 223:884.

Jeong YJ, Lee KS (2008) Pulmonary tuberculosis: up-to-date imaging and management. AJR Am J Roentgenol 191:834-844.

Johnstone J, Majumdar SR, Fox JD, Marrie TJ (2008) Viral infection in adults hospitalized with community-acquired pneumonia: prevalence, pathogens, and presentation. Chest 134:1141-1148.

Jung JI, Kim H, Park SH et al (2001) CT differentiation of pneumonic-type bronchioloalveolar cell carcinoma and infectious pneumonia. Br J Radiol 74:490-494.

Kim EA, Lee KS, Primack SL et al (2002) Viral pneumonias in adults: radiologic and pathologic findings. RadioGraphics 22:S137.

Kollef MH, Shorr A, Tabak YP et al (2005) Epidemiology and outcomes of health-care-associated pneumonia: results from a large US database of culture-positive pneumonia. Chest 128:3854-3862.

Krishnam MS, Suh RD, Tamasian A et al (2007) Postoperative complications of lung transplantation: radiologic findings along a time continuum. RadioGraphics 27:957-974.

Lacombe C, Lewiin M, Monnier-Cholley L et al (2007) Imaging of thoracic pathology in patients with AIDS. J Radiol 88:1145-1154.

Leung AN, Brauner MW, Gamsu G et al (1996) Pulmonary tuberculosis: comparison of CT findings in HIV-seropositive and HIV-seronegative patients. Radiology 198:687.

Leung AN (1999) Pulmonary tuberculosis: the essentials. Radiology 210:307-322.

Lichtenberger III JP, Sharma A, Zachary KC et al (2012) What a differential a virus makes: a practical approach to thoracic imaging findings in the context of HIV infection – Part 1, Pulmonary findings. AJR Am J Roentgenol 198:1295-1304.

Lichtenberger III JP, Sharma A, Zachary KC et al (2012) What a differential a virus makes: A practical approach to thoracic imaging findings in the context of HIV infection – Part 2, Extrapulmonary findings, chronic lung disease, and immune reconstitution syndrome. AJR Am J Roentgenol 198:1305-1312.

Lieberman D, Shvartzman P, Korsonsky I, Lieberman D (2003) Diagnosis of ambulatory community-acquired pneumonia. Comparaison of clinical assessment *versus* chest X-ray. Scand J Prim Health Care 21:57-60.

Lim WS, Baudouin SV, George RC et al (2009) British Thoracic Society guidelines for the management of community acquired pneumonia in adults: update 2009. Thorax 64:1-55.

Little BP, Gilman MD, Humphrey KL et al (2014) Outcome of recommendations for radiographic follow-up of pneumonia on outpatient chest radiography. AJR Am J Roentgenol 202:54-59.

Mabie M, Wunderink RG (2003) Use and limitations of clinical and radiologic diagnosis of pneumonia. Semin Respir Infect 18:72-79.

Mandell LA, Bartlett JG, Dowell SF et al (2003) Update of practice guidelines for the management of community-acquired pneumonia in immunocompetent adults. Clin Infect Dis 37:1405.

Mandell LA, Wunderink RG, Anzueto A et al (2007) Infectious Diseases Society of America/American Thoracic Society consensus guidelines on the management of community-acquired pneumonia in adults. Clin Infect Dis 44 (Suppl 2):S27-S72.

Marchiori E, Zanetti G, Hochhegger B et al (2012) Reversed halo sign on computed tomography: State-of-the-art review. Lung 190: 389-394.

Melbye H (2002) Community pneumonia – more help is needed to diagnose and assess severity. Br J Gen Pract 52:886-888.

Melbye H, Dale K (1992) Interobserver variability in the radiographic diagnosis of adult outpatient pneumonia. Acta Radiol 33:79-83.

Metlay JP, Fine MJ (2003) Testing strategies in the initial management of patients with community-acquired pneumonia. Ann Intern Med 138:109-118.

Metlay JP, Kapoor WN, Fine MJ (1997) Does this patient have community-acquired pneumonia? Diagnosing pneumonia by history and physical examination. JAMA 278:1440-1445.

Mortensen EM, Copeland LA, Pugh MJ et al (2010) Diagnosis of pulmonary malignancy after hospitalization for pneumonia. Am J Med 123:66-71.

Musher DM, Thorner AR (2014) Community-acquired pneumonia. N Engl J Med 371:1619-1628.

Nambu A, Ozawa K, Kobayashi N, Tago M (2014) Imaging of community-acquired pneumonia: Roles of imaging examinations, imaging diagnosis of specific pathogens and discrimination from noninfectious diseases. World J Radiol 6:779-793.

Niederman MS, Mandell LA, Anzueto A et al (2001) American Thoracic Society. Guidelines for the management of adults with community-acquired pneumonia. Diagnosis, assessment of severity, antimicrobial therapy, and prevention. Am J Respir Crit Care Med 163:1730-1754.

Pupaibool J, Limper AH (2013) Other HIV-associated pneumonias. Clin Chest Med 34:243-254.

Primack SL, Hartmann TE, Lee KS, Mueller NL (1994) Pulmonary nodules and the CT halo sign. Radiology 190: 513-515.

Reeders JWAJ, Goodman PC (2001) Differential radiological patterns in AIDS at a glance. In: Reeders JWAJ , Goodman PC (eds) Radiology of AIDS, Springer-Verlag, Heidelberg, pp 293-324.

Reittner P, Müller NL, Heyneman L et al (2000) Mycoplasma pneumoniae pneumonia: radiographic and high-resolution CT. Features in 28 patients. AJR Am J Roentgenol 174: 37-41.

Remund KF, Best M, Egan JJ (2009) Infections relevant to lung transplantation. Proc Am Thorac Soc 6:94-100.

Reynolds JH, McDonald G, Alton H, Gordon SB (2010) Pneumonia in the immunocompetent patient. Br J Radiol 83:998-1009.

Shah RM, Wechsler R, Salazar AM, Spirn PW (1997) Early detection of pneumonia in febrile neutropenic patients: use of thin-section CT. AJR Am J Roentgenol 169:1347-1353.

Sharma S, Maycher B, Eschun G (2007) Radiological imaging in pneumonia: recent innovations. Curr Opin Pulm Med 13: 159-69.

Sider L, Gabriel H, Curry DR, Pham MS (1993) Pattern recognition of the pulmonary manifestations of AIDS on CT scans. RadioGraphics 13:771-784.

Speets AM, Hoes AW, van der Graal Y et al (2006) Chest radiography and pneumonia in primary care: diagnostic yield and consequences for patient management. Eur Resp J 28:933-938.

Syrjala H, Broas M, Suramo I et al (1998) High-resolution computed tomography for the diagnosis of community-acquired pneumonia. Clin Infect Dis 27:358.

Valles J, Martin Loeches I, Torres A et al (2014) Epidemiology antibiotic therapy and clinical outcomes of healthcare-associated pneumonia in critically ill patients: a Spanish cohort study. Intensive Care Med 40:572-581.

Vento S, Cainelli F, Temesgen Z (2008) Lung infections after cancer themotherapy. Lancet Oncol 9:982-992.

Wagner AL, Szabunio M, Hazlett KS et al (1998) Radiologic manifestations of round pneumonia in adults. AJR Am J Roentgenol 170:723.

Winer-Muram HT, Rubin SA, Ellis JV et al (1993) Pneumonia and ARDS in patients receiving mechanical ventilation: diagnostic accuracy of chest radiograph. Radiology 188:479-485.

Wunderink RG, Waterer GW (2014) Clinical practice. Community-acquired pneumonia. N Engl J Med 370:543-551.

Wunderink RG, Woldenberg LS, Zeiss J et al (1992) The radiologic diagnosis of autopsy proven ventilator-associated pneumonia. Chest 101:458-463.

Yeh JJ, Chen SC, Chen CR et al (2014) A high-resolution computed tomography-based scoring system to differentiate the most infectious active pulmonary tuberculosis from community-acquired pneumonia in elderly and non-elderly patients. Eur Radiol 24:2372-2384.

Imaging of Thoracic Trauma

Loren Ketai[1], Caroline Chiles[2]

[1] Department of Radiology, University of New Mexico Health Science Center, Albuquerque, NM
[2] Department of Radiology, Wake Forest University Health Sciences Center, Winston-Salem, NC

Introduction

Each year, approximately 5.8 million people throughout the world die as a result of injuries, accounting for 10% of the world's deaths [1]. Approximately 25% of these are due to motor vehicle accidents. Imaging plays a key role in the diagnosis of cardiothoracic trauma, whether due to blunt force or penetrating trauma. Chest radiography and either computed tomography (CT) or CT angiography are considered complementary in the work-up of individuals with a high-energy mechanism of injury [2]. If cardiac injury is suspected, transthoracic echocardiography is indicated. In patients with a low probability of significant thoracic injury, chest radiography may be sufficient.

Mediastinum

Thoracic Aorta Injury

Thoracic aortic injury is typically the product of deceleration injury or blunt-force trauma to the chest (Table 1). The majority of cases occur as a result of motor vehicle accidents. The severity of the injury depends on the location of the injury within the thoracic aorta and the layers of the aortic wall involved. Injury to the ascending aorta is often fatal, and patients rarely survive long enough to receive medical attention. Radiologists, therefore, more commonly encounter injuries to the descending thoracic aorta and injuries that leave the adventitia intact. Blunt traumatic injury to the aorta can be classified as minimal (intimal tear only or intramural hematoma), aortic pseudoaneurysm, and free rupture [3]. The least severe injury, intimal tear, has only been recognized in the last two decades. It is visible on CT, transesophageal echocardiography, and intravascular ultrasound. On contrast-enhanced CT, intimal tear appears as either a round or triangular intraluminal filling defect attached to the wall of the aorta, or a small (<1 cm), linear filling defect, thought to represent an intimal flap, with or without mediastinal hematoma (Fig. 1). On follow-up imaging, this lesion is typically seen to resolve by 4 weeks and may be managed non-operatively [4]. The term "minimal aortic injury" includes intramural hematoma, which also has a low mortality rate even with conservative management [5]. Intramural hematoma may involve the entire circumference of the aortic wall. On axial CT images, it is seen as a circumferential area of increased attenuation on unenhanced CT; bleeding may also occur within a portion of the aortic wall and appear crescentic in shape.

Injuries that involve more than the intima are regarded as severe aortic injuries. In contained rupture, or aortic pseudoaneurysm, the tear involves both the intima and media, which bulge outwardly, held in place by the intact

Table 1. Traumatic aortic injury

Level of aortic injury	Direct signs	Indirect signs
Minimal aortic injury	Intraluminal thrombus: round or triangular intraluminal filling defect attached to the wall of the aorta Intimal flap: small (<1 cm), thin (linear) filling defect Intramural hematoma: High-attenuation material in the wall of the aorta, which may appear crescentic or circumferential	Mediastinal/periaortic hematoma
Contained rupture	Saccular pseudoaneurysm Fusiform pseudoaneurysm	Mediastinal/periaortic hematoma
Free rupture	Extravasation of contrast material	Mediastinal/periaortic hematoma Hemopericardium if injury involves the ascending aorta

Diseases of the Chest and Heart 2015-2018,
DOI: 10.1007/978-88-470-5752-4_9 © Springer-Verlag Italia 2015

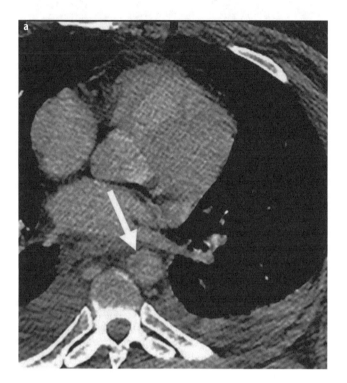

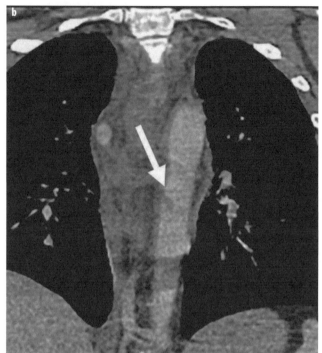

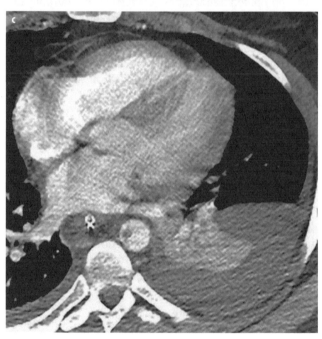

Fig. 1 a-c. Minimal aortic injury. A linear filling defect, likely representing an intimal flap (*arrows*), is seen on axial computed tomography (CT) images (**a**) and on coronal reformats (**b**) in the descending thoracic aorta in a 38-year-old man who was involved in a motor vehicle accident. Three days after the accident, the intimal flap appears more rounded (**c**), possibly due to thrombus formation. On a follow-up CT prior to hospital discharge 3 weeks later, the intraluminal findings had resolved without intervention

adventitia. Adventitial tears may involve 360° of the aortic wall, so that the pseudoaneurysm appears fusiform or barrel-shaped (Fig. 2). When the tear involves only a portion of the adventitia, the pseudoaneurysm bulges eccentrically from the aorta, typically in the region of the aortic isthmus.

The stress placed on the aortic wall during sudden deceleration may result in complete rupture, with disruption of all three layers of the aortic wall – intima, media, and adventitia – with extravasation of blood into the adjacent anatomic compartment (Fig. 3). In some patients with complete rupture of the descending thoracic aorta, mediastinal tissues and the periaortic hematoma can produce a tamponade effect, preventing rapid exsanguination. This is in contrast to free rupture involving the ascending aorta, when blood can rapidly fill the pericardial sac, causing cardiac tamponade and death. It is important to recognize free rupture on imaging and to distinguish it from contained rupture. Although delayed repair may be considered in patients with aortic pseudoaneurysm, or contained rupture, immediate repair is necessary for patients with free aortic rupture.

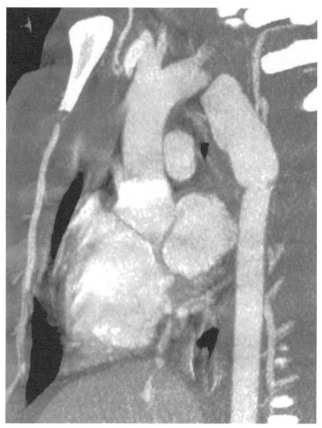

Fig. 2. Contained aortic rupture. A fusiform pseudoaneurysm has formed in the proximal descending thoracic aorta. This occurs when the intima and media are torn and the pseudoaneurysm is contained by the intact adventitia

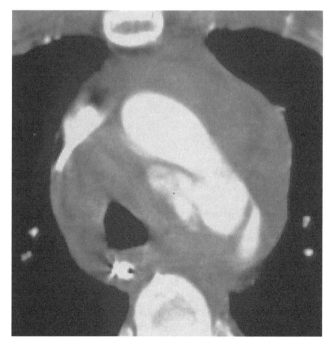

Fig. 3. Free rupture. The extravasation of contrast medium from the transverse thoracic aorta is diagnostic of injury involving all three layers of the aortic wall. Mediastinal hematoma is also present, an indirect sign of aortic injury

In a patient with blunt trauma or deceleration injury, mediastinal hematoma is most commonly due to small venous injury and is therefore considered an indirect sign of aortic injury. Mediastinal hematoma associated with aortic injury is typically adjacent to the transverse and descending thoracic aorta and may dissect superiorly in the extrapleural space to form an "apical cap." Mediastinal hematomas not in contact with the aorta but located in the anterior or posterior mediastinum are more likely to be related to chest wall or spinal fractures [6].

Cardiac Herniation

Cardiac herniation as a result of a traumatic tear of the pericardium is an uncommon occurrence but may be considered in the patient with fluctuating blood pressures after intravenous fluid administration together with tachycardia and dilated jugular veins [7]. Although cardiac-axis deviation may be apparent on a chest radiograph, more specific signs of cardiac herniation are better seen on CT and include the "empty pericardial sac," as air fills the space remaining once the heart is displaced into the hemithorax, and the "collar sign," resulting from the pericardium pinching the heart as it herniates through the pericardial tear. The tear is typically a longitudinal one located along the pericardiophrenic nerve and occurs more commonly on the left side. The mortality of patients with cardiac herniation is high, with death resulting from torsion along the inferior vena cava and great vessels and cardiac strangulation [8].

Hemopericardium

Hemopericardium should raise suspicion of injury to the heart, ascending aorta, or coronary arteries. It is most commonly associated with injury to the aortic root and ascending aorta but may also result from cardiac chamber rupture, myocardial contusion, and coronary artery laceration [8]. Simple fluid should demonstrate attenuation values of 0–10 Hounsfield units (HU) whereas hemopericardium will have attenuation values in the 35-HU range. The rapid accumulation of hemopericardium may result in cardiac tamponade. The latter diagnosis in patients with blunt chest trauma is suggested when CT demonstrates a triad of high-attenuation pericardial effusion, distention of the inferior vena cava and renal veins, and periportal low-attenuation fluid [8].

Esophageal Injury

Esophageal injuries caused by external, non-iatrogenic trauma are rare but potentially catastrophic. Mortality for undiagnosed rupture after 24 h is 10–40%. Chest radiographs may reveal pleural effusions, left sided if the lower third of the esophagus is injured, right sided if the upper two thirds is injured. Pneumomediastinum is also commonly seen but is nonspecific and usually not related to esophageal or tracheobronchial injury (see below):

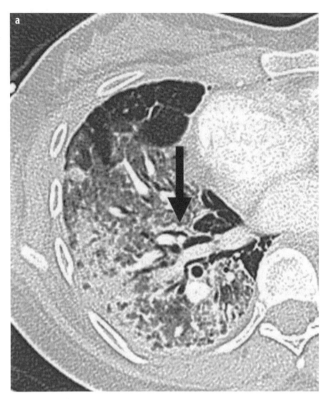
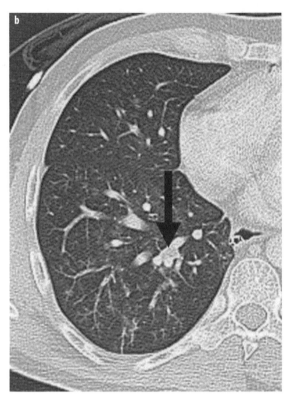

Fig. 4 a, b. Two patient with acute diffuse lung disease. **a** Acute respiratory distress syndrome (ARDS) with dependent consolidation and midlung ground glass opacities. The pneumomediastinum is due to the Macklin effect (*arrow*). **b** Trauma with acute aspiration causing tree in bud opacities and secretions in segmental bronchi (*arrow*)

instead, it represents alveolar rupture and the dissection of air along bronchovascular sheaths to the mediastinum, the so-called Macklin effect (Fig. 4). Fluoroscopic esophagography is moderately sensitive (75%) for esophageal injury and very specific but it can be technically difficult to perform in critically ill patients. In a study of a small group of patients, CT esophagography performed after the ingestion or instillation of contrast and effervescent granules was very accurate in the detection of injury [9]. More recent studies following a similar protocol with the exception of the effervescent granules showed a high specificity but a sensitivity of only 50% [10].

Tracheobronchial Rupture

Tracheobronchial injury as a result of blunt-force trauma is uncommonly seen, as the majority of patients die before reaching the hospital. In a review of 88 surviving patients reported in the literature, the rupture involved the right main bronchus in 41 (47%), and 76% of the injuries were within 2 cm of the carina [11]. The median time until diagnosis was 9 days. Chest radiography may show indirect signs of tracheobronchial rupture, including cervical subcutaneous emphysema, pneumomediastinum, and persistent pneumothorax despite satisfactory positioning of a thoracotomy tube [12]. The "fallen lung sign" describes a collapsed lung lying in a dependent position, tethered to the hilum by pulmonary vessels (Fig. 5) [13].

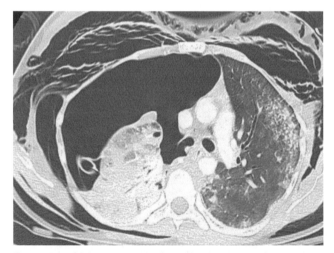

Fig. 5. Bronchial rupture. The lung lies in a dependent position within the right hemithorax, consistent with the "fallen lung sign." Additional evidence of bronchial rupture in this case includes disruption of the bronchus, extensive subcutaneous emphysema, and a large pneumothorax despite satisfactory positioning of a thoracotomy tube

Although originally described on chest radiography, this can also be seen on CT, which may demonstrate disruption in the wall of the trachea or bronchus; however, this is more readily identified at bronchoscopy, which should be performed in any patient with suspected tracheobronchial injury.

Pleural Space

Pneumothorax

Pneumothorax is second only to rib fractures in its prevalence among patients with blunt chest trauma. Rates vary widely, from 5 to 64%, with a recent large series reporting an incidence of 16%. Some patients will develop tension pneumothorax, in which the pleural pressure rises sufficiently to impair venous return, causing hemodynamic instability. A chest radiographic finding of mediastinal shift is not specific for tension pneumothorax; rather, the diagnosis is made on clinical grounds.

Many trauma patients will receive only supine chest radiography, mandating a search for radiographic signs in addition to a pleural line, which may not be visible due to the predilection of pleural air to collect antero-inferiorly in supine patients. The "deep sulcus sign," indicative of an abnormally deep and widened costophrenic sulcus, is the most commonly missed finding of a pneumothorax on supine radiographs. The presence of the "double diaphragm sign," in which air outlines both the dome of the diaphragm and the anterior costophrenic sulcus (seen extending from the seventh costochondral cartilage medially to the 11th rib laterally), may increase the specificity but in general the sensitivity of supine radiographs in detecting pneumothorax remains <25% [14].

The limitations of chest radiography have stimulated the use of bedside ultrasound in the detection of pneumothoraces [15, 16]. In the absence of a pneumothorax, high-frequency probes readily demonstrate the to and fro sliding of the parietal and visceral pleura surfaces, the "sliding lung sign." "B lines", caused by echo reverberations of the air-filled lung, appear as narrow hyperechoic ray-like opacities. While the presence of a sliding lung sign and B lines has a very high negative predictive value, multiple sites in the chest, and not only in the area of the ultrasound probe, must be evaluated. In well-trained hands, the sensitivity of ultrasound for pneumothorax is much greater than that of supine chest radiography, ranging between 50 and 95%.

CT remains the standard for the detection of pneumothoraces against which all other imaging is judged. However, the utility of detecting occult pneumothoraces, whether by CT or ultrasound, is tempered by the more recent surgical literature showing that many of the small pneumothoraces not seen on radiographs have a benign course and may not routinely warrant tube thoracostomy drainage.

Hemothorax

Hemothorax occurs in 30–50% of blunt injuries but more commonly requires surgical intervention following penetrating trauma. On supine radiographs a posterior layering hemothorax can cause hazy opacity of the entire hemithorax through which the pulmonary vasculature is visible. Hemothorax is more easily detected when it is accompanied by a rim of fluid displacing the lung from the lateral and apical chest wall. Hemothorax is readily visible on CT, manifesting as pleural fluid (35–70 HU) and in some cases demonstrating a hematocrit sign in which the densest clot is seen in the dependent pleural space. High attenuation within 10–15 HU of vascular structures is indicative of active hemorrhage, usually arterial.

Following tube thoracostomy, pleural blood loss ⩾250 ml/h or greater >1000–1500 mL often indicates the need for thoracotomy [17, 18]. Initial CT imaging showing a layering hemothorax thicker than 24 mm is a relatively specific indicator that blood loss will exceed this threshold [18]. For patients who do not undergo initial thoracotomy and are instead treated with tube thoracostomy, CT is useful in detecting retained hemothorax. Most patients with a 500-mL retained hematoma require video-assisted thoracoscopy for its evacuation in order to prevent complications, principally empyema. Due to the typical presence of extensive associated parenchymal damage, chest radiography is neither sensitive nor specific for identifying a retained clot. In one series, half of the cases selected for surgical intervention by radiography showed no significant hematoma on chest CT [19].

Extrapleural Hematoma and Chylothorax

When the parietal pleura remains intact, blood may accumulate in the extrapleural space rather than within the pleural space. These extrapleural hematomas can be identified on CT by the inward displacement of extrapleural fat. They are not treated by tube thoracostomy (Fig. 6).

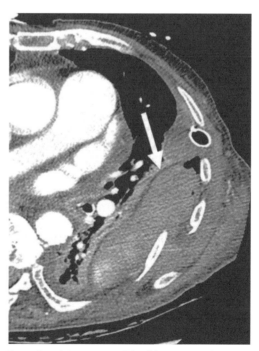

Fig. 6. Extrapleural hematoma. Blood has accumulated in the extrapleural space following blunt force trauma to the left chest wall. Extrapleural fat is displaced inwardly (*arrow*). The biconvex shape and the high-attenuation material within the hematoma suggest an active arterial bleeding source, which may require embolization or surgical intervention

Collections that are biconvex may represent an arterial bleeding source and are more likely to require surgical intervention [20].

Chylothorax is an uncommon complication of chest trauma. It can result from penetrating trauma to the upper mediastinum that injures the thoracic duct as it ascends to the left of the esophagus, resulting in a left sided pleural effusion [21]. Blunt injury to the thoracic duct is often related to hyperextension of the spine and occurs most commonly at the level of the diaphragm, where the duct is located in the right hemithorax, thus giving rise to a right pleural effusion. Pleural fluid from a chylothorax may be lower in attenuation than water due to its fat content but in many cases co-existing protein in the fluid raises its attenuation to that of other pleural effusions.

Pulmonary Injury

Contusion

Pulmonary contusions are defined as the leakage of blood into the alveoli and lung interstitium without the presence of a discrete laceration. CT is more sensitive than radiography but many of the contusions seen on CT alone are not clinically significant. In more extensive injury, CT is useful in differentiating contusion from aspiration or acute respiratory distress syndrome as the etiology of acute lung injury, by showing lung opacities that have geographic borders and cross pleural fissures. These opacities are subpleural but may demonstrate immediate subpleural sparing, particularly in children. If the opacities continue to worsen after 24 h or do not begin to improve after 48–72 h, concurrent volume overload, atelectasis, or super-infection should be suspected.

Laceration

Pulmonary lacerations occur with both blunt and penetrating trauma. When caused by blunt trauma, their location in the lungs can suggest specific mechanisms of injury. For instance, central lacerations are likely caused by shearing forces between the lung and tracheobronchial tree, while peripheral lesions are more commonly related to punctures from overlying fractured ribs [22]. Lacerations from blunt trauma are usually round or oval but vary greatly in size and may be filled by air, blood, or both. Lacerations may become more evident in the first 72 h post-trauma, as the contusion clears, and then resolve slowly over weeks to months. Lacerations do not usually require specific surgical management but can be repaired if associated with bleeding or if surgery is necessary to treat retained hemothorax (see above) [23].

Diffuse Lung Injury

Thoracic trauma can cause diffuse alveolar damage via systemic processes such as shock and hypertransfusion that indirectly damage the lung. Other insults from trauma directly injure the lung parenchyma; these include aspiration, fat emboli, inhalation injury, near drowning, and smoke inhalation. When the extent of injury is severe, damage caused by most mechanisms has a similar radiologic appearance. CT often demonstrates consolidation in the most dorsal lung, ground glass opacities in the mid lung, and nearly normal appearing lung along the ventral surfaces (Fig. 4). Direct pulmonary insults may cause more extensive and asymmetric consolidation than indirect injuries.

In early stages or in less severe cases of alveolar damage, the clinical history and imaging findings may suggest a specific cause. For instance, in cases of acute aspiration pneumonitis, tree-in-bud type centrilobular nodules may co-exist with CT findings of diffuse alveolar damage [24]. In early or mild cases of fat embolization, CT may demonstrate ill-defined nodules <1 cm in size in addition to ground glass opacities and consolidation [25]. The diagnosis of fat emboli, however, is not made radiologically. The presence of bilateral parenchymal opacities is a "major" diagnostic criteria but confirmation requires the presence of non-radiologic "major" criteria (e.g., axillary or subconjunctival petechiae) or multiple "minor" criteria (e.g., fat within the urine, significant hypoxemia).

CT may be more useful in assessing prognosis than in identifying the etiology of lung injury. For example, in burn victims, CT imaging can identify those patients most at risk for diffuse lung damage related to smoke inhalation. The addition of bronchoscopic inspection improves prediction, and at least in theory could be replaced by virtual bronchoscopy [26]. More commonly, CT can be useful in assessing the prognosis of patients with already established diffuse alveolar damage. Development of fibroproliferative changes on CT predicts prolonged mechanical ventilation, the development of barotrauma and ventilator-associated pneumonia [27].

Diaphragm

Diaphragm injuries are less common than pneumothoraces or hemothoraces but their radiologic detection has become more important as the number of trauma patients managed non-operatively has increased. Missed diaphragm injures have been reported in 20% of patients initially managed non-operatively for penetrating trauma. Use of positive pressure ventilation can maintain the viscera within the abdomen despite the presence of a diaphragm laceration, contributing to a delayed diagnosis

Blunt diaphragm injuries are roughly three times more common on the left, are often >10 cm in length, and commonly occur in the posterolateral aspect of the diaphragm [28]. Other laceration sites are reported but the esophageal hiatus is usually spared. Chest radiograph signs of diaphragmatic injury are more commonly appreciated in the setting of left sided injuries. Elevation of the left hemidiaphragm >4 cm above the right strongly

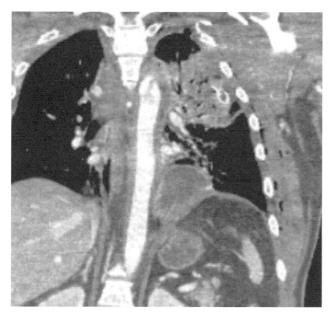

Fig. 7. Diaphragmatic rupture. The stomach has herniated through a left sided diaphragmatic rupture and is pinched by the diaphragm, producing the "collar sign." Additional signs of blunt force trauma in this patient include an aortic tear, hemomediastinum, and laceration/contusion of the left lung

suggests diaphragm injury. This may be accompanied by a U-shaped configuration of the gastric tube, with the abnormally placed gastroesophageal junction (the nadir of the "U") caused by an intact esophageal hiatus.

CT signs of diaphragmatic injury include direct visualization of a diaphragm defect and several different signs based on the abnormal appearance of the upper abdominal viscera [29]. These include herniation of the abdominal viscera into the chest, the collar sign, and the dependent viscera sign. The collar sign describes focal narrowing of an upper abdominal structure that is constricted by the margins of a diaphragm tear (Fig. 7). The dependent viscera sign is caused by the absence of diaphragm restraint on the abdominal viscera, such that the stomach, bowel, or upper third of the liver lie in contact with the posterior chest wall. Each of these signs carries a specificity >90% but a considerably lower sensitivity, mandating a search for multiple signs.

Penetrating diaphragm injuries tend to be considerably smaller than blunt diaphragmatic injuries. Accordingly, radiologic signs based on the constriction or abnormal position of abdominal viscera are generally not helpful. Direct visualization of a diaphragm defect on CT is specific but uncommonly seen. CT demonstration of contiguous injuries on both signs of the diaphragm is the most sensitive CT finding (Fig. 8). Its specificity can be diminished, however, if multiple wounds are present. The absence of this sign remains useful in ruling out penetrating diaphragmatic injury. The construction of double oblique CT images along the trajectory of the knife or bullet can improve the accuracy of diagnosis. Demonstration of a tract extending on both sides of the diaphragm is specific for penetrating diaphragm injury and in many cases is adequate impetus for operative exploration [30].

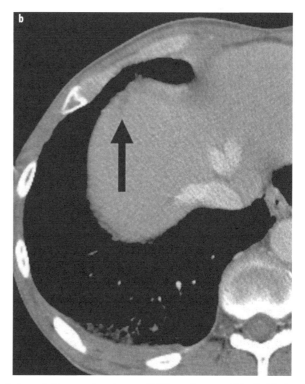

Fig. 8 a, b. Penetrating diaphragm injury. CT sections in a patient stabbed through the anterior chest wall. The trajectory of the knife (*arrows*) can be followed inferiorly through the lung and into the liver parenchyma. The course is indicative of a focal laceration of the diaphragm

Table 2. Chest wall trauma

Fracture/Dislocation	Associated injury	Direct injury
Completely displaced sternal fracture	Traumatic pericardial effusion (40%), spinal fracture (30%)	NA
Manubrium fracture	Thoracic spine (T5–T6) and the thoracolumbar junction (T12–L1)	NA
Type 2 sternomanubrial dislocation	Hyperflexion spinal injury	NA
Type 1 sternomanubrial dislocation	NA	Internal mammary artery
Posterior sternoclavicular joint dislocation	NA	Bracheocephalic vein, aortic arch vessels
Scapulothoracic disassociation	NA	Subclavian/axillary artery, brachial plexus, pseudomeningoceles

NA, not applicable

Chest Wall Trauma

Fracture of the chest wall bones can be clinically significant because of their correlation with overall injury severity or because of the direct anatomic or physiologic impact of the fracture (Table 2). Fractures of the scapula are an example of the former, their presence correlating with more severe chest injury. The association is stronger if more than two separate regions of the scapula are fractured (e.g., scapular body and glenoid neck, scapular spine, and acromion).

Sternal and Rib Trauma

Sternal fractures are also associated with the severity of chest injury, the degree of displacement being the major determinant. Less than 10% of patients with minimally displaced sternal fractures have spinal fractures or traumatic pericardial effusions, but the incidence is much higher in patients with completely displaced sternal fractures. The location of the fracture within the sternum is also significant: those involving the manubrium have the highest association with spinal fractures [31]. Sternomanubrial dislocations share this association with thoracic spine trauma, and specifically type 2 dislocations, in which hyperflexion displaces the manubrium posteriorly with respect to the sternal body. Type 1 sternomanubrial dislocations are those in which the sternal body is displaced posteriorly with respect to the manubrium and are usually the result of a direct blow.

Rib fractures have prognostic significance and can also cause direct physiologic impairment. Mortality increases slightly in patients with two or more rib fractures visible on CT but is high when nine or more are visible. Flail chests, defined as fractures of three or four contiguous ribs in two places, can result in paradoxical motion of a segment of the chest wall, resulting in hypoventilation. Rib fractures now more commonly undergo internal fixation than in the past, although the indications and timing of surgery remain controversial. Patients with a flail chest who require ventilator support but do not have a severe contusion are most likely to benefit [32].

Sternoclavicular Joint and Scapulothoracic Disassociation

Sternoclavicular dislocations are clinically relevant due to potential direct damage to adjacent structures. These injuries are rare because of the extensive ligamentous support, such that forces transmitted along the clavicle are far more likely to fracture the clavicle than dislocate the joint. Anterior dislocations are more common but posterior dislocations are of greater clinical importance due to potential impingement on adjacent structures. Diagnosis of this dislocation without CT is very difficult, even if special radiographic views (e.g., serendipity view) are taken [33].

The sternoclavicular joint may also be disrupted in scapulothoracic disassociations; a severe injury separates the scapula and muscular attachments of the upper extremity from the thorax but without disrupting the overlying skin. Radiographic diagnosis relies on detecting scapular displacement via the scapula index, a measurement easily distorted by differences in arm positioning and by rotation [34]. In suspected cases CT and magnetic resonance imaging are essential for detecting vascular and nerve injuries, respectively.

References

1. World Health Organization (2010) Injuries and violence: The facts. http://whqlibdoc.who.int/publications/2010/9789241599375_eng.pdf
2. Chung JH, Cox CW, Mohammed TL et al (2014) ACR appropriateness criteria blunt chest trauma. J Am Coll Radiol 11:345-351.
3. Azizzadeh A, Valdes J, Miller CC 3rd et al (2011) The utility of intravascular ultrasound compared to angiography in the diagnosis of blunt traumatic aortic injury. J Vasc Surg 53:608-614.
4. Paul JS, Neideen T, Tutton S et al (2011) Minimal aortic injury after blunt trauma: selective nonoperative management is safe. J Trauma 71:1519-1523.
5. Gunn ML, Lehnert BE, Lungren RS et al (2014) Minimal aortic injury of the thoracic aorta: imaging appearances and outcome. Emerg Radiol 21:227-233.
6. Rojas CA, Restrepo CS (2009) Mediastinal hematomas: aortic injury and beyond. J Comput Assist Tomogr 33:218-224.
7. Nassiri N, Yu A, Statkus N, Gosselin M (2009) Imaging of cardiac herniation in traumatic pericardial rupture. J Thorac Imaging 24:69-72.

8. Restrepo CS, Gutierrez FR, Marmol-Velez JA (2012) Imaging patients with cardiac trauma. Radiographics 32:633-649.

9. Fadoo F, Ruiz DE, Dawn SK et al (2004) Helical CT esophagography for the evaluation of suspected esophageal perforation or rupture. AJR Am J Roentgenol 182:1177-1179.

10. Suarez-Poveda T, Morales-Uribe CH, Sanabria A et al (2014) Diagnostic performance of CT esophagography in patients with suspected esophageal rupture. Emerg Radiol 21:505-510.

11. Kiser AC, O'Brien SM, Detterbeck FC (2001) Blunt tracheobronchial injuries: treatment and outcomes. Ann Thorac Surg 71:2059-2065.

12. Kunisch-Hoppe M, Hoppe M, Rauber K et al (2000) Tracheal rupture caused by blunt chest trauma: radiological and clinical features. Eur Radiol 10:480-483.

13. Wintermark M, Schnyder P, Wicky S (2001) Blunt traumatic rupture of a mainstem bronchus: spiral CT demonstration of the "fallen lung" sign. Eur Radiol 11:409-411.

14. Brar MS, Bains I, Brunet G et al (2010) Occult pneumothoraces truly occult or simply missed: redux. J Trauma 69:1335-1337.

15. Hyacinthe AC, Broux C, Francony G et al (2012) Diagnostic accuracy of ultrasonography in the acute assessment of common thoracic lesions after trauma. Chest 141:1177-1183.

16. Yarmus L, Feller-Kopman D (2012) Pneumothorax in the critically ill patient. Chest 141:1098-1105.

17. Bastos R, Baisden CE, Harker L, Calhoon JH (2008) Penetrating thoracic trauma. Semin Thorac Cardiovasc Surg 20:19-25.

18. Shanmuganathan K, Matsumoto J (2006) Imaging of penetrating chest trauma. Radiol Clin North Am 244:225-238, viii.

19. Gignon L, Charbit J, Maury C et al (2014) A simple assessment of haemothoraces thickness predicts abundant transfusion: A series of 525 blunt trauma patients. Injury. doi: 10.1016/j.injury.2014.08.040 [Epub ahead of print].

20. Chung JH, Carr RB, Stern EJ (2011) Extrapleural hematomas: imaging appearance, classification, and clinical significance. J Thorac Imaging 26:218-223.

21. Seitelman E, Arellano JJ, Takabe K et al (2012) Chylothorax after blunt trauma. J Thorac Dis 4:327-330.

22. Sangster GP, Gonzalez-Beicos A, Carbo AI et al (2007) Blunt traumatic injuries of the lung parenchyma, pleura, thoracic wall, and intrathoracic airways: multidetector computer tomography imaging findings. Emerg Radiol 14:297-310.

23. Chou YP, Kuo LC, Soo KM et al (2014) The role of repairing lung lacerations during video-assisted thoracoscopic surgery evacuations for retained haemothorax caused by blunt chest trauma. Eur J Cardiothorac Surg 46:107-111.

24. Prather AD, Smith TR, Poletto DM et al (2014) Aspiration-related lung diseases. J Thorac Imaging 29:304-309.

25. Gallardo X, Castaner E, Mata JM et al (2006) Nodular pattern at lung computed tomography in fat embolism syndrome: a helpful finding. J Comput Assist Tomogr 30:254-257.

26. Koljonen V, Maisniemi K, Virtanen K, Koivikko M (2007) Multi-detector computed tomography demonstrates smoke inhalation injury at early stage. Emerg Radiol 14:113-116.

27. Ichikado K, Muranaka H, Gushima Y et al (2012) Fibroproliferative changes on high-resolution CT in the acute respiratory distress syndrome predict mortality and ventilator dependency: a prospective observational cohort study. BMJ Open 2:e000545.

28. Desir A, Ghaye B (2012) CT of blunt diaphragmatic rupture. Radiographics 32:477-498.

29. Sliker CW (2006) Imaging of diaphragm injuries. Radiol Clin North Am 44:199-211.

30. Dreizin D, Borja MJ, Danton GH et al (2013) Penetrating diaphragmatic injury: accuracy of 64-section multidetector CT with trajectography. Radiology 268:729-737.

31. von Garrel T, Ince A, Junge A et al (2004) The sternal fracture: radiographic analysis of 200 fractures with special reference to concomitant injuries. J Trauma 57:837-844.

32. Leinicke JA, Elmore L, Freeman BD, Colditz GA (2013) Operative management of rib fractures in the setting of flail chest: a systematic review and meta-analysis. Ann Surg 258:914-921.

33. Gyftopoulos S, Chitkara M, Bencardino JT (2014) Misses and errors in upper extremity trauma radiographs. AJR Am J Roentgenol 203:477-491.

34. Brucker PU, Gruen GS, Kaufmann RA (2005) Scapulothoracic dissociation: evaluation and management. Injury 36:1147-1155.

Missed Lung Lesions: Side by Side Comparison of Chest Radiography with MDCT

Nigel Howarth[1], Denis Tack[2]

[1] Institut de Radiologie, Clinique des Grangettes, Geneva, Switzerland
[2] Department of Radiology, EpiCura Hospital, Ath, Belgium

Introduction

Missed lung lesions are one of the most frequent causes of malpractice issues [1-4]. Chest radiography plays an important role in the detection and management of patients with lung cancer, chronic airways disease, pneumonia, and interstitial lung disease. Among all diagnostic tests, chest radiography is essential for confirming or excluding the diagnosis of most chest diseases. However, numerous lesions of a wide variety of disease processes affecting the thorax may be missed on a chest radiograph. For example, the frequency of missed lung carcinoma on chest radiographs can vary from 12 to 90%, depending on study design [5]. Despite the lack of convincing evidence that screening for lung cancer with the chest radiograph improves mortality, chest radiography is still requested for this purpose [6, 7] The chest radiograph will also help in narrowing a differential diagnosis and in determining additional diagnostic measures, in addition to being of use during follow-up. The diagnostic utility of the radiograph will be maximized by integrating the radiological findings with the clinical features of the individual patient [8]. In this chapter, we review the more important radiological principles regarding missed lung lesions in a variety of common chest diseases, with a focus on how the correlation of missed lung lesions with subsequent multi-detector computed tomography (MDCT) can help improve interpretation of the plain chest radiograph.

Reasons for Missed Lung Lesions

The conditions contributing to missed lung lesions, especially carcinomas, have been extensively studied [1, 3, 5, 9-11]. Poor viewing conditions, hasty visual tracking, interruptions, and inadequate image quality, observer inexperience are amongst the most important [9, 10, 12-14]. The features of the lesions themselves, in the case of nodules, such as location, size, border characteristics, and conspicuity, also play a role [10, 12]. Missed lung nodules during the initial reading of a chest radiograph are not uncommon. One estimate is that nearly 30% of lung nodules may be overlooked [15]. Missing a nodule that may represent malignancy will have adverse consequences on patient management, essentially through delayed diagnosis, which may carry medico-legal implications. A number of authors have explored the reasons why lesions are overlooked [16-21]. Specific studies have focused on size [14, 22, 23], contrast gradient [24], conspicuity [25, 26], and anatomic noise during imaging [27].

A more recent study [28] examined the imaging features of non-small-cell lung carcinoma overlooked at digital chest radiography and compared the performances of general and thoracic radiologists with respect to lung carcinoma detection. Frontal and lateral chest radiographs from 30 consecutive patients with lung carcinoma overlooked during the initial reading and from 30 normal controls were submitted to two blinded thoracic radiologists and three blinded general radiologists for retrospective review. The location, size, histopathology, borders, presence of superimposed structures, and lesion density were recorded. Interobserver agreement was calculated and detection performance between thoracic and general radiologists was compared. The average size of carcinomas missed by the thoracic radiologists was 18.1 mm (range 10–32 mm). The average size missed by general radiologists was 27.7 mm (range 12–60 mm). In 71% (5/7) of the cases, the missed lesions were obscured by anatomic superimposition, with 43% located in the upper lobes and 63% identified as adenocarcinomas. Compared with general radiologists, the lesions missed by thoracic radiologists tended to be smaller but also had significantly lower CT density measurements and, more commonly, had ill-defined margins. The clinical stage of the overlooked lesions did not differ between the two groups (p = 0.480). The authors concluded that the size, location, conspicuity, and histopathology of the lesions overlooked on digital chest radiography were similar to those missed on conventional film-screen techniques. Several other studies on the subject have led to similar conclusions [8, 22, 27, 29-32].

Diseases of the Chest and Heart 2015-2018,
DOI: 10.1007/978-88-470-5752-4_10 © Springer-Verlag Italia 2015

The detection of carcinoma on a chest radiograph remains difficult, with implications for patient management. Nowadays, missed detection of a lung carcinoma is by far the most frequent cause of malpractice suits (42% of cases) [4]. Nonetheless, whereas overlooking chronic airways disease, pneumonia, and interstitial lung disease may not have the same potential medico-legal implications, the consequences for patient care could be critical.

By seeking a correlation between MDCT and plain chest radiograph with respect to missed lung lesions, interpretation of the latter imaging modality can be improved. During the course of clinical work, when reporting chest CT, whenever available, every effort should be made to review previous chest radiographs and their reports, as this provides one of the best learning tools for chest radiograph interpretation.

A CT scan can be performed in patients with a negative chest radiograph when there is a high clinical suspicion of chest disease. CT scan, especially high-resolution CT (HRCT), is more sensitive than plain films for the evaluation of interstitial disease, bilateral disease, cavitation, empyema, and hilar adenopathy. CT is not generally recommended for routine use because the data it provides in chronic airways disease and pneumonia are limited, the cost of imaging is high, and there is no evidence that outcome is improved. Thus, a chest radiograph is the preferred method for initial imaging, with CT scan reserved for further characterization (e.g., evaluation of pattern and distribution, detecting of cavitation, adenopathy, mass lesions, or collections).

Many methods have been suggested for the correct interpretation of the chest radiograph, but there is no preferred scheme or recommended system. The clinical question should always be addressed. An inquisitive approach is always helpful and being aware of the areas where mistakes are typically made is essential. Hidden abnormalities can thus be looked for. The difficult "hidden areas" that must be checked are the lung apex, areas superimposed over the heart, around each hilum, and below the diaphragm. In the following, we concentrate on difficult areas, such as lesions at the lung apices or bases or adjacent to or obscured by the hila or heart. For a systematic approach, we divide this review into three sections addressing specific problems: missed nodules, missed consolidations, and missed interstitial lung diseases. Finally, we examine some of the common signs that may help in the detection of lesions located in difficult anatomic areas of the chest.

Specific Problems

Specific problems of missed lung lesions can be divided into missed nodules, missed consolidations, and missed interstitial lung diseases. In the first two, the overlooked pathology may have been detected if special attention had been paid to known difficult "hidden areas." The following examples show how a side-by-side comparison of the chest radiograph and CT images improves our under-

standing of the overlooked lesion. There is no harm done by learning from one's mistakes!

Missed Nodules

Nodular Lesions: Tumors

Nodular lesions are frequently due to lung cancer, which may be primary or secondary. Lung cancer is probably one of the most common lung diseases that radiologists encounter in practice. Berbaum formulated the concept that perception is better if you know where to look and what to look for [33]. Our first example is that of a 53-year-old man who complained of pain in the right axilla for 4 months and underwent chest radiography. The posteroanterior and lateral radiographs were interpreted as showing normal findings (Fig. 1a, 1b). Subsequent MDCT showed a right superior sulcus mass with rib destruction (Fig. 1c, d). Needle biopsy established a diagnosis of bronchogenic carcinoma (adenocarcinoma). Hindsight bias [34] with the information available from the MDCT makes the initial lesion extremely obvious. Careful scrutiny of both apices is essential when reporting a frontal chest radiograph.

Radiological errors can be divided into two types [35]: cognitive, in which an abnormality is seen but its nature is misinterpreted, and perceptual, or the "miss," in which a radiological abnormality is not seen by the radiologist on initial interpretation. The perceptual type is estimated to account for approximately 80% of radiological errors [36].

Our second patient illustrates the complexity of the detection of a lung nodule located close to the hilum. A 77-year-old man with known prostate cancer underwent chest radiography for right upper quadrant abdominal pain (Fig. 2a, b). The radiographs were reported as normal. The coronal and sagittal reformats demonstrated the position of the nodule (Fig. 2c, d), which, with the benefit of hindsight, can be seen clearly on the posteroanterior and lateral chest radiographs.

Nodular Lesions: Infections

Nodular lesions attributed to pulmonary infections are most often seen in nosocomial pneumonias and in immunocompromised patients. They may be caused by bacteria such as *Nocardia asteroides* and *Mycobacterium tuberculosis,* septic emboli, and fungi. *Nocardia asteroides* causes single or nodular infiltrates with or without cavitation. Invasive pulmonary aspergillosis (IPA), mucor, and *Cryptococcus neoformans* may present with single or multiple nodular infiltrates, which often progress to wedge-shaped areas of consolidation. Cavitation is common later in the course of the infiltrate. In the appropriate clinical setting, CT may aid in the diagnosis of IPA by demonstrating the "halo sign." Figure 3 shows the imaging results from a 43-year-old woman with fever after a bone marrow transplant. The posteroranterior radiograph

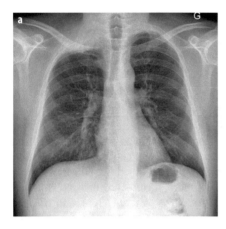
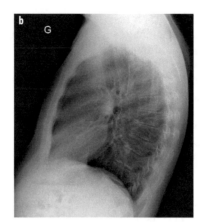
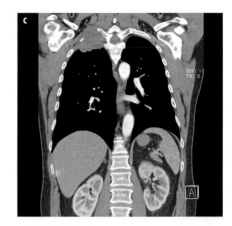
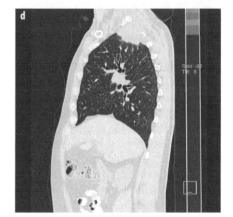

Fig. 1 a-d. A 53-year-old man who underwent chest radiography for pain in the right axilla. Posteroranterior (**a**) and lateral (**b**) radiographs were interpreted as normal. With hindsight bias from MDCT, the right apical mass is obvious. MDCT coronal and sagittal images with soft tissue (**c**) and bone (**d**) windows show a right apical mass with bone destruction

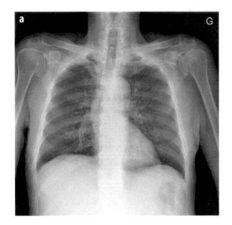
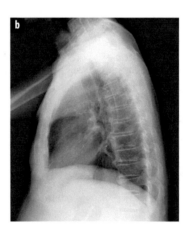
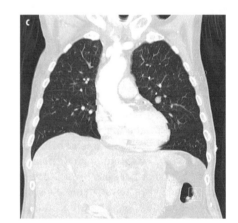
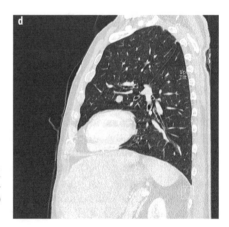

Fig. 2 a-d. A 77-year-old man with right upper quadrant pain. Posteroranterior (**a**) and lateral (**b**) radiographs were interpreted as normal. With hindsight, the 13-mm nodule in the superior segment of the lingula can be seen. Coronal (**c**) and sagittal (**d**) reformats (lung window) show the position of the lingular nodule, close to the hilum

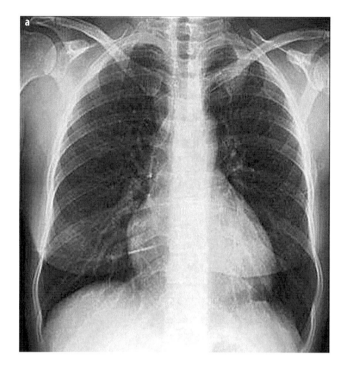

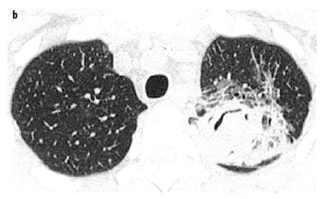

Fig. 3 a, b. A 43-year-old woman with fever after a bone marrow transplant. The posteroranterior radiograph was interpreted as normal (**a**). With hindsight, a subtle infiltrate can be seen at the left apex. Conspicuity is lessened by the overlying clavicle and 1st rib. Also note the in-dwelling catheter from the left brachial vein to the superior vena cava. Axial CT image (lung window) shows nodular consolidation with crescentic cavitation ("air-crescent sign") and a surrounding ground-glass infiltrate ("halo sign") (**b**)

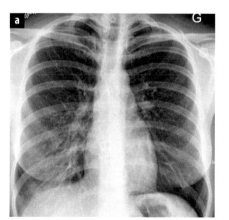
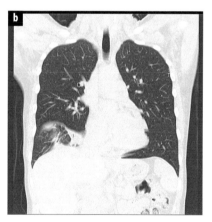
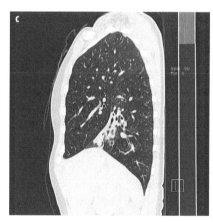

Fig. 4 a-c. A 46-year-old woman with cough and right-sided chest pain. The posteroranterior radiograph was interpreted as normal (**a**). Coronal (**b**) and sagittal (**c**) reformats showing consolidation in the anterior segment of the right lower lobe

was interpreted as normal (Fig. 3a). With hindsight, a subtle infiltrate can be seen at the left apex. Conspicuity is lessened by the overlying clavicle and 1st rib. The axial CT image (Fig. 3b) shows nodular consolidation with crescentic cavitation (the "crescent sign") and a surrounding ground-glass infiltrate (the "halo sign"). These characteristic findings of IPA are best identified on CT.

Missed Consolidations

Airspace Disease

Airspace disease is usually caused by bacterial infections. However, it can be seen in viral, protozoal, and fungal infections as well as malignancy, typically brochioloalveo-

lar carcinoma [37]. Acute airspace pneumonia is characterized by a mostly homogeneous consolidation of lung parenchyma and well-defined borders; it does not typically respect segmental boundaries. An air bronchogram is very common. Progression to lobar consolidation may occur. As with lung nodules, whether consolidation is detected or missed on the plain chest radiograph may depend on a combination of the same factors of size, density, location, and overlying structures. Location is a significant factor for missed consolidations [38, 39]. Consolidations in the middle lobe and both lower lobes can be difficult to diagnose, especially when only the posterioranterior view is obtained [40]. Figure 4 shows the radiographs from a 46-year-old woman with cough and right-sided chest pain. The posteroanterior radiograph was interpreted as normal (Fig. 4a). Due to a clinical

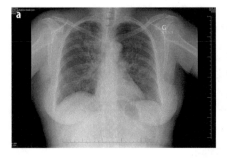 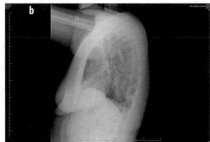 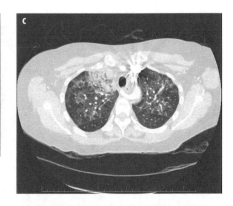

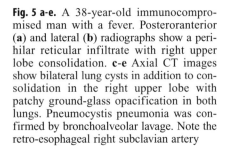 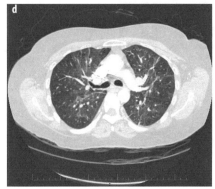 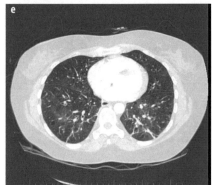

Fig. 5 a-e. A 38-year-old immunocompromised man with a fever. Posteroranterior (**a**) and lateral (**b**) radiographs show a peri-hilar reticular infiltrate with right upper lobe consolidation. **c-e** Axial CT images show bilateral lung cysts in addition to consolidation in the right upper lobe with patchy ground-glass opacification in both lungs. Pneumocystis pneumonia was confirmed by bronchoalveolar lavage. Note the retro-esophageal right subclavian artery

suspicion of pulmonary embolism, MDCT was requested, which showed consolidation in the anterior segment of the right lower lobe. The coronal and sagittal reformats demonstrated the extent of the consolidation (Fig. 4b, c). There were no signs of pulmonary embolism on the contrast medium study. A diagnosis of right lower lobe pneumonia was established and the patient was treated successfully with antibiotics.

Chest radiography is the most frequently performed diagnostic investigation requested by general practitioners in Europe [41]. Chest radiography is considered the gold standard for the diagnosis of pneumonia. It can be used to diagnose pneumonia when an infiltrate is present and to differentiate pneumonia from other conditions that may present with similar symptoms, such as acute bronchitis. The results of the chest radiograph may in some cases suggest a specific etiology (for example, a lung abscess) or reveal a complication (empyema) or coexisting abnormalities (bronchiectasis, bronchial obstruction, interstitial lung disease). Chest radiography remains a valuable diagnostic tool in primary-care patients with a clinical suspicion of pneumonia as it substantially reduces the number of misdiagnosed patients [42]. MDCT can help in differentiating infectious from non-infectious abnormalities and may detect empyema, cavitation, and lymphadenopathy when the chest radiograph cannot. MDCT imaging is useful in patients with community-acquired pneumonia when there is an unresolving or complicated chest radiograph and should be performed in immunocompromised patients with a clinical suspicion

of pneumonia when the chest radiograph is normal. This is especially true when the early diagnosis of pneumonia is critical, as is the case with immunocompromised and severely ill patients [43].

Figure 5 shows the imaging studies from a 38-year-old immunocompromised man with fever. The posteroanterior and lateral radiographs (Fig. 5a, b) were interpreted as showing a peri-hilar reticular infiltrate with right upper lobe consolidation. MDCT was requested to further characterize the infiltrate and revealed ground-glass opacification with bilateral lung cysts (Fig. 5 c-e). Pneumocystis pneumonia was confirmed by bronchoalveolar lavage.

Missed Interstitial Lung Disease

Diffuse (Interstitial or Mixed Alveolar-Interstitial) Lung Disease

Diffuse lung disease presenting with widely distributed patchy infiltrates or interstitial reticular or nodular abnormalities can be produced by a number of disease entities. An attempt is usually made to separate the group of idiopathic interstitial pneumonias from known causes, such as infections, associated systemic disease, or drug-related. The most common infectious organisms are viruses and protozoa. In general, the etiology of an underlying pneumonia cannot be specifically diagnosed because the patterns overlap. It is beyond the aim of this chapter to discuss in detail the contribution of MDCT to the diagnosis of diffuse infiltrative lung disease. The development of HRCT has resulted in markedly improved diagnostic accuracy in acute and chronic diffuse infiltrative lung disease [44-47]. The chest radiograph remains the preliminary radiological investigation of patients with diffuse lung disease but is often non-specific. Pattern recognition in diffuse lung disease has been the subject of controversy for many years. Extensive disease may be required before an appreciable change in radiographic density or an abnormal radiographic pattern can be detected on the plain chest radiograph. At least 10% of patients who are ultimately found to have biopsy-proven diffuse lung disease have an apparently normal chest radiograph [48]. HRCT, and now MDCT, have become integral components of the clinical investigation of patients with suspected or established interstitial lung disease. These techniques have had a major impact on clinical practice [49, 50].

Key Signs for Reducing the Risk of Errors on Chest X-rays

Deep Sulcus Sign

The deep sulcus sign (Fig. 6) is seen on chest radiographs obtained with the patient in the supine position [51]. It represents lucency of the lateral costophrenic angle extending toward the abdomen. The abnormally deep-

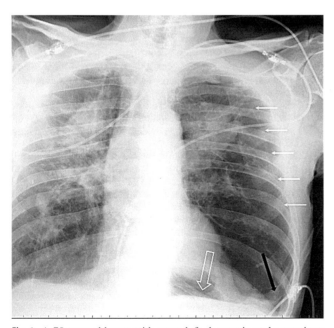

Fig. 6. A 78-year-old man with acute left chest pain and a previous history of pneumoconiosis. Bedside chest radiograph shows a thin white line near the left chest wall (*white arrows*), corresponding to the left lung visceral pleura, and indicating a pneumothorax. The deep lucency of the left lateral costophrenic angle extending towards the abdomen is an indirect sign of pneumothorax (*black arrow*). The continuous diaphragmatic sign is also seen as air separating the diaphragm from the heart (*white hollow arrow*)

ened lateral costophrenic angle may have a sharp, angular appearance. In the supine patient, air in the pleural space (pneumothorax) collects anteriorly and basally within the nondependent portions of the pleural space; when the patient is upright, the air collects in the apicolateral location. If air collects laterally rather than medially, it deepens the lateral costophrenic angle and produces the deep sulcus sign. In Fig. 6, a deep sulcus sign is seen on the left, in addition to a continuous diaphragmatic sign, present when there is air between the diaphragm and the heart.

Spine Sign

On the normal lateral chest radiograph, the attenuation decreases (the lucency increases) as one progresses down the thoracic vertebral bodies [52]. If the attenuation increases, locally or diffusely, there must be a posteriorly located lesion (Fig. 7). This lesion might not be seen on the frontal view, as it might be hidden by the heart or the hila.

Silhouette Sign

In a chest X-ray, non-visualization of the border of an anatomic structure that is normally visualized shows that the area neighboring this margin is filled with tissue or material of the same density [53]. The silhouette sign is an important indicator of the presence and localization of a lesion.

Take-Home Messages

Despite the increasing use of CT imaging in the diagnosis of patients with chest disorders, chest radiography is still the primary imaging method in patients with suspected chest disease. The presence of an infiltrate on a chest radiograph is considered the gold standard for diagnosing pneumonia. Extensive knowledge of the radiographic appearance of pulmonary disorders is essential when diagnosing pulmonary disease. Chest radiography is also the imaging tool of choice in the assessment of complications and in the follow-up of patients with pulmonary diseases.

MDCT plays an increasing role in the diagnosis of chest diseases, especially in patients with unresolving symptoms. CT will aid in the differentiation of infection and non-infectious disorders. The role of CT in suspected or proven chest disease can be summarized as follows:

1. CT is valuable in the early diagnosis of chest disease, especially in patients in whom an early diagnosis is important (immunocompromised patients, critically ill patients)
2. CT may help with the characterization of pulmonary disorders
3. CT is an excellent tool in assessing the complications of chest disease

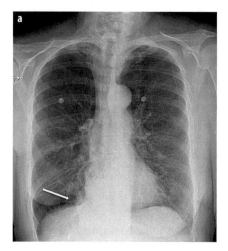
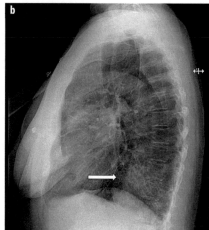
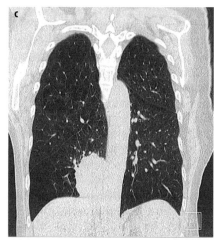
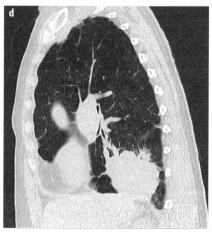

Fig. 7 a-d. A 69-year-old woman with chronic obstructive pulmonary disease and hemoptysis. The posteroanterior chest radiograph **(a)** shows an opacity next to the right border of the heart (*arrow*) and obliterating the right side of the spine. This "silhouette sign" of the right posterior mediastinal border indicates that the lesion is in a posterior location in the right lower lobe. Lateral view **(b)** shows an increased density (*arrow*) of the lower spine compared with the upper and middle thoracic spine ("spine sign"). This increased density is due to a large mass in the right lower lobe. Coronal CT image **(c)** shows the right lower lobe mass obliterating the border of the mediastinum. The sagittal CT image **(d)** shows the posterior location of the mass

4. CT is required in the investigation of patients with a persistent or recurrent pulmonary infiltrate.

A side-by-side comparison between the chest radiograph and MDCT images when confronted with a missed lung lesion is very instructive. The radiologist should be able to understand the reasons for missing certain lesions. By adopting this inquisitive approach, both cognitive and perceptual errors can be reduced.

References

1. Berlin L (1986) Malpractice and radiologists: an 11.5-year perspective. AJR Am J Roentgenol 147:1291-1298.
2. Berlin L (1995) Malpractice and radiologists in Cook County, IL: trends in 20 years of litigation. AJR Am J Roentgenol 165:781-788.
3. Potchen EJ, Bisesi MA (1990) When is it malpractice to miss lung cancer on chest radiographs? Radiology 175:29-32.
4. Baker, SR, Patel RH, Yang L et al (2013). Malpractice suits in chest radiology: an evaluation of the histories of 8265 radiologists. Journal of Thoracic Imaging 28:388-391.
5. Quekel LG, Kessels AG, Goei R et al (1999) Miss rate of lung cancer on the chest radiograph in clinical practice. Chest 115:720-4.
6. Melamed MR (2000) Lung cancer screening results in the National Cancer Institute New York study.
7. Marcus PM (2001) Lung cancer screening: an update. J Clin Oncol 19:83S-86S. Cancer 89:2356-2362.
8. Aideyan UO, Berbaum K, Smith WL (1995) Influence of prior radiologic information on the interpretation of radiographic examinations. Acad Radiol 2:205-208.
9. Carmody DP, Nodine CF, Kundel HL (1980) An analysis of perceptual and cognitive factors in radiographic interpretation. Perception 9:339-344.
10. Austin JH, Romney BM, Goldsmith LS (1992) Missed bronchogenic carcinoma: radiographic findings in 27 patients with a potentially resectable lesion evident in retrospect. Radiology 182:115-122.
11. Turkington PM, Kennan N, Greenstone MA (2002) Minsinterpretation of the chest x-ray as a factor in the delayed diagnosis of lung cancer. Postgrad Med J 78:158-160.
12. Woodring JH (1990) Pitfalls in the radiologic diagnosis of lung cancer. AJR Am J Roentgenol 154:1165-1175.
13. Monnier-Cholley L, Arrive L, Porcel A et al (2001) Characteristics of missed lung cancer on chest radiographs: a French experience. Eur Radiol 11:597-605.
14. Krupinski EA, Berger WG, Dallas WJ et al (2003) Searching for nodules: what features attract attention and influence detection? Acad Radiol 10:861-868.
15. Samei E, Flynn MJ, Eyler WR (1999) Detection of subtle lung nodules: relative influence of quantum and anatomic noise on chest radiographs. Radiology 213:727-734.
16. Kundel HL, Nodine CF, Krupinski EA (1989) Searching for lung nodules. Visual dwell indicates locations of false-positive and false-negative decisions. Invest Radiol 24:472-478.
17. Samuel S, Kundel HL, Nodine CF et al (1995) Mechanism of satisfaction of search: eye position recordings in the reading of chest radiographs. Radiology 194:895-902.
18. Quekel LG, Goei R, Kessels AG et al (2001) Detection of lung cancer on the chest radiograph: impact of previous films,

clinical information, double reading, and dual reading. J Clin Epidemiol 54:1146-1150.

19. Tsubamoto M, Kuriyama K, Kido S et al (2002) Detection of lung cancer on chest radiographs: analysis on the basis of size and extent of ground-glass opacity at thin-section CT. Radiology 224:139-144.

20. Shah PK, Austin JH, White CS et al (2003) Missed non-small cell lung cancer: radiographic findings of potentially resectable lesions evident only in retrospect. Radiology 226:235-241.

21. Samei E, Flynn MJ, Peterson E, Eyler WR (2003) Subtle lung nodules: influence of local anatomic variations on detection. Radiology 228:76-84.

22. Kelsey CA, Moseley RD, Brogdon BG et al (1977) Effect of size and position on chest lesion detection. AJR Am J Roentgenol 129:205-208.

23. Kimme-Smith C, Hart EM, Goldin JG et al (1996) Detection of simulated lung nodules with computed radiography: effects of nodule size, local optical density, global object thickness, and exposure. Acad Radiol 3:735-741.

24. Kundel HL, Revesz G, Toto L (1979) Contrast gradient and the detection of lung nodules. Invest Radiol 14:18-22.

25. Kundel HL (1975) Peripheral vision, structured noise and film reader error. Radiology 114:269-273.

26. Revesz G, Kundel HL (1977) Psychophysical studies of detection errors in chest radiology. Radiology 123:559-562.

27. Kundel HL, Revesz G (1976) Lesion conspicuity, structured noise, and film reader error. AJR Am J Roentgenol 126:233-238.

28. Wu M-H, Gotway MB, Lee TJ et al (2008) Features of non-small cell lung carcinomas overlooked at digital chest radiography. Clin Radiol 63:518-528.

29. Herman PG, Hessel SJ (1975) Accuracy and its relationship to experience in the interpretation of chest radiographs. Invest Radiol 10:62-67.

30. Bass JC, Chiles C (1990) Visual Skill. Correlation with detection of solitary pulmonary nodules. Invest Radiol 25:994-998.

31. Sone S, Li F, Yang ZG et al (2000) Characteristics of small lung cancers invisible on conventional chest radiography and detected by population based screening using spiral CT. Br J Radiol 73:137-145.

32. Yang ZG, Sone S, Li F et al (2001) Visibility of small peripheral lung cancers on chest radiographs: influence of densitometric parameters, CT values and tumour type. Br J Radiol 74:32-41.

33. Berbaum KS (1995) Difficulty of judging retrospectively whether a diagnosis has been « missed ». Radiology 194:582-583.

34. Berlin L (2000) Hindsight bias. AJR Am J Roentgenol 175:597-601.

35. Berlin L (2001) Defending the « missed » radiographic diagnosis. AJR Am J Roentgenol 176:317-322.

36. Berlin L, Hendrix RW (1998) Perceptual errors and negligence. AJR Am J Roentgenol 170:863-867.

37. Jung JI, Kim H, Park SH et al (2001) Differentiation of pneumonic-type bronchioloalveolar cell carcinoma and infectious pneumonia. Br J Radiol 74:490-494.

38. Melbye H, Dale K (1992) Interobserver variability in the radiographic diagnosis of adult outpatient pneumonia. Acta Radiol 33:79-83.

39. Albaum MN, Hill LC, Murphy M (1996) Interobserver reliability of the chest radiograph in community-acquired pneumonia. Chest 110 :343.

40. Chotas HG, Ravin CE (1994) Chest radiography: estimated lung volume and projected area obscured by the heart, mediastinum, and diaphragm. Radiology 193:403-404.

41. Woodhead M, Gialdroni Grassi G, Huchon GJ et al (1996) Use of investigations in lower respiratory tract infection in the community: a European survey. Eur Respir J 9:1596-1600.

42. Speets AM, Hoes AW, van der Graaf Y et al (2006) Chest radiography and pneumonia in primary care: diagnostic yield and consequences for patient management. Eur Respir J 28:933-938.

43. Heussel CP, Kauczor HU, Ullmann AJ (2004) Pneumonia in neutropenic patients. Eur Radiol 14:256-271.

44. Mathieson JR, Mayo JR, Staples CA et al (1989) Chronic diffuse inflitrative lung disease: comparison of diagnostic accuracy of CT and chest radiography. Radiology 171:111-116.

45. Grenier P, Valeyre D, Cluzel P et al (1991) Chronic diffuse interstitial lung disease: diagnostic value of chest radiography and high-resolution CT. Radiology 179:123-132.

46. Padley SPG, Hansell DM, Flower CDR et al (1991) Comparative accuracy of high resolution computed tomography and chest radiography in the diagnosis of chronic diffuse inflitrative lung disease. Clin Radiol 44:222-226.

47. Webb WR, Müller NL, Naidich DP (2001) High-resolution CT of the lung, 3rd Ed. Lippincott Williams & Wilkins, Philadelphia, PA.

48. Epler GR, McLoud TC, Gaensler EA et al (1978) Normal chest roentgenograms in chronic diffuse inflitrative lung disease. N Engl J Med 298:934-939.

49. Aziz ZA, Wells AU, Bateman ED et al (2005) Interstitial lung disease: effects of thin-section CT on clinical decision making Radiology 238:725-733.

50. Flaherty KR, King TE Jr, Raghu G et al (2004) Idiopathic interstitial pneumonia: what is the effect of a multi-disciplinary approach to diagnosis? Am J Respir Crit Care Med 170:904-910.

51. Kong A (2003) The deep sulcus sign. Radiology 228:415-416.

52. Ely JW, Berbaum KS, Bergus GR et al (1996) Diagnosing left lower lobe pneumonia: usefulness of the 'spine sign' on lateral chest radiographs. J Fam Pract 43:242-248.

53. Algın O, Gökalp G, Topal U (2011) Signs in chest imaging. Diagnostic and Interventional Radiology, 17:18-29.

Plain Film and HRCT Diagnosis of Interstitial Lung Disease

Sujal R. Desai[1], Jeffrey R. Galvin[2]

[1] King's College Hospital NHS Foundation Trust, London, UK
[2] Departments of Radiology and Internal Medicine, University of Maryland School of Medicine, Baltimore, MD, USA

Introduction

There is little doubt that imaging tests have a central role in the investigation of patients with suspected and established diffuse interstitial lung diseases (DILD). In most cases, physicians who manage patients with DILD will request a plain chest radiograph. However, high-resolution computed tomography (HRCT) is usually indicated, particular at initial review. HRCT, for a variety of reasons discussed below, is superior to plain radiography. In many cases where, historically, biopsy might have been considered mandatory, there has been a paradigm shift because of HRCT. For example, in some patients with idiopathic pulmonary fibrosis (characterized by the histological pattern of usual interstitial pneumonia), the HRCT appearances may be characteristic enough for biopsy to be unnecessary [1–3]. In instances in which a radiological diagnosis is not possible, HRCT may provide guidance as to the best site for surgical biopsy. More recently, HRCT has moved into the realms of prognostic evaluation and disease staging [4–9].

The HRCT Technique

In the era of multi-detector row CT machines, a brief summary of the HRCT technique is perhaps pertinent. The two technical features that differentiate HRCT imaging from conventional CT are, first, the narrow X-ray beam collimation, which significantly improves spatial resolution, and, second, the use of a dedicated reconstruction algorithm [10]. The "high-frequency" algorithm effectively exaggerates the naturally high contrast milieu of the lungs (i.e., aerated lung vs. more solid elements) [10]. The conspicuities of vessels, small bronchi, and interlobular septa are increased compared to conventional (thick-section) CT images [11]. An important downside of high-frequency algorithms is the increased visibility of image noise although, in practice, this generally does not hamper radiological interpretation.

HRCT in Diffuse Interstitial Lung Disease

The term DILD is a convenient catch-all for a heterogeneous group of disorders [2]. The DILDs have been subcategorized as follows: (1) DILDs that have a known etiology (e.g., secondary to exposure to certain drugs or a connective tissue disorder); (2) the idiopathic interstitial pneumonias (which themselves have undergone classification [12] and a more recent update [13]; (3) the granulomatous DILDs; and (4) a group of diffuse lung diseases that include Langerhans cell histiocytosis and lymphangioleiomyomatosis.

In patients with established diffuse lung disease, HRCT will not only detect but also characterize parenchymal abnormalities with greater accuracy than plain chest radiography. One important caveat is that in patients with nodular infiltrates, traditional "interspaced" HRCT images may mislead; on thin section images the dimensions of nodules and pulmonary vessels may be comparable, making the distinction difficult [14]. This is unlikely to be an issue on thin-section volumetric acquisitions. In practice, the range of CT features that commonly indicate the presence of ILD is relatively limited. Thus, radiologists will typically encounter some combination of reticulation, ground-glass opacification, honeycombing, dilatation of airways in regions of reticulation and ground-glass opacification ("traction bronchiectasis"), nodules, and thickening of interlobular septa [15, 16].

Findings at HRCT generally reflect the *macroscopic* abnormalities seen by the pathologist. This was elegantly demonstrated in the very early days of HRCT by Müller and colleagues, who showed that the morphologic features in patients with idiopathic pulmonary fibrosis (at that time still known as cryptogenic fibrosing alveolitis) reflected the histopathological changes [17]. A reticular pattern was seen in seven out of nine patients and corresponded to areas of irregular fibrosis at microscopy.

Not surprisingly, because there is no anatomical superimposition, the sensitivity of HRCT is better than that of chest radiography. However, a more important issue than sensitivity is the confidence and accuracy with which the diagnosis can be made. In the oft-quoted landmark study by Mathieson and colleagues, experienced chest radiologists were asked to independently indicate up to three diagnoses based on evaluations of the chest radiographs and CT scans of 118 patients with a variety of biopsy-confirmed ILDs [18]. Importantly, for the first-choice diagnosis, the readers were asked to assign a level of confidence. The first important finding of this study (which effectively put HRCT on the map) was that, compared with chest radiography, a confident diagnosis was made nearly *twice* as often using HRCT. The second, and perhaps more striking, message was that when experienced radiologists were confident of the diagnosis on HRCT, they were almost always correct [18]. However, a confident diagnosis on chest X-ray (which, incidentally, was offered in only 25% of the cases), was associated with a significantly lower rate of correct diagnoses.

The results of subsequent studies have not always mirrored those of the initial study by Mathieson [18, 19]. However, because of study design, the majority of the comparative studies in HRCT probably undervalued its true utility [1]. Firstly, there was no recourse to pre-test probabilities for observers in early series and, therefore, these do not accurately reflect clinical practice. Secondly, radiologists (and specifically those with an interest in thoracic disease) have become increasingly familiar with the spectrum of HRCT patterns and disease. This, almost certainly, would be associated with a proportionate increase in the confidence of *experienced* observers in making HRCT diagnoses, were such a study to be repeated today. Some justification for this last statement comes from a study that addressed the clinically vexing issue of "end-stage" lung disease [20], in which two experienced thoracic radiologists independently made correct first-choice diagnoses in just under 90% of cases, with nearly two-thirds of those diagnoses made with high confidence. On first inspection, these data seem less than impressive. However, the results of open lung biopsy (the supposed "gold-standard" for a diagnosis of DILD) are not infrequently inconclusive, no doubt in part relating to the degree of observer variability between pathologists [21].

An Approach to HRCT Diagnoses

It must be acknowledged that HRCT interpretation can be difficult, even for trained thoracic radiologists! This is not surprising given the sheer numbers of documented DILDs. These broad-ranging disorders manifest with a relatively small number of histopathological patterns (e.g., fibrosis, consolidation, intra-alveolar hemorrhage) which, in turn, are reflected by a similarly select group of HRCT features (reticulation, ground-glass opacification, nodularity, thickening of interlobular septa). However, with a systematic approach to HRCT interpretation the observer should, in time, be able to offer a sensible (and

manageably short) list of differential diagnoses. To this end, a proposed schema, presented in the form of questions that the observer should ask (in roughly the order given), is as follows.

Is There a "Real" Abnormality?

This is a crucial first question: the radiologist must first determine whether what is shown on HRCT represents real disease. CT features attributable to technical factors/normal variation (for instance, caused by a poor inspiratory effort, inadequate mAs, regions of physiologically dependent atelectasis) must not be overinterpreted and reported as disease. Making the distinction between normality and abnormality can also be difficult when there is apparently minimal disease or, conversely, when there is diffuse abnormality, as may occur with subtle but widespread decreased attenuation (mosaicism) or increased (ground-glass opacity) attenuation.

If There Is an Abnormality, What Is/Are the Predominant HRCT Pattern(s)?

Having decided that there is a definite abnormality on HRCT, the observer should attempt to identify the dominant pattern(s) using only the standard radiological terms [15]. The use of non-standard, terminology (e.g., patchy opacification, parenchymal opacities) or descriptive terms in which there is an implied pathology (e.g., interstitial pattern or alveolitis) is misleading and best avoided.

What Is the Distribution of the Disease?

Since many DILDs have a predilection for certain zones, an evaluation of the dominant distribution is of diagnostic value. For instance, it is known that in the majority of patients with idiopathic pulmonary fibrosis (IPF) the disease tends to be most obvious in the mid- to lower zones. This contrasts with fibrosis in patients with sarcoidosis, which typically has a predilection for the upper lobes. In addition, the radiologist should take note of the axial distribution (central vs. peripheral) which, in contrast with chest X-ray, can readily be made on HRCT. The potential value can be demonstrated by again using the example of IPF and sarcoidosis: the former is commonly peripheral (subpleural) whereas in the latter the distribution tends to be central (and bronchocentric). A final example is seen in patients with organizing pneumonia, in which consolidations may have a striking perilobular predilection [22].

Are There Any Ancillary Findings?

Ancillary HRCT features may suggest or, indeed, exclude certain diagnoses. Thus, the presence or absence of the following may be of diagnostic value in specific cases:
a. Pleural thickening/effusions /plaques (± calcification) may suggest asbestos-related lung disease as opposed to IPF as a possible cause of lung fibrosis.

b. Reactive intrathoracic nodal enlargement (hilar/mediastinal) is "normal" in fibrotic DILDs. However, symmetrical hilar nodal enlargement may suggest a diagnosis of sarcoidosis or occupational lung disease. Intrathoracic nodal enlargement is uncommon in pulmonary vasculitides (e.g., Wegener's granulomatosis).

c. Bronchiectasis with co-existent suppurative airways disease in a patient with established pulmonary fibrosis may point to a diagnosis of an underlying connective tissue disease, such as rheumatoid arthritis.

d. The demonstration of intrapulmonary cysts in the appropriate clinical context suggests a range of diagnoses, including Langerhans cell histiocytosis, lymphangioleiomyomatosis, and lymphocytic interstitial pneumonia.

e. Consolidation indicative of organizing pneumonia may co-exist with signs of fibrosis and parenchymal distortion in patients with connective-tissue-disease-related lung disease.

What Is the Likely Pathology?

Knowledge of the relationships between the HRCT appearances and the possible histopathological correlates is crucial. Thus, in a patient with predominant consolidation it is reasonable to conclude that the dominant pathology involves the air spaces, whereas in a patient with reticulation the likely pathological process affects the interstitium.

What Is the Clinical Background?

Clinical data must always be integrated when formulating a radiological opinion. However, it is often advisable to review the clinical information *after* evaluation of the radiological features. This is particularly true at the very start of HRCT interpretation, when the radiologist is deciding whether or not there is a "real" abnormality (see above). Specific clinical features that may be of importance in HRCT interpretation include basic demographic data (age, gender, ethnicity), smoking history, time course of the illness (i.e., have symptoms developed over hours and days or weeks and months?), and any relevant past medical history.

HRCT Appearances in Select DILDs

A working knowledge of the relationship between histopathological changes and HRCT patterns and the typical appearance of common DILDs is of value in day-to-day practice. The following sections briefly consider the HRCT appearances of a few DILDs.

Idiopathic Pulmonary Fibrosis/Usual Interstitial Pneumonia

IPF is a chronic progressive fibrosing interstitial lung disease associated with a histologic and/or HRCT pattern of usual interstitial pneumonia (UIP) [23]. At low-power microscopy, there is temporally heterogeneous fibrosis admixed with areas of unaffected lung [2]. In areas of fibrosis, there will be characteristic honeycombing. The disease has a striking basal and subpleural predilection.

To make a diagnosis of a *UIP pattern* on HRCT, the radiologist must therefore look for the following: (1) a reticular pattern, (2) honeycombing (with or without traction bronchiectasis), and (3) a subpleural, basal, disease distribution [23] while ensuring that features *inconsistent with a UIP pattern* (i.e., mid/upper zone predominance, a bronchovascular distribution, ground-glass opacification more extensive than reticulation, widespread micronodularity, multiple cysts away from areas of honeycombing, a mosaic attenuation pattern in three or more lobes, and consolidation) are absent. In the absence of honeycombing (but with the other features in the list), an HRCT diagnosis of *possible UIP* can be made.

The presence of a UIP pattern on HRCT is accurate and obviates histologic confirmation [3, 24]. However, typical appearances may not be present in over half of patients with biopsy-proven disease [24, 25].

(Cryptogenic) Organizing Pneumonia

Organization is a common response to lung injury and is part of the normal process of lung repair. It is represented on histology by plugs of fibroblastic tissue that fill the alveolar spaces. This same fibroblastic tissue may be identified in respiratory and terminal bronchioles, explaining the use of the older term "bronchiolitis obliterans organizing pneumonia," but which has been replaced by "organizing pneumonia" (OP) [12]. OP was first recognized in 1923 as a response to unresolved pneumonia [26]. Most cases are likely to be post-infectious; however, the organism is rarely recovered. The OP pattern is also a common feature in a wide range of other diseases, including collagen-vascular disease, hypersensitivity pneumonitis, chronic eosinophilic pneumonia, drug reaction, and radiation-induced lung injury. The appearance of OP on imaging is highly variable, depending on the prior injury and the stage at which it is imaged [27]. A minority of patients present with solitary pulmonary nodules or focal areas of consolidation. However, the dominant finding in OP is bilateral consolidation that is peripheral, often with sparing of the subpleural portion of the lung. Opacities are often perilobular and may be associated with septal lines. In some patients, OP may progress to an non-specific interstitial pneumonia pattern of fibrosis (see below). Although many cases of OP will clear with steroids, a substantial minority of patients are left with significant disability due to pulmonary fibrosis [27-29].

Non-specific Interstitial Pneumonia

After UIP, non-specific interstitial pneumonia (NSIP) is the most common pattern of idiopathic interstitial pneumonias (IIP) and linked with a better survival [13, 24, 30]. This pattern of IIP may be idiopathic but more commonly it is seen in a variety of clinical contexts, including connective tissue disorders (especially systemic sclerosis) and as a consequence of drug-related toxicity. At the histologic level there are varying amounts of interstitial inflammation and fibrosis, which, in stark contrast to what is seen in UIP, has a temporally and spatially uniform appearance.

On HRCT, one of the key findings is ground-glass opacification which is typically bilateral and symmetrically distributed in the lower zones [30, 31]. In some patients, the extent of ground-glass may decrease over time and become replaced by reticulation (i.e., with UIP-like features) [32]. Reticulation (generally without significant honeycombing) is usually also present.

Respiratory Bronchiolitis/Respiratory Bronchiolitis Interstitial Lung Disease/Desquamative Interstitial Pneumonia and Pulmonary Langerhans Cell Histiocytosis

Respiratory bronchiolitis (RB), of variable severity, is an almost invariable pathologic finding in all smokers [33]. Importantly, this lesion is asymptomatic and not associated with physiologic impairment in the vast majority of individuals. However, in a small minority, there will be the clinical manifestations of an interstitial lung disease. It is this clinico-pathologic/radiologic entity that has been called respiratory bronchiolitis interstitial lung disease (RBILD). The cardinal HRCT signs of RB/RBILD include "soft" centrilobular nodules, ground-glass opacification, smooth thickening of interlobular septa, and lobular foci of decreased attenuation [34-36].

Desquamative interstitial pneumonia (DIP) was first described by Leibow in 1965. Dypsneic patients with DIP were found to have numerous inflammatory cells in alveolar spaces [37]. The cells were thought to be desquamated pneumocytes but are now recognized as the same macrophages identified in patients with RB and RBILD. The majority of patients with DIP are heavy smokers and the disease is now considered part of the spectrum of inflammatory lung disease related to the inhalation of cigarette smoke [34]. Patients with DIP suffer an increased incidence of pulmonary fibrosis that fits the histologic pattern of NSIP [38, 39]. Imaging in patients with DIP is typified by homogeneous or patchy areas of ground glass opacity in the mid and lower lung zones [39, 40].

Langerhans' cell histiocytosis (LCH) is confined to the lungs in approximately 90% of patients. Although the pathogenesis is unknown, most if not all of the patients are cigarette smokers. Pulmonary LCH (PLCH) is characterized by bronchiolocentric collections of Langerhans cells admixed with a variety of other inflammatory cells forming a stellate nodule [41]. Over time infiltration of the airway wall results in its damage and subsequent dilatation [42]. In the late stage of PLCH, small stellate scars are surrounded by emphysematous spaces. Imaging reflects the histologic progression, with early bronchiolocentric nodules in the upper lobes progressing to a combination of bizarrely shaped cysts and nodules [43, 44].

In the final stages, the appearance may be indistinguishable from severe bullous emphysema.

It is important to recognize that findings of RB, DIP, PLCH and the NSIP pattern of fibrosis commonly coexist in biopsies of dypneic smokers. Some of the histologic changes are reflected on imaging, while others are below the resolution of chest CT.

Cigarette Smoking-Related Fibrosis

The relationship between cigarette smoke and fibrosis remains contentious [36, 45–50]. Niewoehner's original description of RB did not include fibrosis of the alveolar wall [33].However, there is substantial support for a relationship between cigarette smoke exposure and a pattern of alveolar wall fibrosis other than UIP [46, 51-55]. In our experience there is a group of dyspneic cigarette smokers who, as seen on CT, present with a combination of well-formed cystic spaces that follow the typical upper-lobe-predominant distribution of smoking-related emphysema, with variable surrounding ground glass opacity and reticulation that may extend into the lower lung zones [48]. These patients commonly present with strikingly normal flows and volumes on pulmonary function testing and a low diffusing capacity. The unexpectedly normal flows and volumes are the result of the opposing effects of emphysema and fibrosis [56].

Sarcoidosis

Non-caseating epithelioid-cell granulomata are the histopathologic hallmark of sarcoidosis [57]. Since the granulomata have a tendency to distribute along the lymphatics, the lymphatic pathways that surround the axial interstitium that invests bronchovascular structures and those located subpleurally (including the subpleural lymphatics along the fissures) are typically involved. Not surprisingly, a nodular infiltrate (presumably reflecting conglomerate granulomata) with a propensity to involve the bronchovascular elements is a characteristic CT finding [58, 59]. Subpleural nodularity is also commonly seen. In the later stages of the disease there may be obvious signs of established lung fibrosis with upper zone volume loss, parenchymal distortion, and traction bronchiectasis. Because of the bronchocentric nature of the disease, signs of small-airways disease are seen at CT in some patients with sarcoidosis [60].

Hypersensitivity Pneumonitis

Exposure to a range of organic antigens will cause lung disease in some patients, probably due to an immunologically mediated response [57]. In the subacute stage, there is an interstitial infiltrate comprising lymphocytes and plasma cells with a propensity to involve the small airways (bronchioles). Scattered non-caseating granulomata may be seen. Predictably, at CT, there is diffuse ground-glass opacification, ill-defined centrilobular nodules, and lobular areas of decreased attenuation on images performed at end-expiration [61, 62]. The CT appearances of subacute hypersensitivity pneumonitis may be identical to those of RBILD [36]. Consideration of the smoking history may help in the differentiation: a history of smoking is the norm in the vast majority of patients with RBILD, whereas cigarette smoke appears to protect against the development of hypersensitivity pneumonitis.

References

1. Wells AU (1998) Clinical usefulness of high resolution computed tomography in cryptogenic fibrosing alveolitis. Thorax 53:1080-1087.
2. King TE Jr., Costabel U, Cordier JF et al (2000) Idiopathic pulmonary fibrosis: diagnosis and treatment. International consensus statement. Am J Respir Crit Care Med 161:646-664.
3. Hunninghake GW, Zimmerman MB, Schwartz DA et al (2001) Utility of a lung biopsy for the diagnosis of idiopathic pulmonary fibrosis. Am J Respir Crit Care Med 164:193-196.
4. Goh NSL, Desai SR, Veeraraghavan S et al (2008) Interstitial lung disease in systemic sclerosis: a simple staging system. Am J Respir Crit Care Med 177:1248-1254.
5. Wells AU, Antoniou KM (2014) The prognostic value of the gap model in chronic interstitial lung disease: the quest for a staging system. Chest 145:672-674.
6. Walsh SLF, Wells AU, Sverzellati N et al (2014) An integrated clinico-radiological staging system for pulmonary sarcoidosis: a case-control study. Lancet Respiratory Medicine 2:123-130.
7. Ryerson CJ, Vittinghoff E, Ley B et al (2014) Predicting survival across chronic interstitial lung disease: the ILD-GAP model. Chest 145:723-728.
8. Walsh SLF, Sverzellati N, Devaraj A et al (2014) Connective tissue disease related fibrotic lung disease: high-resolution computed tomographic and pulmonary function indices as prognostic determinants. Thorax 2014:216-222.
9. Edey AJ, Devaraj A, Barker RP et al (2011) Fibrotic idiopathic interstitial pneumonias: HRCT findings that predict mortality. Eur Radiol 21:1586-1593.
10. Mayo JR, Webb WR, Gould R et al (1987) High-resolution CT of the lungs: an optimal approach. Radiology 163:507-510.
11. Murata K, Khan A, Rojas KA, Herman PG (1988) Optimization of computed tomography technique to demonstrate the fine structure of the lung. Invest Radiol 23:170-175.
12. Travis WD, King TE, Jr., and the Multidisciplinary Core Panel (2002) American Thoracic Society/European Respiratory Society international multidiscplinary consensus classification of idiopathic interstitial pneumonias. Am J Respir Crit Care Med 165:277-304.
13. Travis WD, Costabel U, Hansell DM et al (2013) An official American Thoracic Society/European Respiratory Society statement: update of the international multidisciplinary classification of the idiopathic interstitial pneumonias. Am J Respir Crit Care Med 188:733-748.
14. Remy-Jardin M, Remy J, Deffontaines C, Duhamel A (1991) Assessment of diffuse infiltrative lung disease: comparison of conventional CT and high-resolution CT. Radiology 181:157-162.
15. Hansell DM, Bankier AA, MacMahon H et al (2008) Fleischner society: glossary of terms for thoracic imaging. Radiology 246:697-722.
16. Hansell DM, Lynch DA, McAdams HP, Bankier AA (2010) Basic patterns in lung disease. In: Hansell DM, Lynch DA, McAdams HP, Bankier AA, Eds. Imaging of Diseases of the Chest, 5th Ed. Mosby Elsevier, pp 83-151.
17. Müller NL, Miller RR, Webb WR et al (1986) Fibrosing alveolitis: CT-pathologic correlation. Radiology 160:585-588.
18. Mathieson JR, Mayo JR, Staples CA, Müller NL (1989) Chronic diffuse infiltrative lung disease: comparison of diagnostic accuracy of CT and chest radiography. Radiology 171:111-116.
19. Padley SPG, Hansell DM, Flower CDR, Jennings P (1991) Comparative accuracy of high resolution computed tomography and chest radiography in the diagnosis of chronic diffuse infiltrative lung disease. Clin Radiol 44:222-226.
20. Primack SL, Hartman TE, Hansell DM, Müller NL (1993) End-stage lung disease: CT findings in 61 patients. Radiology 189:681-686.
21. Nicholson AG, Addis BJ, Bharucha H et al (2004) Inter-observer variation between pathologists in diffuse parenchymal lung disease. Thorax 59:500-505.
22. Ujita M, Renzoni EA, Veeraraghavan S et al (2004) Organizing pneumonia: perilobular pattern at thin-section CT. Radiology 232:757-761.
23. Raghu G, Collard HR, Egan J et al (2011) An official ATS/ERS/JRS/ALAT statement: idiopathic pulmonary fibrosis - evidence-based guidelines for diagnosis and management. Am J Respir Crit Care Med 183:788-824.
24. Flaherty KR, Thwaite EL, Kazerooni EA et al (2003) Radiological versus histological diagnosis in UIP and NSIP: survival implications. Thorax 58:143-148.
25. Sverzellati N, Wells AU, Tomassetti S et al (2010) Biopsy-proved idiopathic pulmonary fibrosis: spectrum of nondiagnostic thin-section CT diagnoses. Radiology 254:957-964.
26. Symmers D, Hoffman AM (1923) The increased incidence of organizing pneumonia. JAMA 81:297-298.
27. Kligerman SJ, Franks TJ, Galvin JR (2013) Organization and fibrosis as a response to lung injury in diffuse alveolar damage, organizing pneumonia, and acute fibrinous amd organizing pneumonia. Radiographics 33:1951-1975.
28. Akira M, Inoue Y, Arai T et al (2011) Long-term follow-up of high-resolution CT findings in non-specific interstitial pneumonia. Thorax 66:61-65.
29. Lee JW, Lee KS, Lee HY et al (2010) Cryptogenic organizing pneumonia: serial high-resolution CT findings in 22 patients. AJR Am J Roentgenol 195:916-922.
30. Flaherty KR, Martinez FJ, Travis W, Lynch JP, III (2001) Nonspecific interstitial pneumonia (NSIP). Semin Respir Crit Care Med 22:423-434.
31. MacDonald SLS, Rubens MB, Hansell DM et al (2001) Nonspecific interstitial pneumonia and usual interstitial pneumonia: comparative appearances at and diagnostic accuracy of thin-section CT. Radiology 221:600-605.
32. Silva CIS, Müller NL, Hansell DM et al (2008) Nonspecific interstitial pneumonia and idiopathic pulmonary fibrosis: changes in pattern and distribution of disease over time. Radiology 247:251-259.
33. Niewoehner DE, Kleinerman J, Rice DB (1974) Pathologic changes in the peripheral airways of young cigarette smokers. N Engl J Med 291:755-758.
34. Heyneman LE, Ward S, Lynch DA et al (1999) Respiratory bronchiolitis, respiratory bronchiolitis-associated interstitial lung disease, and desquamative interstitial pneumonia: different entities or part of the spectrum of the same disease process? AJR Am J Roentgenol 173:1617-1622.
35. Moon J, du Bois RM, Colby TV et al (1999) Clinical significance of respiratory bronchiolitis on open lung biopsy and its relationship to smoking related interstitial lung disease. Thorax 54:1009-1014.
36. Desai SR, Ryan SM, Colby TV (2003) Smoking related interstitial lung diseases: histopathological and imaging perspectives. Clin Radiol 58:259-268.
37. Liebow AA, Steer A, Billingsley JG (1965) Desquamative interstitial pneumonia. Am J Med 39:369-404.
38. Wells AU, Nicholson AG, Hansell DM (2007) Smoking-induced diffuse interstitial lung diseases. Thorax 62:904-910.

39. Craig PJ, Wells AU, Doffman S et al (2004) Desquamative interstitial pneumonia, respiratory bronchiolitis and their relationship to smoking. Histopathology 45:275-282.
40. Hartman TE, Primack SL, Kang E-Y et al (1996) Disease progression in usual interstitial pneumonia compared with desquamative interstitial pneumonia: assessment with serial CT. Chest 110:378-382.
41. Vassallo R, Ryu JH, Colby TV et al (2000) Pulmonary Langerhans'-cell histiocytosis. N Engl J Med 342:1969-1978.
42. Kambouchner M, Basset F, Marchal J et al (2002) Three-dimensional characterisation of pathologic lesions in pulmonary langerhans cell histiocytosis. Am J Respir Crit Care Med 166:1483-1490.
43. Leatherwood DL, Heitkamp DE, Emerson RE (2007) Pulmonary Langerhans cell histiocytosis. Radiographics 27:265-268.
44. Abbott GF, Rosado-de-Christenson ML, Franks TJ et al (2004) Pulmonary Langerhans cell histiocytosis. Radiographics 24:821-841.
45. Wright JL, Tazelaar HD, Churg A (2011) Fibrosis with emphysema. Histopathology 58:517-524.
46. Katzenstein AL, Mukhopadhyay S, Zanardi C, Dexter E (2010) Clinically occult interstitial fibrosis in smokers: classification and significance of a surprisingly common finding in lobectomy specimens. Hum Pathol 41:316-325.
47. Churg A, Müller NL, Wright JL (2010) Respiratory bronchiolitis/interstitial lung disease: fibrosis, pulmonary function, and evolving concepts. Arch Pathol Lab Med 134:27-32.
48. Galvin JR, Franks TJ (2009) Smoking-related lung disease. J Thorac Imaging 24:274-284.
49. Kawabata Y, Hoshi E, Murai K et al (2008) Smoking-related changes in the background lung of specimens resected for lung cancer: a semiquantitative study with correlation to postoperative course. Histopathology 53:707-714.
50. Yousem SA, Colby TV, Gaensler EA (1989) Respiratory bronchiolitis-associated interstitial lung disease and its relationship to desquamative interstitial pneumonia. Mayo Clin Proc 64:1373-1380.
51. Lang MR, Fiaux GW, Gillooly M (1994) Collagen content of alveolar wall tissue in emphysematous and non-emphysematous lungs. Thorax 49:319-326.
52. Adesina AM, Vallyathan V, McQuillen EN et al (1991) Bronchiolar inflammation and fibrosis associated with smoking: a morphologic cross-sectional population analysis. Am Rev Respir Dis 143:144-149.
53. Frasca JM, Auerbach O, Carter HW, Parks VR (1983) Morphologic alterations induced by short-term cigarette smoking. Am J Pathol 111:11-20.
54. Niewoehner DE, Hoidal JR (1982) Lung fibrosis and emphysema: divergent responses to a common injury? Science 217:359-360.
55. Auerbach O, Garfinkel L, Hammond EC (2014) Relation of smoking and age to findings in lung parenchyma: a microscopic study. Chest 65:29-35.
56. Washko GR, Hunninghake GW, Fernandez IE et al (2011) Lung volumes and emphysema in smokers with interstitial lung abnormalities. N Engl J Med 364:897-906.
57. Colby TV, Carrington CB (1995) Interstitial lung disease. In: Thurlbeck WM, Churg AM (Eds) Pathology of the lung, 2nd Ed. Thieme Medical Publishers, New York, pp 589-737.
58. Lynch DA, Webb WR, Gamsu G et al (1989) Computed tomography in pulmonary sarcoidosis. J Comput Assist Tomogr 1989;13(3):405-10.
59. Brauner MW, Grenier P, Mompoint D et al (1989) Pulmonary sarcoidosis: evaluation with high-resolution CT. Radiology 172:467-471.
60. Hansell DM, Milne DG, Wilsher ML, Wells AU (1998) Pulmonary sarcoidosis: morphologic associations of airflow obstruction at thin-section CT. Radiology 209:697-704.
61. Remy-Jardin M, Remy J, Wallaert B, Müller NL (1993) Subacute and chronic bird breeder hypersensitivity pneumonitis: sequential evaluation with CT and correlation with lung function tests and bronchoalveolar lavage. Radiology 189:111-118.
62. Hansell DM, Wells AU, Padley SPG, Müller NL (1996) Hypersensitivity pneumonitis: correlation of individual CT patterns with functional abnormalities. Radiology 199:123-128.

A Systematic Approach to Chest Radiographic Diagnosis

Melissa L. Rosado-de-Christenson[1], Jeffrey S. Klein[2]

[1] Department of Radiology, Saint Luke's Hospital of Kansas City, MO, USA; Department of Radiology, University of Missouri-Kansas City, MO, USA
[2] Department of Radiology, University of Vermont College of Medicine, VT, USA

Introduction

Chest radiographs are frequently obtained for the assessment of patients who present with a variety of thoracic complaints. In addition, asymptomatic patients undergoing a physical exam, a hospital admission, or a preoperative assessment may also undergo chest radiography.

Accurate interpretation of chest radiographs requires knowledge of imaging anatomy, as obscuration of normally visualized structures may be the only clue to the presence of an abnormality. Radiography allows the visualization and assessment of the lungs, central airways, pulmonary vasculature, mediastinum, heart, great vessels, and chest wall (including skeletal and soft-tissue structures). The superimposition of complex structures of various radiographic densities (air, water, calcium, metal, fat) makes radiographic interpretation challenging. Radiologists must work with technologists to achieve proper patient positioning and optimal radiographic technique. Unusual opacities must be assessed to determine whether they are intrinsic or extrinsic to the patient and to exclude artifacts and foreign bodies. In addition, the radiologist must carefully evaluate all visualized medical devices for appropriate course and position.

A Systematic Assessment

Here we present a systematic approach to the analysis of chest radiographs. An orderly assessment of each anatomic region and structure will yield a comprehensive imaging evaluation, allow identification of subtle abnormalities, and decrease interpretive errors. The following must be evaluated in each and every chest radiograph: patient positioning, radiographic technique, medical devices (if present), lungs (volume, opacities, vasculature), airways, hila, mediastinum (cardiomediastinal silhouette, great vessels), pleura, and chest wall.

Lungs

Lung Volume

In normal subjects, postero-anterior (PA) chest radiographs obtained at full inspiration or total lung capacity (TLC) result in the visualization of the ten posterior ribs above the diaphragm. Lung volume may be increased in patients with obstructive diseases such as emphysema and reduced in those with restrictive diseases such as pulmonary fibrosis.

Atelectasis may involve the entire lung, a lung lobe, or a pulmonary segment [1]. Obstructive (resorption) atelectasis is characterized by the absence of intrinsic air bronchograms. As it may result from endoluminal obstruction, a centrally obstructing neoplasm such as lung cancer must be excluded (Fig. 1). Relaxation (passive) atelectasis often results from mass effect, commonly from pleural effusion. Cicatricial atelectasis is related to pulmonary fibrosis. Rounded atelectasis occurs adjacent to pleural thickening in which subpleural atelectatic lung "folds" upon itself.

Direct signs of atelectasis include fissural displacement, bronchovascular crowding, and shift of calcified granulomas. Indirect signs include increased pulmonary opacity, ipsilateral mediastinal shift, hilar displacement, ipsilateral hemidiaphragm elevation, and compensatory hyperinflation of the adjacent lung [2].

Parenchymal Opacities

Parenchymal opacities include alveolar and interstitial processes. Pneumonia typically manifests with consolidation due to alveolar filling by purulent material and may be lobar or sublobar, or it may manifest with patchy pulmonary opacities. Consolidation often exhibits intrinsic air bronchograms and may also result from alveolar edema or hemorrhage (Table 1).

A pulmonary nodule is defined as a round or ovoid density <3 cm in diameter [3]. A benign pattern of intrinsic calcification allows the confident diagnosis of

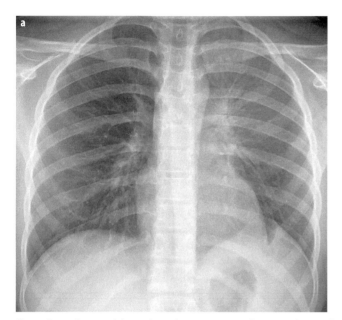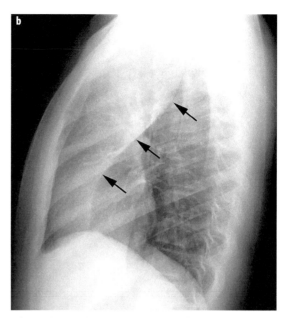

Fig. 1 a, b. Left upper lobe atelectasis. Postero-anterior (PA) chest radiograph (**a**) shows left upper lobe atelectasis manifesting as a vague left upper lung zone opacity with elevation of the left hemidiaphragm. The lateral chest radiograph (**b**) shows the opaque atelectatic left upper lobe and anterosuperior displacement of the major fissure (*arrows*). The etiology of the atelectasis was a left upper lobe lung cancer

Table 1. Differential diagnosis of air space opacification (ASO)

Finding(s)	Disease
Focal/segmental ASO	Pneumonia, contusion, infarct, lung cancer (adenocarcinoma)
Lobar ASO	Pneumonia, endogenous lipoid pneumonia, adenocarcinoma
Patchy ASO	Infection, cryptogenic organizing pneumonia, adenocarcinoma, metastases, emboli
Diffuse ASO	Edema, hemorrhage, pneumonia
Perihilar ASO	Edema, hemorrhage
Peripheral ASO	Eosinophilic pneumonia, acute respiratory distress syndrome, contusion
Rapidly changing/resolving ASO	Edema, eosinophilic pneumonia, hemorrhage

Table 2. Differential diagnosis of the solitary pulmonary nodule

Finding(s)	Disease
Granuloma	
Primary malignancy: Lung cancer, carcinoid tumor	
Solitary metastasis	
Hamartoma	
Focal organizing pneumonia	
Hematoma	

granuloma, for which further evaluation is not required. However, many pulmonary nodules are indeterminate on radiography and require further assessment and characterization with computed tomography (CT) to exclude malignancy (Fig. 2 and Table 2).

A pulmonary mass is a round or ovoid pulmonary opacity ≥3 cm in diameter and is highly suspicious for malignancy, typically lung cancer. The radiologist should look for pertinent ancillary findings of malignancy including other lung nodules, lymphadenopathy, pleural effusion, and chest wall involvement.

Interstitial opacities may manifest with reticular, linear, and/or small nodular opacities. As the normal interstitium is not visible on radiography, visualization of peripheral subpleural reticular opacities is always abnormal. A reticulonodular pattern occurs when abnormal linear opacities are superimposed on micronodular opacities.

Table 3. Ancillary findings in patients with interstitial lung disease and differential diagnostic considerations

Finding(s)	Disease
Hilar lymph node enlargement	Sarcoidosis, lymphangitic carcinomatosis, viral pneumonia
Clavicular/osseous erosions	Rheumatoid associated ILD (UIP, NSIP)
Pleural effusion	Infection, edema
Pleural plaques	Asbestosis
Hyperinflation	PLCH, end-stage sarcoidosis, lymphangioleiomyomatosis, emphysema with UIP
Esophageal dilatation	Scleroderma associated ILD (UIP, NSIP), recurrent aspiration
Conglomerate masses	Silicosis, sarcoidosis, talcosis
Basilar sparing	PLCH, sarcoidosis
Basilar predominance	UIP, aspiration

ILD, interstitial lung disease; UIP, usual interstitial pneumonia; NSIP, nonspecific interstitial pneumonia; PLCH, pulmonary Langerhans cell histiocytosis

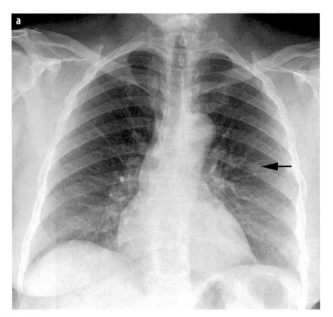
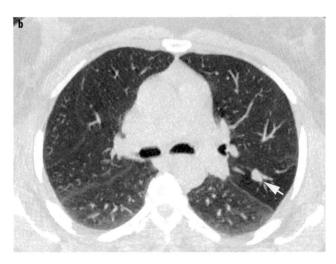

Fig. 2 a, b. Solitary pulmonary nodule. **a** PA chest radiograph shows a nodule in the left mid lung zone (*arrow*). **b** Unenhanced chest computed tomography (CT) (lung window) shows a lobular soft-tissue nodule (*arrow*) in the left upper lobe. Typical carcinoid tumor was diagnosed by CT-guided needle biopsy

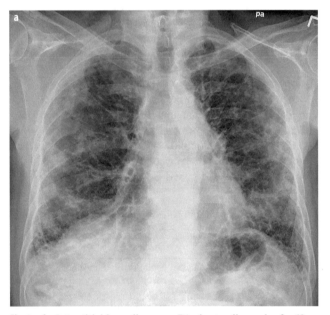
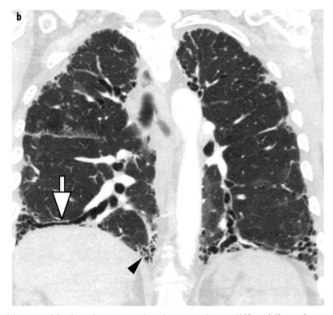

Fig. 3 a, b. Interstitial lung disease. **a** PA chest radiograph of a 62-year-old man with chronic progressive dyspnea shows diffuse bilateral peripheral reticular interstitial opacities and low lung volumes. **b** Coronal contrast-enhanced chest CT shows subpleural reticulation, traction bronchiectasis (*arrow*), and honeycomb cysts (*arrowhead*), consistent with usual interstitial pneumonia

Interstitial opacities frequently result from interstitial edema characterized by perihilar haze, peribronchial thickening, septal thickening, and subpleural edema often associated with cardiomegaly and pleural effusion [4]. Associated radiographic findings can help limit the differential diagnosis (Table 3).

Cells and fibrosis may also infiltrate the pulmonary interstitium, producing reticular and reticulonodular interstitial opacities in diseases such as sarcoidosis, siliciosis, and lymphangitic carcinomatosis.

The idiopathic interstitial pneumonias are a distinct group of disorders often characterized by basilar predominant pulmonary fibrosis associated with volume loss. The diagnosis usually requires further imaging with high-resolution chest CT to assess for the presence or absence of honeycombing (Fig. 3).

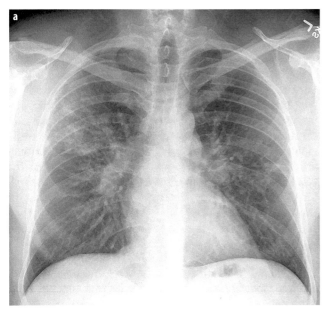
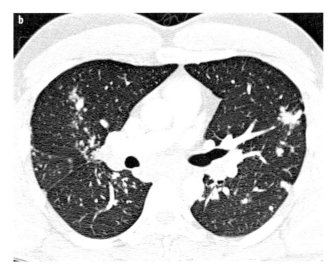

Fig. 4 a, b. Lymphadenopathy. **a** PA chest radiograph shows bilateral hilar, right paratracheal, and aortopulmonary window lymph node enlargement associated with reticulonodular opacities in the upper and mid lung zones. **b** Contrast-enhanced chest CT shows bilateral hilar and subcarinal lymphadenopathy and multifocal perilymphatic pulmonary nodules, consistent with suspected sarcoidosis

Airways

The trachea and bronchi should be assessed for size, patency, and course. Tracheal narrowing may be focal or diffuse. Focal tracheal narrowing or stenosis often results from mucosal damage from prolonged intubation. Airway neoplasms may manifest as endoluminal soft-tissue nodules that may be associated with volume loss. Endotracheal tumors may grow to obstruct up to 75% of the airway lumen before symptoms ensue. Airway neoplasms may also manifest as focal or diffuse airway stenosis and must be differentiated from inflammatory processes that may produce airway stenosis. Bronchiectasis is defined as irreversible bronchial dilatation and may result from infection, cystic fibrosis, primary ciliary dyskinesia, or allergic bronchopulmonary fungal disease [5].

Hila

On normal frontal chest radiographs, the right hilum is lower than the left in 97% of cases, and the hila are at the same level in 3% of cases. Alterations of these relationships should suggest volume loss. The right hilum is anterior to the left on lateral chest radiography. The intermediate stem line, visible on lateral chest radiography, represents the posterior walls of the right mainstem bronchus and bronchus intermedius and should be assessed for abnormal thickening, which may be seen in interstitial edema and in central malignancies.

Hilar enlargement may result from a central neoplasm, lymphadenopathy (Fig. 4), or enlarged central pulmonary arteries, such as in pulmonary hypertension. The "hilum

Table 4. Etiologies of hilar enlargement

Unilateral	Bilateral
Lung cancer	Sarcoidosis
Infection (granulomatous)	Metastatic lymphadenopathy
Metastatic lymphadenopathy	Pulmonary hypertension
Bronchogenic cyst	Lymphoma
Valvular pulmonic stenosis (left)	Infection (granulomatous)

convergence sign" refers to enlarged vessels coursing towards the enlarged hilum and signifies a vascular etiology. The "hilum overlay sign" refers to visualization of the normal hilar vasculature through a mediastinal soft-tissue mass that projects over the hilum (Table 4) [6].

Mediastinum

The mediastinum is the space between the mediastinal pleural reflections bound anteriorly by the sternum and posteriorly by the thoracic vertebrae. It extends from the thoracic inlet superiorly to the diaphragm inferiorly. It contains the heart, pericardium, central great vessels, esophagus, trachea, carina and proximal mainstem bronchi, the thoracic duct, lymph nodes, and mediastinal fat. The radiologist must be familiar with the normal mediastinal contours and its normal lines, stripes, and interfaces in order to identify subtle abnormalities.

Heart

The right cardiac border is formed by the right atrium, and the left cardiac border by the left ventricle inferiorly and a small portion of the left atrial appendage superiorly. The right ventricle projects anteriorly and inferiorly on the lateral chest radiograph. The posterior cardiac border is formed by the left ventricle inferiorly and the left atrium superiorly.

The heart must be assessed for its shape and size. The normal pericardium is not visible on radiography. Enlargement of the cardiac silhouette may result from cardiac enlargement and/or pericardial effusion. When the volume of the latter is large, a "water bottle heart" morphology may be seen on frontal chest radiographs or an "epicardial fat pad sign" on lateral radiography. In the "epicardial fat pad sign," the pericardial effusion appears as a curvilinear band of soft tissue >2 mm thick and outlined by mediastinal fat anteriorly and by subepicardial fat posteriorly. Constrictive pericarditis may manifest with linear pericardial calcification. Cardiac calcifications may correspond to coronary artery, valvular, or annular calcifications or curvilinear calcification in a left ventricular aneurysm secondary to myocardial infarction.

Systemic Arteries

The normal aortic arch is readily visible on radiography and characteristically produces an indentation on the left inferior tracheal wall. With increasing aortic atherosclerosis and ectasia, a larger portion of the aorta is visible and may exhibit intimal atherosclerotic calcification. The left para-aortic interface projects through the left heart and courses vertically towards the abdomen. The left subclavian artery is seen as a concave left superior mediastinal interface on frontal chest radiography. A right aortic arch is usually associated with a right descending thoracic aorta. In the absence of associated congenital heart disease, it is also frequently associated with non-mirror image branching characterized by an aberrant left subclavian artery, which may be seen as an indentation on the posterior trachea on lateral chest radiography [7].

Systemic Veins

The azygos arch is visible at the right tracheobronchial angle and normally measures <1 cm in diameter when the patient is in the upright position. The azygos arch may be contained within an accessory azygos fissure, as an anatomic variant. Enlargement of the azygos arch may occur in azygos continuation of the inferior vena cava, in which the vertical portion of the azygos vein manifests as a vertically oriented right-sided mediastinal interface [7].

Pulmonary Arteries

Enlargement of the pulmonary arteries may represent pulmonary hypertension and is typically associated with enlargement of the pulmonary trunk. The pulmonary trunk is visible as a left mediastinal interface located above the heart and below the aortopulmonary window on frontal radiography.

Lines, Stripes, and Interfaces

The anterior and posterior junction lines represent the interfaces between the right and left upper lobes, and may be thickened by fat, lymphadenopathy, or mediastinal masses. The paravertebral stripes may be thickened by lymphadenopathy or fat. An abnormal convex contour of the upper azygoesophageal recess may result from subcarinal lymphadenopathy or a bronchogenic cyst, while hiatus hernia often produces convexity of the lower one-third of the azygoesophageal recess. Convexity of the aortopulmonary reflection may be caused by mediastinal fat, lymphadenopathy, anterior mediastinal masses, or anomalous vasculature [7].

Mediastinal Masses

Mediastinal masses include primary and secondary neoplasms, mediastinal cysts, vascular lesions, glandular enlargement (thyroid and thymus), and herniations (hiatus and Morgagni). Since 10% of mediastinal masses are vascular in their etiology, a vascular lesion should always be considered in a patient with a mediastinal contour abnormality.

The first step in the assessment of a mediastinal mass is determining that there is indeed a mediastinal abnormality. Focal unilateral mediastinal masses are typically primary neoplasms, enlarged lymph nodes, cysts, and vascular aneurysms or anomalous vessels. While diffuse symmetric mediastinal widening without mass effect can be seen in mediastinal lipomatosis, when lobulated or asymmetric it should suggest lymphadenopathy in a patient with advanced lung cancer, metastatic disease, or lymphoma (Fig. 5).

The mediastinal mass should then be localized within a radiographic mediastinal compartment (anterior, middle or posterior) based on the lateral chest radiograph. Ancillary findings should be noted, such as benign pressure erosion in patients with paravertebral masses (typical of neurogenic neoplasms). The "cervicothoracic sign" can be used to localize superior mediastinal and thoracic inlet masses. Clinical factors such as age, gender, and presence or absence of symptoms allow the radiologist to provide a focused differential diagnosis prior to proceeding to cross-sectional imaging. Mediastinal widening in the setting of trauma may represent hemorrhage from traumatic vascular injury (Table 5) [8].

Pleura

Pleural abnormalities are those that involve the pleural space, such as gas (pneumothorax) or fluid (pleural effusion), or the pleural surfaces, including thickening (pleural plaques, neoplasms) with or without pleural calcification (pleural plaques, fibrothorax).

Pneumothorax manifests with visualization of a pleural line and may be traumatic, iatrogenic, or spontaneous.

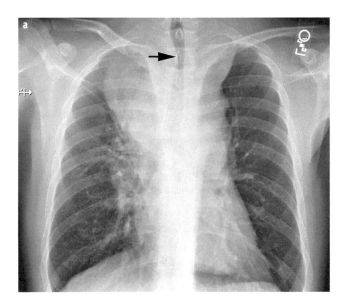

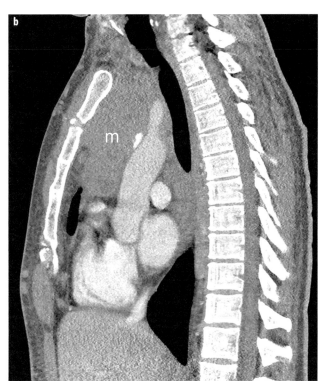

Fig. 5 a, b. Mediastinal mass. **a** PA chest radiograph shows bilateral lobular mediastinal widening with mass effect on the trachea (*arrow*) and findings of supraclavicular lymph node involvement. **b** Sagittal reformatted CT shows an anterior mediastinal mass (*m*). CT-guided core tissue biopsy showed non-Hodgkin lymphoma

Table 5. Differential diagnosis of mediastinal masses

Anterior	Middle	Posterior
Lymphoma	Lung cancer	Neurogenic neoplasm
Thymic neoplasm	Lymphadenopathy (lymphoma, metastases)	Aneurysm
Germ cell neoplasm	Foregut cyst	Extramedullary hematopoiesis
Thyroid goiter	Hiatus hernia	

Spontaneous pneumothorax is categorized as primary (no visible underlying lung disease) and secondary (underlying lung disease).

Pleural effusion is categorized as transudative or exudative, and manifests as blunting of the costophrenic angle, producing a meniscus. Transudative pleural effusions are usually secondary to heart failure. Exudative effusions are often secondary to infection, malignancy, or pulmonary infarction. Pleural effusions may exhibit loculation, which should raise the suspicion of empyema in

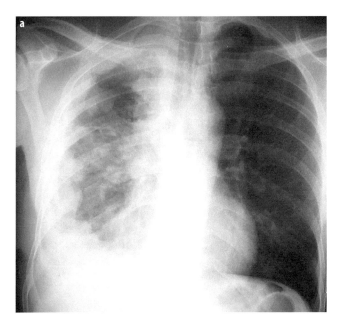

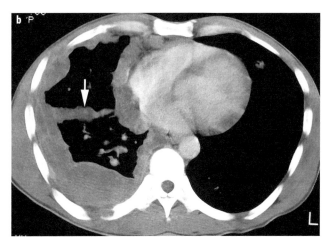

Fig. 6 a, b. Malignant pleural mesothelioma. **a** PA chest radiograph shows circumferential, nodular right pleural thickening. **b** Axial contrast-enhanced chest CT shows encasement of the right lung by a circumferential nodular pleural thickening extending into the major fissure (*arrow*)

a patient with signs and symptoms of infection. An air-fluid level in the pleural space in the absence of prior intervention is diagnostic of a bronchopleural fistula. Massive pleural effusions and pleural effusions with associated pleural nodules should suggest malignancy. Circumferential nodular pleural thickening is virtually diagnostic of malignancy. The differential diagnosis includes metastatic disease, malignant pleural mesothelioma (Fig. 6), and lymphoma [9, 10].

Diffuse pleural calcification may reflect a fibrothorax and can result from prior hemothorax or tuberculous empyema. Multifocal bilateral discontinuous pleural calcifications are typical of pleural plaques in asbestos-related pleural disease [10].

Chest Wall

The symmetry of normal chest wall structures such as the breast shadows in women and the ribs and scapulae should be analyzed to detect chest wall abnormalities. Nonsurgical absence of a portion of a rib or vertebral body may be instrumental in making the diagnosis of malignancy. Rib destruction adjacent to a thoracic mass is indicative of chest wall involvement [11]. Benign pressure erosion is characteristic of neurogenic neoplasms and chest wall vascular abnormalities. Soft-tissue calcification may indicate prior trauma (myositis ossificans), collagen vascular disease (dermatomyositis), or the presence of a vascular lesion (hemangioma) or a bone-forming malignancy (chondrosarcoma). Gas within the chest wall could indicate an air leak in the setting of trauma, pneumomediastinum or pneumothorax.

References

1. Ashizawa K, Hayashi K, Aso N et al (2001) Lobar atelectasis: diagnostic pitfalls on chest radiography. Br J Radiol 74:89-97.
2. Abbott GA (2012) Approach to atelectasis and volume loss. In: Rosado-de-Christenson ML (ed) Diagnostic imaging – Chest. Amirsys, Salt Lake City, UH, pp 1-56.
3. Hodnett PA, Ko JP (2012) Evaluation and management of indeterminate pulmonary nodules. Radiol Clin North Am 50:895-914.
4. Cardinale L, Priola AM, Moretti F et al (2014) Effectiveness of chest radiography, lung ultrasound and thoracic computed tomography in the diagnosis of congestive heart failure. World J Radiol 6:230-237.
5. Boiselle P (2008) Imaging of the large airways. Clin Chest Med 41:617-626.
6. Felson B (1973) Localization of intrathoracic lesions. In: Felson B (ed) Chest roentgenology. Saunders, Philadelphia, PA, pp 39-41.
7. Gibbs JM, Chandrasekhar CA, Ferguson EC (2007) Lines and stripes: Where did they go? – From conventional radiography to CT. Radiographics 27:33-48.
8. Whitten CR, Khan S, Munneke GJ et al (2007) A diagnostic approach to mediastinal abnormalities. Radiographics 27:657-671.
9. Cardinale L, Ardissone F, Asteggiano F et al (2013) Diffuse neoplasms of the pleural serosa. Radiol Med 118:366-378.
10. Gallardo X, Castaner E, Mata JM (2000) Benign pleural diseases. Eur J Radiol 34:87-97.
11. Tateishi U, Gladish GW, Kusumoto M et al (2003) Chest wall tumors: Radiologic findings and pathologic correlation. Radiographics 23:1491-1508.

Diseases of the Chest Wall, Pleura, and Diaphragm

Aine Kelly[1], Nicola Sverzellati[2]

[1] University of Michigan Hospital System, Ann Arbor, MI, USA
[2] Department of Surgical Sciences, Section of Radiology, University of Parma, Parma, Italy

Introduction

Chest radiography is useful to evaluate the chest wall, pleura, and diaphragm, while magnetic resonance imaging (MRI) provide high-quality studies of the extraparenchymal extent of lesions residing in the superior sulcus (apical) region. As skeletal abnormalities are very difficult to detect, the individual bones must be carefully examined. Normal variants, unlike abnormalities, are often bilateral and reasonably symmetric, such that a side by side comparison is helpful. To help distinguish a lung mass from an extraparenchymal (pleural, diaphragmatic, or chest wall) mass, determination of the angle between the mass and the lung edge is often informative: acute for lung and obtuse for extraparenchymal (Fig. 1). With extraparenchymal lesions, it may be difficult to distinguish those originating in the pleura from those arising in the chest wall, as the shape can be similar; however, the presence of bone destruction indicates an extrapleural origin.

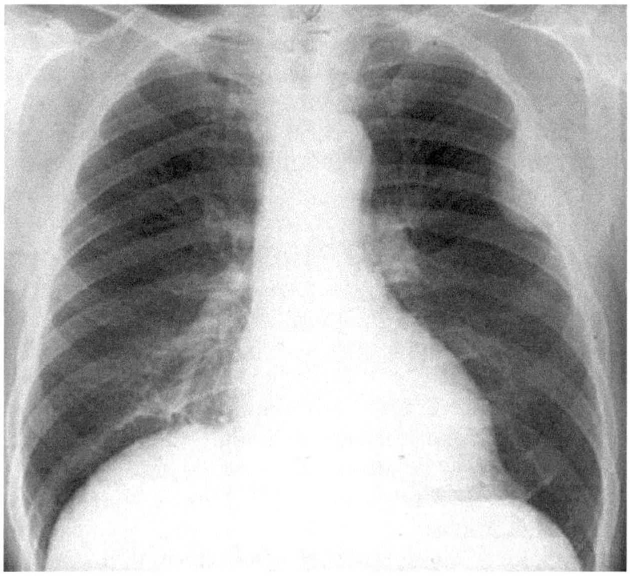

Chest Wall Disease

The normal chest wall is symmetric. The most common causes of asymmetry are rotation and kyphoscoliosis. On chest radiography, the side to which the patient is rotated is more radiolucent (in a left anterior oblique/right posterior oblique position the right side is more lucent). Chest radiography is useful to evaluate skeletal disease, calcifications, and subcutaneous emphysema.

Calcifications

Calcifications deposited in soft tissues may be metastatic or dystrophic. Metastatic calcifications occur with elevated serum calcium, in which case calcium hydroxyapatite crystals are deposited in multiple locations, including the lung, stomach, kidney, and vascular system [1]. Dystrophic calcifications in altered, necrotic, or dead tissues are seen in patients with normal serum calcium and phosphorus levels and occur in association with connective tissue disorders, in subcutaneous tissues, muscles, and fascial planes as calcification universalis.

Soft-Tissue Masses

These must first be differentiated from asymmetries arising from patient positioning, contralateral surgery (mastectomy), and atrophy (poliomyelitis and stroke). Primary tumors are rare. Malignancies include fibrosarcoma and malignant fibrohistiocytoma, with lipomas as the most common benign primary tumor. Neurogenic tumors, such as neurofibromas, arise from intercostal nerves or the paraspinal ganglia and can be found at multiple sites in neurofibromatosis type 1 (von Recklinghausen disease).

Fig. 1. Extraparenchymal mass forms an obtuse angle with the chest wall in a patient with a solitary plasmacytoma. Note the bone destruction indicating the origin of the tumor outside the lung and pleura

Diseases of the Chest and Heart 2015-2018,
DOI: 10.1007/978-88-470-5752-4_13 © Springer-Verlag Italia 2015

Inflammatory Diseases of the Chest Wall

Bacterial infection of the chest wall is rare and typically involves the ribs and sternum. Osteomyelitis can spread hematogenously or directly from an adjacent infectious process, typically *Staphylococcus aureus* or *Pseudomonas aeruginosa*. Radiography may demonstrate soft-tissue swelling overlying rib destruction and a periosteal reaction in chronic cases but computed tomography (CT) and MRI are much more sensitive and specific. CT is limited in its detection of bone marrow abnormalities, while MRI allows the early detection of osteomyelitis by showing bone marrow edema on T2 and marrow hypointensity on T1 images. However, CT is more sensitive than MRI in showing cortical destruction and a periosteal reaction.

Chest wall involvement with tuberculosis (TB) is uncommon, occurring via hematogenous spread or, more rarely, by direct extension from the underlying lung or pleura; the latter is referred to as empyema necessitans. Chest wall involvement in TB manifests as osseous and cartilaginous destruction and soft-tissue masses with calcifications and rim enhancement [2]. Fungal infections of the chest wall occur in immunocompromised patients, with *Aspergillus* accounting for 80–90% of cases [3]. In 15% of the cases of thoracic actinomycosis, the fungus invades the chest wall, creating fistulas and empyema necessitans. Postoperative patients are at risk of *Nocardia* infection.

Congenital Diseases of the Chest Wall

Poland syndrome is characterized by aplasia of the pectoralis major muscles, and occasionally by hypoplasia of the ipsilateral chest wall, scapula, and ribs. Imaging reveals a smaller and more lucent hemithorax, while cross sectional imaging demonstrates the absence of the pectoral muscles and a smaller, hypoplastic hemithorax [4].

Pectus Excavatum

In this variant in chest wall development (incidence 1/400–1/1000), the sternum is depressed relative to the anterior chest (ribs) and often tilts rightward, with the mediastinum leftward [3, 5]. In most cases, it is a cosmetic issue only, but in severe cases, it can lead to pain, dyspnea, and restrictive lung disease. On radiographs, the right side of the mediastinum is indistinct, simulating middle lobe airspace disease. The depressed sternum is visible on the lateral projection [3].

Injuries to the Thoracic Skeleton, Rib Fractures, and Trauma

Upper rib fractures suggest severe trauma, and a search should be made for associated injury of the aorta, great vessels, and brachial plexus [6]. Fractures of the medial clavicle and sternum are also associated with vascular and cardiac injury. Sternal fractures are very difficult to visualize on frontal chest radiographs and may be seen on the lateral view, but nearly all are visible by CT, which will demonstrate any adjacent hematoma. Significantly displaced sternal fractures should lead one to look for associated cardiac injury. Lower rib fractures can be associated with hepatic, renal, or splenic injury. Abdominal radiographs are helpful to depict fractures of the lower ribs, as they are better visualized.

A flail chest (or segment) occurs with five or more consecutive rib fractures (or three or more ribs fractured in two places). The flail segment moves paradoxically during respiration, with resultant ventilatory compromise. Fractures of the thoracic spine account for 15–30% of all spinal fractures. The most vulnerable segment is at the thoracolumbar junction (T9–T12). Most (~70%) thoracic spine fractures are visible on radiographs, but CT shows almost all of them and, more importantly, will demonstrate the displacement or retropulsion of bone fragments into the spinal canal and cord.

Bone Masses

The most common non-neoplastic tumor of the thoracic skeleton is fibrous dysplasia, which accounts for 30% of the benign bone tumors of the chest wall [7]. These slow-growing tumors often occur in the posterolateral ribs and are usually asymptomatic unless pressure symptoms or pathologic fractures occur. Fibrous dysplasia manifests as an expansile lytic lesion with a hazy or ground glass appearance. Plasmacytoma and multiple myeloma are the most common malignant neoplasms of the thoracic skeleton and can present as extraparenchymal masses with bone destruction, similar in appearances to other metastases [8]. Bone lesions are well defined; they have a punched out appearance. In advanced cases there is marked erosion as well as areas of expansion and destruction of bone cortex, sometimes with thick ridging around the periphery, giving a "soap bubble" appearance.

Thalassemia

With extramedullary hematopoiesis, hematopoietic tissues outside the bone marrow produce blood cells. This occurs mostly in the chronic hemolytic anemias, with thalassemia being the most common. Normal marrow tissue can expand outside the medulla through permeative erosions or by the reactivation of previously dormant hematopoietic tissues [9]. Ineffective erythropoiesis leads to expansion of the bone marrow space in the ribs, long bones, vertebral column, skull, and, characteristically, facial bones, and may lead to osteoporosis. Paravertebral and rib lesions are most often seen incidentally but can occasionally cause mass effect on the spinal canal and cord compression. On radiography, bilateral lobulated paravertebral masses and rib expansion are seen.

Pleural Disease

When assessing for pleural effusion or pneumothorax, the patient's positioning for the radiograph should be taken into account, as air moves upwards and fluid moves downwards within the pleural space. In the critically ill supine patient, air will rise to be anterior and fluid will layer posteriorly and over the apex as a cap. Intraperitoneal gas rises to the highest point, under the diaphragm dome on upright radiographs. Even ill patients can roll onto their side for a decubitus view; in those with effusions place the effusion side down to allow the fluid to layer along the ribs. For suspected pneumothorax, the abnormal side should be up, to allow the air to rise.

Pleural Effusion

On upright studies, pleural fluid produces a meniscus sign, displacing the affected lung away from the costophrenic sulci and blunting the angle. Evaluate the posterior costophrenic sulcus (the lowest point) on upright chest radiographs for small pleural effusions. On the frontal view, evaluate the lateral costophrenic angle or sulcus, keeping in mind that a subpulmonic effusion may be present with the lateral costophrenic angle unblunted. With subpulmonic fluid, the ipsilateral hemidiaphragm will be of uniform attenuation. There will be a lack of visibility of the posterior lung vessels through the hemidiaphragm on the frontal view, and lateral displacement of the apparent dome of the hemidiaphragm (with a more sharply sloping lateral aspect). On supine radiographs, free flowing pleural fluid layers posteriorly, possibly obscuring the meniscus or borders (with lung or normal pleura). If the effusion is large enough, there may be an apical pleural cap, as fluid caps the apex of the lung.

Pleural fluid may be loculated in the presence of adhesions or scars. It can track into fissures even if not loculated and is often recognizable because of its tapering cigar-shaped appearance. A "pseudotumor" can occur when the fluid has a more rounded shape; a homogeneous density with a different shape on two orthogonal projections is a clue to its nature (as is a comparison between old and follow up radiographs showing a change in size).

With large pleural effusions, mediastinal structures will deviate to the opposite side. Another important effect of large pleural effusions is diaphragmatic inversion. When this occurs, the two hemidiaphragms move in opposite directions during respiration. As a result, air may move over and back between the two lungs (pendelluft or pendulum respiration), with the net effect being increased dead space and significant dyspnea. Thoracentesis with removal of enough fluid to restore the affected hemidiaphragm to its normal position may provide marked relief of symptoms. Left hemidiaphragm inversion is easier to diagnose, since it results in mass effect in the left upper quadrant, displacing the gas-filled stomach.

In hospitalized patients, pleural effusions may arise as a consequence of congestive cardiac failure or post-surgically. Congestive heart failure effusions are usually bilateral and typically symmetric, although occasionally they are unilateral or more asymmetric, with the right larger than the left. With unilateral effusions (or left larger than the right) in a non-surgical patient, other causes include pneumonia, infarction, neoplasm, trauma, and connective tissue disorders (especially systemic lupus erythematosus and rheumatoid arthritis). With pulmonary embolus, radiographs may reveal small unilateral or bilateral hemorrhagic pleural effusions and atelectasis.

Adjacent upper abdominal abnormalities can cause effusion (most often unilateral), with the most common etiologies including splenic trauma, subdiaphragmatic abscess, pancreatitis, and ascites. Here, the clinical history is very helpful, while thoracentesis can be diagnostic (e.g., elevated amylase with pancreatitis). With ascites (e.g., due to liver failure), pleural effusions can develop because of ascites leaking through the diaphragm. When a right subdiaphragmatic abscess is suspected, ultrasound can be very helpful, but for suspected left upper quadrant fluid collections CT is better.

Trauma can result in pleural effusion, more commonly unilateral. This is obvious with multiple rib fractures but less apparent with, for example, aortic laceration in the absence of fractures. Another less obvious case is a malpositioned vascular catheter or feeding tube. Inadvertent placement of a feeding tube into the lung is usually benign, as long as it is discovered before a feeding is given. However, pleural placement is not similarly benign, as tension pneumothorax and empyema are among its important consequences.

Empyema

Pneumonia patients commonly have uninfected pleural fluid (sympathetic effusion). Infection of the pleura (empyema) can occur as a complication, with organisms such as TB and fungi having a particular predilection for the pleural space. The differentiation of empyema from lung abscess can generally be accomplished by chest X-ray alone and corroborated by thoracic ultrasound. Empyemas typically make right or obtuse angles with the adjacent chest wall, while lung abscesses usually demonstrate acute angles only. In addition, empyemas are usually oval or lenticular in shape and therefore are larger on one of two orthogonal projections, while lung abscesses are more spherical in shape and thus more similar in size on two orthogonal projections. CT can help by demonstrating the empyema as more mass-like, deflecting vessels and bronchi in its path, while lung abscess is more destructive of lung structures but less mass-like. The smoother margins of a pleural abnormality and the CT "split pleura sign" of enhancing visceral and parietal pleura around an empyema can also aid in the differential diagnosis (Fig. 2).

Neither chest X-ray nor CT alone can establish the presence or absence of infection in the lung or pleural space; rather, clinical findings (such as fever and elevated

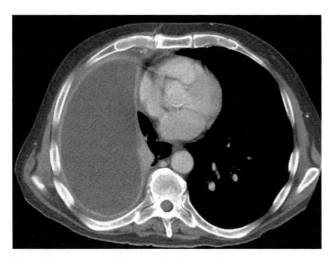

Fig. 2. Right pleural effusion with thickened visceral and parietal pleura ("split pleura sign")

white blood cell count) are important in raising the possibility of infection. The role of imaging is to localize the infection to the lung or pleura. The final etiology of pleural effusion is sometimes established on clinical grounds alone. In difficult cases, diagnosis generally relies on thoracentesis and an analysis of the pleural fluid. Ultrasound imaging and marking of the adjacent chest wall can be helpful to guide thoracentesis.

Pneumothorax

Air can enter the pleural space as a result of lung, tracheobronchial or esophageal injury. Pneumothorax is seen in 15-40% of acute chest trauma patients. Upright frontal radiography is preferred for detecting pneumothorax, as air tends to rise up within the pleural space. However, lateral decubitus radiography with the suspected side of the pneumothorax up is an alternative. Many small and even moderate-sized pneumothoraces not visible on supine radiographs are readily identified at CT.

Pneumothorax is best diagnosed by visualization of the lung edge outlined by pleural air. Apical lucency and absence of vessels are less reliable and can be produced by bullae. As for pleural effusions, the detection of pneumothorax becomes difficult with supine patients, with the non-dependent portion of the pleural space near the anterior hemidiaphragm. Lucency near the lung bases should raise suspicion, particularly in the presence of the deep sulcus sign, even when no lung edge is visualized. Pneumothorax can track into fissures with air in the minor fissure considered as another sign of supine pneumothorax.

A tension pneumothorax is a medical emergency, as mediastinal structures can be compressed, causing decreased venous return to the heart and hemodynamic instability. With increasing intrapleural pressure, mediastinal structures deviate contralaterally, with ipsilateral hemithorax hyperexpansion and hemidiaphragm depression.

The differential diagnosis for pneumothorax is far less extensive than that for pleural effusion. Most cases follow trauma but can occur secondary to ruptured blebs, with the latter typically found in aesthenic young males. Interstitial lung disease is another potential cause and honeycombing or lung cysts increase the risk of pneumothorax, particularly in males with eosinophilic granuloma and in females with lymphangioleiomyomatosis.

Other potential causes, in which the radiograph is normal, include subpleural abnormalities that tend to cavitate, such as tuberculosis and metastases. Squamous primary neoplasms account for most cavitary metastases, but cavitation is also a feature of sarcomas. Increased intrathoracic pressure (e.g., asthma or pregnancy) is another potential explanation for pneumothorax with an otherwise normal or nearly normal radiograph. A persistent pneumothorax after chest tube insertion and suction suggests either a malfunctioning chest tube, bronchial injury, or bronchopleural fistula.

A special category of pneumothorax is the pneumothorax ex vacuo, which is a complication of lobar collapse [10]. In this condition, the collapse results in a sudden increase in negative intrapleural pressure surrounding the collapsed lobe. As a result, gas from the ambient tissues and blood is drawn into the pleural space while the seal between the visceral and parietal pleura of the adjacent lobe or lobes remains intact. The pneumothorax resolves as soon as the bronchial obstruction is relieved and the collapsed lobe re-expands. Recognition of this entity is critical as appropriate treatment is to relieve the bronchial obstruction rather than insert a pleural drainage catheter.

Hemothorax

Bleeding from low-pressure pulmonary vessels is usually self-limiting; however, injury to large central pulmonary vessels, systemic thoracic veins or arteries, or lacerated viscera can lead to a large, potentially life-threatening hemothorax requiring surgical intervention. As for pneumothorax, hemothorax can be difficult to detect on supine radiographs, due to dependent posterior layering. Signs of hemothorax on a supine chest radiograph include apical cap, hazy increased opacity projected over the hemithorax, and confluent lateral pleural thickening. A hemothorax should always be considered when rib fractures are found. CT is the most accurate way to detect even small amounts of pleural fluid. On CT, hemothorax is suggested when the pleural fluid measures >35–40 HU. In some cases, dependent layering of the higher-attenuation hematocrit can be seen in the pleural space. The delayed or late appearance of pleural fluid that continues to slowly accumulate over several days, particularly following a penetrating injury or recent thoracic surgery, raises the possibility of a chylous effusion secondary to thoracic duct disruption.

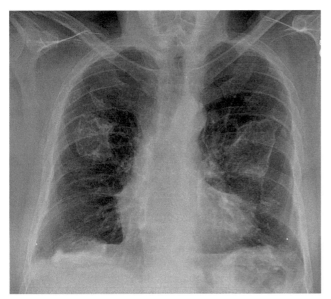

Fig. 3. "Holly leaf" appearance of bilateral calcified pleural plaques, seen en face, in a patient with a history of asbestos exposure (he had worked in a shipyard). Note the calcified plaques also on the hemi-diaphragmatic surface

Pleural Plaques or Thickening

Unlike pleural fluid or air, pleural implants or plaques are often better seen with CT than on chest X-ray. Pleural plaques are common in patients exposed to asbestos (asbestos-related pleural plaques), are usually bilateral, and are sometimes visibly calcified. A characteristic location is at the diaphragmatic domes and under the lower posterolateral ribs [11]. With plaques visualized en face, the imaging appearances are often irregularly shaped, poorly marginated opacities. Calcified pleural plaques en face often have scalloped outlines, giving a "holly leaf"-like appearance (Fig. 3). A clue to their extraparenchymal (pleural) location is that the long axis of pleural plaques is not parallel that of the underlying pulmonary vasculature.

Unilateral pleural plaques can also occur with asbestos exposure, but in this setting other possibilities, such as prior empyema or trauma, should be raised. Untreated hemothorax or TB may result in a small hemithorax with extensive pleural calcification (fibrothorax).

Pleural Implants and Masses

Pleural implants may be seen with metastatic disease but metastatic disease more commonly causes pleural effusion. Many pleural masses are obscured on chest radiography (and even on CT) by surrounding pleural effusion. However, not all pleural masses are accompanied by effusions. In these cases, CT may reveal soft-tissue implants, suggesting the malignant nature of the effusion. Contrast-enhanced CT is generally better able to distinguish solid elements of pleural masses from effusion.

With chronic pleural hematoma, dependent layering of the higher-attenuation hematocrit component may occur. It is usually visible on CT, simulating a malignant effusion. Malignant thymoma often causes unilateral multifocal pleural implants, but these are generally not associated with effusion.

Benign fibrous tumor of the pleura (benign mesothelioma) often presents as a single pleural mass, ranging in size from small to enormous [12]. Lesions may be pedunculated, such that the mass may change position by twisting around its pedicle. Even large benign fibrous tumors are generally distinguishable from malignant mesothelioma by their focal nature (malignant mesothelioma being typically more widespread) and the lack of associated pleural effusion. Benign fibrous tumors are generally easily recognized as pleural lesions by their shape, except when located in a pleural fissure, in which case the lesion may be round and sharply marginated. This lesion might raise concern for malignancy but CT localization of the "mass" to the pleural fissure makes benign fibrous tumor the more likely diagnosis. Clinical clues are sometimes also useful in diagnosing benign fibrous tumor, such as associated hypertrophic pulmonary osteoarthropathy and, less commonly, hypoglycemia. In a third of cases, malignant degeneration occurs, necessitating excision.

Pleural metastases are far more common than primary pleural neoplasms. Many neoplasms metastasize to the pleura, with those closest more likely (bronchogenic and breast). In a patient with a pleural mass and a known primary neoplasm elsewhere, metastases should still be considered even if the malignancy is not frequently associated with pleural disease. Ovarian cancer frequently spreads to the peritoneum and can give rise to pleural effusions when malignant ascites passes through hemidiaphragm defects. Pleural metastases from ovarian cancer are referred to as Meigs syndrome. Patients with pleural metastases may have unilateral or bilateral effusions.

Malignant mesothelioma is the most common primary neoplasm, typically appearing as lobulated pleural masses associated with pleural effusion, often unilateral. A history of asbestos exposure (or bilateral calcified pleural plaques) can be a helpful clue but asbestos exposure is only documented in about half of mesothelioma patients. In some patients, the lack of mediastinal shift away from the side of extensive pleural abnormality is a clue to the diagnosis of malignant mesothelioma [13, 14]. Metastatic adenocarcinoma closely mimics malignant mesothelioma, with circumferential nodular pleural masses often including the medial pleura (Fig. 4).

Diaphragmatic Disease

The right hemidiaphragm is usually a rib interspace higher than the left, with its upper border at the 5th anterior rib through the 6th–7th anterior rib interspace level on the posteroanterior radiograph. The diaphragm is inseparable

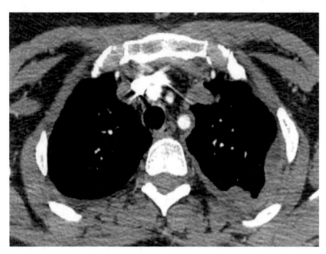

Fig. 4. Nodular thickening of the left pleura, including the mediastinal aspect, in a 43-year-old patient with malignant mesothelioma

from the abdominal structures on radiographs. Multiplanar CT is ideally suited to visualize the diaphragm due to its differential attenuation from adjacent intraperitoneal fat and aerated lung. CT shows the diaphragm as a smooth soft-tissue attenuation band-like structure that is thicker at the edges and thinner (sometimes imperceptibly) towards the central tendon [15]. Folds or bundles of muscles (slips) run obliquely along the inferior surface, are often asymmetric, and can have a mass like appearance if they are seen in cross-section, especially in males, where they are more prominent. Multiple slips can give the diaphragm a scalloped appearance where the muscle bulges upwards on either side of them. Defects and hernias may be congenital (Bochdalek, Morgagni or eventration) or acquired (hiatus hernia, trauma, or paralysis). Predisposing conditions for all abdominal hernias include pregnancy, trauma, obesity, chronic constipation, and chronic cough.

Bochdalek Hernia

In adults, 90% of congenital hernias are Bochdalek hernias. These hernias are more common on the left because of the protective effect of the liver on the right posteriorly [16]. Bochdalek hernias occur posterolaterally due to the persistence of a gap between the costal and vertebral portions of the diaphragm, through which peritoneal fat and, less commonly, kidney and other solid organs or bowel protrude [17]. Neonates and young children under a year may present with respiratory symptoms, while older children and adults more likely present with acute or chronic gastrointestinal symptoms, if any. Rarely, patients can present with bowel incarceration, strangulation, perforation, or shock. However, nowadays, most Bochdalek hernias are discovered incidentally on CT imaging, as small defects, particularly in patients with longstanding obstructive lung disease. For incidentally discovered hernias, no further action is needed. Imaging appearances of

Bochdalek hernia include discontinuity of the posterior or posteromedial diaphragm with protrusion of peritoneal or retroperitoneal fat through the defect. Less commonly, colon, small bowel, liver, spleen, or kidney may also herniate into the thoracic cavity. On CT, discontinuity of the diaphragm is usually easily visualized [15]. On chest radiography, the differential diagnosis will include lipomas, lung or diaphragmatic tumors, neurogenic tumors, pulmonary sequestrations, or intrathoracic kidney.

Morgagni Hernia

Less than 10% of congenital hernias are Morgagni hernias. They arise anteromedially due to the failed fusion of the sternal and costal portions of the hemidiaphragm [18, 19]. They are more common in females and occur more frequently on the right, possibly due to greater support provided by the pericardial attachments on the left. In adults, protrusion of omentum is the most common form, and only rarely, bowel, stomach or liver. On imaging, Morgagni hernia will appear as a fatty mass in the right cardiophrenic angle that can be difficult to differentiate from a prominent epicardial fat pad. The differential diagnosis will include lipoma, teratoma, thymoma, thymolipoma, or liposarcoma. Detection of displaced curvilinear omental vessels within the "mass" or coursing across the diaphragmatic defect, characteristic of Morgagni hernia, is best appreciated on coronal CT or MRI.

Diaphragmatic Eventration

An eventration is a congenital circumscribed area of diaphragmatic muscular aplasia or thinning that allows bulging of the abdominal contents towards the thorax, due to the relative pressure gradient between the peritoneum and the thorax [17]. Unlike a true hernia, the abdominal contents are still confined by a layer of pleura, diaphragmatic tendon and peritoneum [15]. Symptoms are rare and include tachypnea, dyspnea, recurrent pneumonia, and failure to thrive. These cases can be treated with surgical plication (folding or tucking and suturing). Eventration occurs most commonly on the right side anteromedially and can become more pronounced with increasing intra-abdominal pressure, usually as a result of obesity. Imaging shows an anterior elevation of the hemidiaphragm, since the thinning and weakening involve this portion, with a normal posterior position. With diaphragmatic paralysis, the posterior portion will also be elevated. On CT, there may be relative thickening of the muscle at the edge of the eventration. In some cases the edges are undercut, with upwards ballooning of the eventrated portion [17].

Esophageal Hiatus Hernia

The esophageal hiatus is at the T10 level and contains the esophagus, vagus nerve, and sympathetic nerve branches [16]. This ring functions as an anatomic sphincter by constricting upon inspiration and helping to prevent gastroesophageal reflux. In hiatal hernia, there is herniation of part of or, rarely, the entire stomach, or another abdominal organ or fat. Obesity, aging, and general weakening of the musculofascial structures may cause enlargement of an esophageal hiatus. Esophageal hiatal hernias can be sliding or rolling (para-esophageal) or a combination of these two. Sliding hernias comprise 90% of esophageal hernias, with displacement of the gastroesophageal junction and a portion of (or the entire) stomach upwards into the thoracic cavity, with loss of the usual anti-reflux mechanism. With the para-esophageal type, a portion (or all) of the stomach or other abdominal contents, such as the spleen or intestines, roll up past the gastroesophageal junction into the thoracic cavity. On chest radiography, herniation of the stomach will be visible as an opacification behind the heart on the lateral view and obliteration of the azygoesophageal line on a frontal view [19].

Traumatic Diaphragmatic Rupture or Hernia

Diaphragmatic rupture occurs in about 5% of patients with blunt trauma [20]. Mechanisms of injury include lateral impact, which distorts the chest wall with shearing forces across the diaphragm, and frontal impact, which causes increased intra-abdominal pressure and "blows out" the diaphragm. Most diaphragmatic ruptures are associated with significant intra-abdominal injuries. Left and right diaphragmatic ruptures are thought to occur equally frequently, but right sided ruptures may be more clinically occult due to protection from the liver. Left ruptures tend therefore to be reported in most (75–90%) cases, with the majority of tears occurring posterolaterally, at the musculotendinous junction, i.e., the weakest portion. Most diaphragmatic tears resulting from blunt trauma are >2 cm in length with many left tears being >10 cm long.

Visceral organ herniation occurs in about half of the cases of diaphragmatic rupture, with the stomach and colon herniating most commonly on the left side, and sometimes small bowel, spleen, and kidney. On the right side, the liver most commonly herniates and occasionally the colon. Herniation can be complicated by strangulation, leading to ischemia, infarction, or obstruction. In some cases, herniation can be delayed after diaphragmatic rupture, but the relatively increased intra-abdominal pressure will cause the defect to increase in size, increasing the likelihood of herniation of the intra-abdominal contents into the thorax. The progression may be prevented if patients need positive pressure ventilation after their injury, which eliminates or reverses the pressure gradient. The delay period between injury and herniation is known as the latent phase and can go for months or years, but most cases of strangulation declare themselves within 3 years of the trauma.

Chest radiography can show the secondary signs of herniation including: apparent hemidiaphragm elevation;

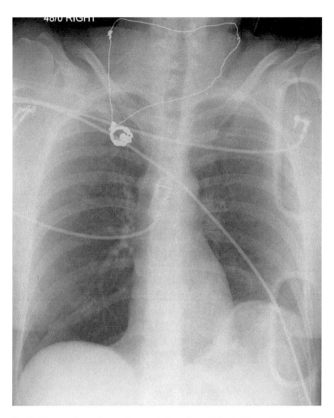

Fig. 5. Unusual configuration and elevation of the left hemidiaphragm in a trauma patient. A large tear in the left hemidiaphragm was found at surgery

irregularity/obscuration (Fig. 5) or discontinuous contour; contralateral mediastinal shift; air-containing viscera above the hemidiaphragm; and basilar opacification and an abnormal U-shaped configuration of a gastric tube with an elevated tip. However, these signs are nonspecific and can also be seen with atelectasis, lung contusion, subpulmonic pleural effusion, post-traumatic lung cysts, pneumothorax, hiatal hernia, and phrenic nerve paralysis. Diaphragmatic eventration can also simulate injury, in which case comparison with old radiographs may be helpful. CT is better than radiography, with the advantage of multiplanar viewing. CT signs of diaphragmatic injury include: focal discontinuity of the diaphragm; non-visualization of the diaphragm (absent "hemi-diaphragm sign") or a large gap between the torn ends of the diaphragm (perhaps with muscular contraction at torn ends; the "curled diaphragm" sign; Fig. 6); herniation of peritoneal fat, omentum, bowel, or an organ; focal constriction of bowel or an organ at the site of herniation ("collar sign") and herniated organs or bowel not supported posteriorly because of the ruptured diaphragm falling dependently, abutting the posterior ribs ("dependent viscera sign"). Other signs include concomitant pneumothorax and pneumoperitoneum and/or hemothorax and hemoperitoneum. Coronal T2-weighted MRI can be used to document diaphragmatic injuries in the non-acute setting.

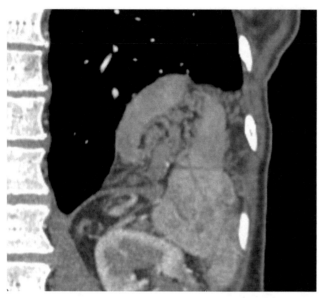

Fig. 6. Coronal contrast-enhanced computed tomography. Traumatic left hemidiaphragmatic hernia, through which the spleen and vessels are partially herniating. The thickened medial portion of the left hemidiaphragm is visible

Penetrating injuries of the diaphragm are more common than blunt injuries. The site of injury is more random, depending on the trajectory of the penetrating object. These injuries tend to be smaller, most being <2 cm and many <1 cm, related to the size of the penetrating object. Visceral herniation is uncommon with these smaller injuries. Penetrating injuries are usually diagnosed clinically, relying on the entry site and direction of the wound. Patients with these injuries commonly undergo exploratory surgery, at which time the diaphragmatic injury is diagnosed and repaired. Imaging findings include pneumothorax, hemothorax, or radiopaque material associated with the projectile near the diaphragm or indicating the path through the diaphragm.

Diaphragmatic Weakness or Paralysis

There are many causes of weakness or paralysis, including central nervous disease or phrenic nerve damage from thoracic surgery or invasion by tumors [21]. Thoracic imaging is not usually rewarding when it comes to diagnosing the causes, except for direct invasion by tumors in the chest. Bilateral diaphragmatic paralysis is usually symptomatic, often presenting with respiratory failure. Diaphragmatic paralysis is more commonly unilateral, often asymptomatic, and usually discovered incidentally on imaging.

On radiography, bilateral paralysis manifests as the smooth elevation of the hemidiaphragms and decreased lung volumes. The costophrenic and costovertebral sulci will be deep and narrow. The lateral view reveals a smooth contour and elevated diaphragmatic position.

Linear atelectasis may also be present, usually at the lung bases. The differential diagnosis of bilateral diaphragmatic elevation includes poor inspiratory effort, obesity with decreased chest wall compliance, subpulmonic pleural effusions, subdiaphragmatic processes such as ascites, ileus, and organomegaly, and pleural adhesions. With a unilateral elevated hemidiaphragm, the left hemidiaphragm may lie at the level of or above the right, or the right hemidiaphragm will lie more than the usual one interspace higher than the left side. A paralyzed hemidiaphragm will be elevated in its entirety, including the posterior take off point, which helps differentiate it from eventration.

Fluoroscopic sniff testing can be helpful in cases of unilateral diaphragmatic weakness or paralysis, with the weak side moving more slowly downwards (caudal) or paradoxically upwards (with paralysis) during quiet inspiration, deep inspiration, and sniffing [21]. The sniff test can be falsely positive in normal individuals and it is not as useful in patients with bilateral paralysis. Ultrasonography has also been used to diagnose paralysis, following the same principles as the fluoroscopic sniff test to assess diaphragmatic movement. CT is very useful to evaluate processes that can contribute to dysfunction or cause diaphragmatic elevation, including obstructive airways disease, pleural effusion, subdiaphragmatic abscess, ascites, organomegaly, or ileus. Dynamic T2-weighted MRI in the coronal (or sagittal) plane can be used to assess paralysis, with the diaphragm depicted as a low-T2-signal structure. MRI can also allow quantitative evaluation, including the excursion, synchronicity, and velocity of diaphragmatic motion.

Tumors of the Diaphragm

Primary tumors are rare and more than half are benign [22]. Benign tumors are resected if they are symptomatic or if there is diagnostic doubt [22, 23]. The most common primary malignant lesion is rhabdomyosarcoma, followed by fibrosarcoma [8]. Direct involvement of the diaphragm from lung cancer and other intra-abdominal or intrathoracic tumors, including mesothelioma and esophageal and hepatic carcinomas, can occur. Drop metastases may also be seen in thymoma and, with intraperitoneal spread, in ovarian cancer. The diaphragm can also be involved by metastases due to benign processes such as endometriosis.

Conclusion

For evaluation of the chest wall, pleura, and diaphragm, a combination of different imaging modalities coupled with a good clinical history (especially trauma and known malignancy) and knowledge of imaging principles (air, water, blood and soft tissue) can give valuable diagnostic clues.

References

1. Stewart VL, Herling P, Dalinka MK (1983) Calcification in soft tissues. JAMA 250:78-81.
2. Jeung MY, Gangi A, Gasser B et al (1999) Imaging of chest wall disorders. Radiographics 19:617-637.
3. Baez JC, Lee EY, Restrepo R, Eisenberg RL (2013) Chest wall lesions in children. AJR Am J Roentgenol 200:W402-419.
4. Mutlu H, Sildiroglu O, Basekim CC, Kizilkaya E (2007) A variant of Poland syndrome associated with dextroposition. J Thorac Imaging 22:341-342.
5. Donnelly LF (2001) Use of three-dimensional reconstructed helical CT images in recognition and communication of chest wall anomalies in children. AJR Am J Roentgenol 177:441-445.
6. Miller LA (2006) Chest wall, lung, and pleural space trauma. Radiol Clin North Am 44:213-224, viii.
7. Hughes EK, James SL, Butt S et al (2006) Benign primary tumours of the ribs. Clin Radiol 61:314-322.
8. Tateishi U, Gladish GW, Kusumoto M et al (2003) Chest wall tumors: radiologic findings and pathologic correlation: part 2. Malignant tumors. Radiographics 23:1491-1508.
9. Orphanidou-Vlachou E, Tziakouri-Shiakalli C, Georgiades CS (2014) Extramedullary hemopoiesis. Semin Ultrasound CT MR 35:255-262.
10. Woodring JH, Baker MD, Stark P (1996) Pneumothorax ex vacuo. Chest 110:1102-1105.
11. Walker CM, Takasugi JE, Chung JH et al (2012) Tumorlike conditions of the pleura. Radiographics 32:971-985.
12. Rosado-de-Christenson ML, Abbott GF, McAdams HP et al (2003) From the archives of the AFIP: localized fibrous tumor of the pleura. Radiographics 23:759-783.
13. Wang ZJ, Reddy GP, Gotway MB et al (2004) Malignant pleural mesothelioma: evaluation with CT, MR imaging, and PET. Radiographics 24:105-119.
14. Truong MT, Viswanathan C, Godoy MB et al (2013) Malignant pleural mesothelioma: role of CT, MRI, and PET/CT in staging evaluation and treatment considerations. Semin Roentgenol 48:323-334.
15. Sandstrom CK, Stern EJ (2011) Diaphragmatic hernias: a spectrum of radiographic appearances. Curr Probl Diagn Radiol 40:95-115.
16. Taylor GA, Atalabi OM, Estroff JA (2009) Imaging of congenital diaphragmatic hernias. Pediatr Radiol 39:1-16.
17. Nason LK, Walker CM, McNeeley MF et al (2012) Imaging of the diaphragm: anatomy and function. Radiographics 32:E51-70.
18. Anthes TB, Thoongsuwan N, Karmy-Jones R (2003) Morgagni hernia: CT findings. Curr Probl Diagn Radiol 32:135-136.
19. Eren S, Ciri F (2005) Diaphragmatic hernia: diagnostic approaches with review of the literature. Eur J Radiol 54:448-459.
20. Eren S, Kantarci M, Okur A (2006) Imaging of diaphragmatic rupture after trauma. Clin Radiol 61:467-477.
21. Kharma N (2013) Dysfunction of the diaphragm: imaging as a diagnostic tool. Curr Opin Pulm Med 19:394-398.
22. Kim MP, Hofstetter WL (2009) Tumors of the diaphragm. Thorac Surg Clin 19:521-529.
23. Tateishi U, Gladish GW, Kusumoto M et al (2003) Chest wall tumors: radiologic findings and pathologic correlation: part 1. Benign tumors. Radiographics 23:1477-1490.

Pulmonary Manifestations of Systemic Diseases

Cornelia Schaefer-Prokop[1], Brett M. Elicker[2]

[1] Department of Radiology, Meander Medical Centre, Amersfoort en Radboud University, Nijmegen, The Netherlands
[2] Department of Radiology and Biomedical Imaging, University of California, San Francisco, CA, USA

Introduction

Lung involvement in systemic disease may be a manifestation of the underlying pathological process, a complication of the underlying disease, or related to treatment. In certain diseases, such as sarcoidosis or Wegener's granulomatosis, lung involvement is a predominant feature where in others, such as Henoch-Schönlein purpura, it is only rarely present.

Lung involvement has a profound effect on prognosis but it may be challenging to accurately diagnose. Imaging often plays a central role when it is suspected clinically. In the following, we focus on the more common systemic disorders in which pulmonary abnormalities develop, including sarcoidosis, connective tissue diseases, and vasculitis. While a comprehensive review of the lung manifestations of all systemic diseases is not possible, a few selected rare disorders (inflammatory bowel disease, amyloidosis, Erdheim-Chester disease, and IgG$_4$-related sclerosing disease) are also discussed.

Pulmonary Sarcoidosis

Sarcoidosis is a systemic disorder of unknown origin. It is characterized by non-caseating epithelioid cell granulomas in multiple organs, but morbidity and mortality are closely related to pulmonary manifestations, occurring in >90% of patients. The computed tomography (CT) appearance of pulmonary sarcoidosis varies greatly and mimics that of many other diffuse lung diseases; conversely, the CT features of several diseases can resemble those of sarcoidosis.

The histology of pulmonary sarcoidosis consists of noncaseating granulomas with a rim of lymphocytes and fibroblasts in a perilymphatic distribution, which may either resolve or cause fibrosis. The disease can occur at any age, but mostly affects individuals between 20 and 40 years of age and only rarely occurs in those over 65 years of age. The prognosis is mostly good, with disease reso-lution often occurring in <2 years. Mortality is between 1 and 5%.

Staging (Siltzbach classification) is based on chest X-ray findings, described in the following:

Stage 0   normal chest radiograph
Stage I   bilateral hilar and paratracheal lymphadeno-pathy
Stage II   lymphadenopathy and nodular opacities
Stage III   nodular opacities without lymphadenopathy or signs of fibrosis
Stage IV   fibrosis.

This classification scheme is purely descriptive and does not indicate disease activity.

Pulmonary findings include small, well-defined nodules in a characteristic perilymphatic distribution in relation to the subpleural surface, adjacent to the major fissures, along thickened interlobular septa, and adjacent to vessels in the lobular core. The nodules may be evenly distributed throughout both lungs, predominantly in the upper and middle lung zones; however, they may be also clustered in the perihilar and peribronchovascular regions with relative sparing of the lung periphery, or they may be grouped in small areas. The confluence of granulomas results in larger nodules (1-4 cm, nodular sarcoid, "galaxy sign") or ill-defined opacities (ground glass or consolidations, up to 10 cm, alveolar sarcoidosis). On CT, lymphadenopathy is seen in up to 50% patients and is accompanied by calcifications, either eggshell or with an amorphous cloudlike pattern.

Up to 25% of patients develop irreversible pulmonary fibrosis with architectural distortion, septal displacement, traction bronchiectasis, honeycombing, and bullae (stage IV). Conglomerate masses occur mostly in a perihilar location and represent areas of fibrosis with characteristic traction bronchiectasis. Volume loss of the upper lobes is associated with hilar retraction.

Airway abnormalities include airway compression, caused by the surrounding lymphadenopathy, and traction

Diseases of the Chest and Heart 2015-2018,
DOI: 10.1007/978-88-470-5752-4_14 © Springer-Verlag Italia 2015

Table 1. Typical and atypical features of pulmonary sarcoidosis at high-resolution computed tomography

Typical features

Lymphadenopathy: hilar, mediastinal, bilateral symmetric, well defined

Nodules: micronodules (2- to 4-mm), well defined, larger coalescing nodules

Perilymphatic distribution: subpleural, interlobular septa, peribronchovascular

Fibrosis: reticular densities, architectural distortion, traction bronchiectasis, volume loss

Distribution: predominance of parenchymal abnormalities in upper lobes and perihilar areas

Atypical features

Lymphadenopathy: unilateral, isolated, in atypical mediastinal locations

Airspace consolidations: conglomerate masses, confluent alveolar opacities (alveolar sarcoidosis)

Linear opacities: interlobular septal thickening

Fibrocystic changes: cysts, bullae, honeycomb like opacities, upper lobe predominance

Airway involvement: atelectasis, mosaic pattern

Pleural disease: effusion, chylo/hemothorax, pneumothorax, pleural plaques

bronchiectasis, due to the surrounding fibrosis. Granulomas within the bronchial walls lead to irregular bronchial wall thickening with narrowing of the large and small airways.

The latter results in a mosaic pattern on expiration CT that may even precede the appearance of other parenchymal abnormalities and is considered an early sign of extralymphatic disease spread.

Sarcoidosis may present with very characteristic high-resolution CT (HRCT) features that secure the diagnosis and obviate further invasive procedures. However, sarcoidosis is also known to present with less typical features (Table 1).

Especially in advanced disease stages with fibrosis, the differential diagnosis between sarcoidosis and other fibrosing diseases can be very challenging. Table 2 summarizes the imaging findings that are helpful in differentiating several diseases.

Complications include the development of aspergillomas and pulmonary hypertension. Mycetomas are a typical complication of stage IV sarcoidosis: they present as a soft-tissue mass located in a preexisting cavitation in patients with fibrotic sarcoidosis. Life-threatening hemoptysis may require immediate interventional therapy (embolization of the bronchial arteries). Pulmonary hypertension occurs in patients with end-stage fibrosis but may be also caused by mediastinal fibrosis, extrinsic compression of the pulmonary arteries by lymphadenopathy, or intrinsic sarcoid vasculopathy, including features of pulmonary veno-occlusive disease.

Table 2. Diseases with imaging features that overlap with sarcoidosis

Differential diagnosis	Overlapping finding	Suggestive of sarcoidosis
Lymphangitic carcinomatosis	• Irregular "beaded" thickening of the interlobular septa	• Upper lobe predominance • Absence of pleural effusion • Less central bronchial cuffing
Silicosis/Pneumoconiosis	• Pleural pseudoplaques • Eggshell calcifications of lymph nodes • Perihilar fibrotic masses	• No calcifications in pseudoplaques • Pseudoplaques consist of confluent nodules • The perihilar fibrotic masses extend directly from the hilar structures and move posteriorly (upper lobe volume loss)
Chronic EAA/chronic HP and UIP/IPF	• Honeycombing • Traction bronchiectasis • Architectural distortion • Lobular distribution of areas with air trapping (in the presence of obliterative bronchiolitis) and fibrosis	• UIP pattern predominantly in upper lobes or perihilar region • Thickened interlobular septa • Lymph node calcifications • Fibrosis and traction bronchiectasis tend to run from the hilar structures dorsolaterally
Lymphoproliferative disorders	• Lymphadenopathy	• Usually but not always symmetric • Presence of typical parenchymal findings (caveat: biopsy may be necessary)
Chronic beryllium disease	• Nodular pattern	• Large hilar lymphadenopathy • No exposure to beryllium • Other organ involvement
Tuberculosis	• Nodular pattern (normally random versus perilymphatic nodules, however, sarcoidosis may occasionally show a random pattern)	• Egg shell or disperse calcifications as opposed to rough TB calcifications • Symmetric calcifications (in TB frequently asymmetric) • Clinical symptoms of acute infection in patients with miliary TB
CVID	• Nodules in perilymphatic distribution • Ill-defined nodules in mid-lower predominance	• Different clinical history (in CVID recurrent bacterial infection) • Different histological features

EAA, exogenic allergic alveolitis; HP, hypersensitivity pneumonitis; UIP; usual interstitial pneumonia; IPF, idiopathic pulmonary fibrosis; TB, tuberculosis; CVID, common variable immune deficiency

Collagen Vascular Diseases

Collagen vascular diseases are characterized primary on clinical grounds, namely, typical clinical complaints and physical examination findings. The presence of specific autoantibodies may greatly assist in the correct diagnosis. Involvement of the respiratory system is often seen in collagen vascular diseases and results in significant morbidity and mortality. It is important to note that lung abnormalities may precede the other clinical manifestations, sometimes by more than 5 years.

Lung injury from collagen vascular disease can affect each portion of the lung, the pleura, alveoli, interstitium, vasculature, lymphatic tissue, and both the large and small airways. Commonly, more than one compartment is involved. Many of the parenchymal manifestations of collagen vascular disease are similar to those of the idiopathic interstitial pneumonias and can be classified using the same system.

Lung biopsy is rarely obtained in patients with a defined connective tissue disease. For this reason, HRCT often determines the predominant pattern of injury, which in turn is important in determining treatment and prognosis.

While many patterns of injury are associated with the particular collagen vascular diseases, certain patterns are more representative than others. For instance, nonspecific interstitial pneumonia is the most common pattern in patients with scleroderma. It is also important to note that more than one pattern of injury may be present in the same patient.

Rheumatoid Arthritis

Most patients with rheumatoid arthritis (RA) have abnormalities on HRCT. However, CT-detected abnormalities are often not associated with symptoms. Airways abnormalities such as bronchial wall thickening (12–92%) or bronchial dilation (30–40%) are more common than parenchymal changes, including reticular abnormality (10–20%), ground-glass opacity (15–25%), honeycombing (10%), and consolidation (5%). Nodular changes and pleural disease, the latter preceding parenchymal changes, are also seen.

Airways disease appears to be the earliest manifestation of RA in the lung. Bronchiectasis and air trapping are common findings. There is a recognized association between rheumatoid disease and obliterative bronchiolitis (constrictive bronchiolitis), in which the bronchioles are destroyed and replaced by scar tissue. The characteristic CT finding is mosaic perfusion with expiratory air trapping often associated with bronchial dilation. Follicular bronchiolitis is a second type of small-airway disorder recognized in rheumatoid lung disease. The major CT finding is centrilobular nodules and areas of ground glass opacity.

Rheumatoid lung fibrosis is substantially more common in males than in females. The two most frequently occurring patterns of lung fibrosis are usual interstitial pneumonia (UIP) and nonspecific interstitial pneumonia (NSIP). Of all connective tissue diseases, RA is the most common to present with a UIP pattern. The CT findings in interstitial pneumonia associated with RA are often indistinguishable from those of the idiopathic varieties; however, other findings, such as nodules, pulmonary arterial enlargement, or pleural abnormality, may provide a clue to the underlying diagnosis. UIP and NSIP both typically demonstrate a subpleural and basilar distribution of findings. A confident diagnosis of UIP may be made when honeycombing and reticulation is also present. In NSIP there is an absence of honeycombing and subpleural sparing is present.

The introduction of a new generation of biologic agents used to treat RA has resulted in a new array of potential pulmonary side effects. The most important of these is the impaired immunity related to the use of anti-tumor necrosis factor (TNF) antibodies (etanercept, infliximab, and adalimumab), which has resulted in a substantially increased incidence of tuberculosis (sometimes disseminated or extraarticular) and of nontuberculous mycobacterial infection.

Low-dose methotrexate may be associated with subacute hypersensitivity pneumonitis in 2–5% of patients. Pre-existing radiographic evidence of interstitial lung disease in patients with RA suggests a predisposition to the development of methotrexate pneumonitis. Infections, such as pneumocystis pneumonia, are another potential complication of therapy.

Scleroderma (Progressive Systemic Sclerosis)

Parenchymal lung involvement is very common in patients with scleroderma. At autopsy, the lungs are abnormal in at least 80% of cases. Lung fibrosis is the most common pattern of abnormality, with NSIP being much more common (>90%) than UIP. Pulmonary hypertension, either isolated or in association with lung fibrosis, is another frequent finding. Pulmonary hypertension develops especially in patients with limited scleroderma (CREST syndrome). Esophageal dilation is seen on CT in up to 80% of cases.

The CT findings in scleroderma reflect the dominant NSIP histology. Cellular NSIP presents with ground glass opacity and/or a fine reticular pattern, often in posterior and subpleural distributions. Fibrotic NSIP shows irregular reticulation and traction bronchiectasis as the predominant findings. Honeycombing is often absent, but when present it is limited in extent. Cellular and fibrotic NSIP often co-exist such that the findings may overlap. Subpleural sparing is particularly suggestive of a NSIP pattern.

The lung fibrosis associated with scleroderma is associated with a much better prognosis than that found in idiopathic lung fibrosis, probably due in part to the predominant NSIP histology. Fibrotic changes may remain stable for many years. In a large treatment study, the extent of lung fibrosis identified on baseline CT was an important independent predictor of physiologic progression and of the response to treatment.

Pulmonary arterial hypertension usually causes enlargement of the main and proximal pulmonary arteries, as seen on chest radiograph or CT, but normal-sized pulmonary arteries do not exclude the diagnosis. The presence of pericardial thickening or fluid in patients with scleroderma is also a strong predictor of echocardiographic pulmonary hypertension.

There is an increased prevalence of lung cancer in patients with scleroderma, especially in those with lung fibrosis. The relative risk of malignancy ranges from 1.8 to 6.5.

Systemic Lupus Erythematosus

Pleuritis is the most commonly seen pleuropulmonary manifestation of systemic lupus erythematosus (SLE), found in 40–60% of patients, and may or may not be associated with pleural effusion.

Fibrotic interstitial lung disease is less frequent in SLE than in the other collagen vascular diseases. While pulmonary infection is said to be the most common pulmonary complication of lupus, acute pulmonary hemorrhage is also an important pulmonary complication of this condition, characterized radiologically by diffuse or patchy consolidation and ground glass abnormality.

In patients with lupus, acute lupus pneumonitis is a poorly defined entity, characterized by a variable degree of respiratory impairment accompanied by focal or diffuse pulmonary consolidation. It is now believed that most cases previously identified as lupus pneumonitis probably represented acute interstitial pneumonia with or without pulmonary hemorrhage. It is mostly associated with renal infiltration and multi-organ failure.

Other complications of lupus may include diaphragmatic dysfunction, pulmonary hypertension, and pulmonary thromboembolism, which may be related to the presence of antiphospholipid antibodies. Diaphragmatic dysfunction, thought to be due to a diaphragmatic myopathy, is manifested by reduced lung volumes ("shrinking lungs" with plate-like atelectasis).

Polymyositis/Dermatomyositis

The presence of interstitial lung disease (ILD) in polymyositis/dermatomyositis (PM/DM) correlates strongly with the presence of anti-Jo-1 antibodies. Between 50% and 70% of patients who are anti-Jo-1 positive have ILD whereas the frequency of ILD falls to about 10% if antibodies are absent. ILD may antedate myositis in patients with anti-Jo-1 antibodies.

The most common pathological findings are NSIP and organizing pneumonia (OP), often occurring in combination. As with other collagen vascular diseases, the occurrence of interstitial pneumonia may precede the development of clinical myositis.

Lung disease associated with PM/DM or with the antisynthetase syndrome, a closely related entity, often has a typical CT appearance consisting of confluent ground glass opacity and consolidation in the lower lobes superimposed on a background of reticular abnormality with traction bronchiectasis. This pattern reflects the characteristic histologic combination of OP and fibrotic NSIP. On serial evaluation, the changes of consolidation, ground glass abnormality, reticular abnormality, and traction bronchiectasis may all be partially reversible with treatment. Consolidation may also progress to reticular abnormality.

PM/DM can be associated with other collagen vascular diseases (SLE, scleroderma, RA, Sjögren syndrome). There is an increased risk for malignancy (especially breast lung, ovary, and stomach malignancies), which in up to 20% of patients is concurrently diagnosed within 1 year of follow-up.

Sjögren Syndrome (SS)

CT provides substantial information regarding the patterns of pulmonary involvement by Sjögren syndrome (SS). These may be divided into airway abnormality, interstitial fibrosis, pulmonary hypertension, and those suggestive of lymphoid interstitial pneumonia.

Airway-related abnormalities consist of bronchial wall thickening, bronchiectasis, bronchiolectasis, and the tree-in-bud pattern. Small-airway disease may manifest as a mosaic attenuation pattern and expiratory air trapping.

NSIP and lymphoid interstitial pneumonia (LIP) are the most common patterns of parenchymal lung disease. NSIP resembles that seen in scleroderma. LIP is characterized by ground glass abnormality due to the homogeneous lymphocytic infiltration. Peribronchovascular, centrilobular, and subpleural nodules may also be seen, and cysts measuring 5–30 mm are often present. These cysts frequently contain thin septa; they may be associated with soft-tissue nodules sitting either close to them or in their walls. Similar cysts may be found in follicular bronchiolitis. These changes are ascribed to bronchiolar obstruction on the basis of lymphocytic wall infiltration. Cysts are helpful in distinguishing LIP from lymphoma.

Lymphoma should be suspected if consolidation, large nodules (>1 cm), mediastinal lymphadenopathy or effusions are present. However, similar large, "pseudo-alveolar," poorly defined nodules were found in four patients with combined amyloidosis and LIP. In contrast to other cystic lung diseases, such as lymphangioleiomyomatosis, the cysts of LIP show a peribronchovascular and lower lung predominance.

Mixed Connective Tissue Disease

Mixed connective tissue disease (MCTD) is an overlap syndrome that is a distinct clinicopathological entity. The principal characteristics are the presence of: (1) features of SLE, scleroderma, and PM/DM, occurring together or evolving sequentially during observation; and (2) antibodies to an extractable nuclear antigen (RNP).

Pulmonary involvement is common in MCTD. A study of 144 unselected patients found CT evidence of infiltrative

Table 3. The most recent classification of systemic vasculitis: from the 2012 Chapel Hill Consensus conference

	Vasculitis	Pulmonary-renal syndrome	Pulmonary hemorrhage	Pulmonary hypertension
Small-vessel vasculitis, ANCA-associated	GPA (formerly Wegener's)	Pulmonary involvement 90% Renal involvement 80%	In about 10%	–
	Eosinophilic granulomatous vasculitis with polyangiitis GPA(Church Strauss)	up to 25%	Rare	–
	Microscopic polyangiitis	Frequently associated with necrotizing glomerulonephritis	Frequent	–
Small vessel vasculitis, immune-complex type	Cryoglobulinemic IgA (Henoch Schoenlein) HUV Anti-GBM (formerly Goodpasture's)			
Medium-vessel vasculitis	PAN	–	Very rare idiopathic, associated with hepatitis B; part of RA, SLE	–
Large-vessel vasculitis	Kawasaki syndrome			
	GCA	–	Rare, focal	Rare
	Takayasu arteritis	–	Rare, focal	Rare
Collagen vascular diseases	RA	–	Very rare, diffuse	Up to 60%
	SS	–	Rare, diffuse with necrotizing vasculitis	10–60%
	MCTD	–	Rare, diffuse	Up to 45%
	SLE	Up to 60%, late	In at least 4%, diffuse	5–45%

ANCA, anti-neutrophil cytoplasmic antibody; GPA, granulomatous vasculitis with polyangiitis; HUV, hypocomplementemic vasculitis; GBM, glomerular basement membrane; PAN, polyarteritis nodosa; GCA, giant cell arteritis; RA, rheumatoid arthritis; SS, Sjögren syndrome; MCTD, mixed connective tissue disease; SLE, systemic lupus erythematosus

lung disease in 67%. Many affected patients are asymptomatic. The pulmonary abnormalities resemble those seen in SLE, SS, and PM/DM. Thus, pleural thickening and pleural and pericardial effusions are common. Ground glass attenuation is the most frequent parenchymal abnormality. The CT pattern corresponds most closely to that of NSIP. Less frequent findings include honeycombing, consolidation, and poorly defined centrilobular nodules.

Other important complications of MCTD are pulmonary arterial hypertension, and esophageal dysmotility, with sequelae of recurrent aspiration.

Undifferentiated Connective Tissue Disease (or Interstitial Lung Disease with Autoimmune Features)

Not all patients with interstitial lung disease meet the criteria of having a collagen vascular disease. Among patients with histologically proven UIP or NSIP whose disease was originally diagnosed as idiopathic, because it did not fulfill the criteria of one of the established collagen vascular diseases, subgroups of patients with one or more serological features of an autoimmune process have been subsequently identified. Several terms have been suggested to describe the condition detected in these subgroups, including undifferentiated connective tissue disease (UCTD), interstitial lung disease with autoimmune features, and lung-dominant CTD. Whether these patients have a better prognosis than patients without these autoimmune features or even a prognosis comparable to that of patients with

established collagen vascular diseases is not yet known.

The term "lung-dominant CTD" has been proposed for the subgroup of patients with: (1) NSIP, UIP, LIP, OP, or diffuse alveolar damage in the lung determined by histology or HRCT; (2) insufficient extrathoracic features of a definite collagen vascular disease but a combination of serologic features suggesting an autoimmune process; and (3) no identifiable alternative cause for interstitial pneumonia.

Pulmonary Vasculitis/Diffuse Alveolar Hemorrhage

The pulmonary vasculitides encompass a clinically, radiologically, and histopathologically heterogeneous group of diseases that are usually associated with a systemic vasculitis. The clinical symptoms and radiologic signs suggestive of pulmonary vasculitis include diffuse alveolar hemorrhage (DAH), acute glomerulonephritis, upper-airways disease, lung or cavitary nodules, mononeuritis multiplex, and palpable purpura.

The classification of systemic vasculitis remains controversial. In the most recent classification, the Chapel Hill Consensus Conference (CHCC) of 2012 (Table 3), the main consideration remained the predominant vascular size involved, but the presence of ANCA (anti-neutrophil cytoplasmic antibody) was newly added. Small vessel vasculitis (SVV) is divided into ANCA-associated vasculitis (AAV) and immune complex SVV. AAV represents necrotizing vasculitis with only few or no immune deposits predominantly affecting the small vessels; patients are MPO-ANCA or PR3 ANCA positive but in a minority of cases ANCA-negative. ANCA specificity should be indicated because it appears to identify distinct categories of disease.

The combined involvement of the lungs and kidneys by some of these diseases accounts for their description as pulmonary-renal syndrome. Note that capillaritis/vasculitis can also manifest in the setting of the various collagen vascular diseases.

ANCA-Associated Granulomatous Vasculitis with Polyangiitis (GPA, Formerly Wegener's Disease)

Granulomatous vasculitis with polyangiitis is the most common of the AAV. It affects the sinuses, kidneys, and lungs, resulting in the classic triad of symptoms comprising sinusitis and/or tracheobronchitis, pathological chest X-ray (with or without hemoptysis), and microhematuria. However, any part of the body may be involved. Females and males are affected equally and at any age (mostly age 40–55 years). Airway involvement is more frequent in males. The most common cause of death is renal failure. With treatment, the 24-month survival is 80%. The factors initiating disease are unknown, but current data support the involvement of (recurrent) infection for GPA. Up to 80% of patients are (in the course of disease) ANCA-positive (mostly PR3-ANCA). Histologic findings include necrotizing granulomatous vasculitis of the small to medium vessels without associated infection.

The most frequently seen pulmonary abnormalities are multiple nodules with or without a CT halo sign (perinodular hemorrhage). They tend to involve the subpleural regions, but there is no predilection for upper or lower lung zones. Although the nodules can be as large as 10 cm, most are smaller. Cavitations have thick walls. Peripheral wedge-shaped consolidations resemble infarcts and may also cavitate. Diffuse consolidations or ground glass opacities represent pulmonary hemorrhage. Fibrotic changes reflect preexisting disease.

In addition there may be a concentric thickening of the tracheal or bronchial walls with diameter reduction, potentially causing atelectasis. Bronchial abnormalities mainly involve the segmental and subsegmental bronchi. Involvement of the subglottic trachea is most typical.

Churg-Strauss Syndrome

Eosinophilic granulomatous disease with polyangiitis (Churg-Strauss syndrome, CSS) is caused by a small-vessel systemic vasculitis that almost exclusively occurs in patients with asthma and is characterized by a marked serum eosinophilia. Clinically, radiologically, and pathologically it combines features of GPA and eosinophilic pneumonia (=allergic granulomatosis and angiitis). Many other organs may be involved including the heart (up to 47%), the skin (up to 40%), and the musculoskeletal sys-

tem (up to 50%). Involvement of the peripheral nerves is more frequent while glomerulonephritis (GN) and pulmonary hemorrhage are less common than in GPA.

Up to 30% of patients are ANCA-positive, mostly MPO-ANCA. Histology demonstrates small vessel (arteries and veins) vasculitis with eosinophilic infiltrates, and vascular and extravascular granulomas. Five-year survival is reported in up to 80% of patients; 50% of the deaths are related to cardiac involvement.

Upper-airways disease and pulmonary abnormalities are seen in up to 70% of patients with CSS. The most common pulmonary findings include transient, multifocal, and non-segmental consolidations without zonal predilection. The presence of (non-cavitating) small nodules or diffuse reticular densities has also been reported. If located subpleurally, the consolidations mimic eosinophilic pneumonia. Diffuse consolidations or ground glass attenuation reflect hemorrhage.

Airway abnormalities are also an important thoracic manifestation and include wall thickening, dilatation, small nodules, and mosaic perfusion. Increased interlobular septa may reflect edema caused by cardiac and/or renal involvement or eosinophilic infiltration of the septa. Eosinophilic pleural effusion is seen in up to 50% of patients.

Airway changes consisting of tree-in-bud, bronchial wall thickening, and bronchial dilatation are likely related to asthma and develop in almost patients. Wall thickening can also be caused by eosinophilic involvement.

Microscopic Polyangiitis/Diffuse Alveolar Hemorrhage

Microscopic polyangiitis is a systemic necrotizing small-vessel vasculitis with granulomatous inflammation. Clinically, it is characterized by a long prodromal phase with weight loss and fever followed by a rapidly progressive GN. Microscopic polyangiitis is the most common cause of pulmonary-renal syndrome: rapidly progressive GN is seen in up to 90%, pulmonary involvement in up to 50%. More than 75% of patients are ANCA-positive in the course of disease, mostly MPO ANCA.

Microscopic polyangiitis is characterized by the combination of GN and diffuse alveolar hemorrhage (DAH). Imaging findings include patchy, bilateral, or diffuse airspace opacities. The opacity can show features of consolidations and ground glass, depending on the amount of alveolar filling by blood. The opacifications may be diffuse or more pronounced in the dependent lower parts of the lungs. A halo surrounding a consolidation or nodule underlines the character of the hemorrhage. During the phase of resorption, interlobular lines ("crazy paving") are increasingly seen.

Repeated hemorrhage leads to fibrosis, with honeycombing, reticulation, and traction bronchiectasis.

Goodpasture Syndrome/DAH

Goodpasture syndrome describes the clinical triad of circulating anti-glomerular basement membrane antibody, DAH, and (necrotizing) GN. Presenting symptoms comprise an acute onset of dyspnea and hemoptysis.

Histologically, there is a linear deposition of IgG along the glomerular basement membranes, such that renal biopsy is used to establish the diagnosis. The serology comprises c-ANCA or p-ANCA positivity in 30% and anti-basement membrane antibodies in >90% of patients. Young males are more often affected than females (M:F=9:1), although the condition is also seen in elderly females. With treatment, the prognosis is good. Recurrent episodes cause pulmonary fibrosis.

Imaging features consists of diffuse or patchy ground glass or consolidations based on alveolar hemorrhage that typically resolve within days. The subpleural space is usually spared, with predominance instead of the perihilar areas in the mid and lower lung zones. Pleural effusion is uncommon. After recurrent episodes, traction bronchiectasis, a reticular pattern, and honeycombing may evolve.

DAH caused by pulmonary capillaritis (Table 3) needs to be differentiated from bland pulmonary hemorrhage (e.g., coagulation disorders, mitral stenosis, drug-induced, etc.) and hemorrhage associated with diffuse alveolar damage (drug-induced, acute respiratory distress syndrome, bone marrow transplantation, or crack cocaine inhalation).

Miscellaneous Systemic Disorders

Inflammatory Bowel Disease

Ulcerative colitis and Crohn disease are associated with a wide variety of pulmonary complications, which may precede the diagnosis of inflammatory bowel disease (IBD) or may occur years after the initial diagnosis, and even after complete colectomy for ulcerative colitis. Indeed there is some suggestion that pulmonary complications may be more common after surgical treatment, perhaps because anti-inflammatory treatment is withdrawn. Both Crohn disease and ulcerative colitis can be associated with tracheobronchitis and airway stenosis. Bronchiectasis and bronchial wall thickening are also common. Small-airway involvement can have a pattern of panbronchiolitis. Parenchymal abnormalities associated with IBD include OP, pulmonary hemorrhage, and, in Crohn disease, granulomatous infiltration.

Amyloidosis and Light-Chain Deposition Disease

These rare disorders are characterized by the extracellular deposition of proteins in one or more organs. They share clinical, radiographic, and pathological features. The main difference between these two entities is the Congo red staining pattern and the fibrillar structure seen on electron microscopy of amyloidosis. Both entities may be associated with a plasma cell dyscrasia.

Three radiographic manifestations of amyloidosis are described: nodular parenchymal, diffuse alveolar septal, and tracheobronchial. The nodular parenchymal form presents radiographically as one or more solid lung nodules, often found incidentally. These may be confused with malignancy, particularly when spiculated borders are present. A slow growth rate is typical, and calcification may be present. The diffuse alveolar septal form is characterized by the presence of widespread deposits throughout the lungs. The most common findings are small nodules (typically in a perilymphatic distribution), consolidation, ground glass opacity, and reticulation. The presence of calcification associated with these abnormalities may be particularly suggestive. The tracheobronchial form shows extensive thickening of the trachea and/or bronchi with or without calcification.

The imaging findings of light-chain deposition disease are less well described. There are two types: nodular and diffuse. The nodular type presents with scattered solid nodules, often associated with cysts. The nodules are typically located within or adjacent to the wall of the cysts. The diffuse type may show diffuse small nodules, resembling the diffuse alveolar septal type of amyloidosis.

Erdheim-Chester Disease

Erdheim-Chester disease is an infiltrative disorder in which non-Langerhans cell histiocytes are found in one or more organ systems. The primary organs affected include bones, brain, kidneys, and the cardiovascular system. Middle-aged males are most commonly affected. While pathology is helpful in excluding lymphoproliferative malignancies, the pathological findings may be nonspecific; thus typical radiographic features are a key to the correct diagnosis. Characteristic imaging findings in the chest include peri-adventitial aortic soft-tissue thickening that may involve the aorta and its main branches diffusely, giving rise to the term "coating" of the aorta. The most common lung finding is smooth interlobular septal thickening, resembling pulmonary edema. The most characteristic finding outside of the chest is circumferential perinephric soft tissue, resembling lymphoma.

IgG$_4$-Related Sclerosing Disease

This disorder was originally thought to be isolated to the pancreas and thus was previously called lymphoplasmocytic sclerosing pancreatitis. However, it is now realized that IgG$_4$-related sclerosing disease is a systemic order associated with IgG4 plasma cells and with fibrosclerosis in multiple organ systems. The primary organs involved include the pancreas, hepatobiliary system, salivary glands, and lymph nodes. The findings in the chest are variable and may include nodules, lymphadenopathy, airway thickening, and pleural abnormalities. IgG4-related sclerosing disease may account for a proportion of the idiopathic interstitial pneumonias.

Acknowledgment. D.A. Lynch, Dept. of Radiology, NJH Denver, CO, US, for his contribution to the preparation of this manuscript.

Suggested Reading

Sarcoidosis

Brauner MW, Lenoir S, Grenier P et al (1993) Pulmonary sarcoidosis: CT assessment of lesion reversibility. Radiology 182:349-354.

Criado E, Sanchez M, Ramirez J et al (2010) Pulmonary sarcoidosis: typical and atypical manifestations at high resolution CT with pathologic correlation. Radiographics 30:1567-1586.

Handa T, Nagai S, Fushimi Y et al (2006) Clinical and radiographic indices associated with airflow limitations in patients with sarcoidosis. Chest 130:1851-1856.

Nakatsu M, Hatabu H, Morikawa K et al (2002) Large coalescent nodules in pulmonary sarcoidosis: "sarcoid galaxy sign". AJR Am J Roentgenol 178:1389-1393.

Spagnolo P, Sverzellati N, Well AU, Hansell DM (2014) Imaging aspecys of the diagnosis of sarcoidosis. Eur Radiol 24:807.

Collagen vascular diseases

American Thoracic Society/European Respiratory Society International Multidisciplinary Consensus (2002) Classification of the Idiopathic Interstitial Pneumonias. Am J Respir Crit Care Med 165:277-304.

Hwang JH, Misumi S, Sahin H et al (2009) Computed tomographic features of idiopathic fibrosing interstitial pneumonia: comparison with pulmonary fibrosis related to collagen vascular disease. J Comput Assist Tomogr 33:410-415.

Kim EA, Lee KS, Johkoh T et al (2002) Interstitial lung diseases associated with collagen vascular diseases: radiologic and histopathologic findings. RadioGraphics 22:S151-165.

Lynch DA (2009) Lung disease related to collagen vascular diseases. J Thorac Imag 24:299-309.

Rheumatoid arthritis

Aquino SL, Webb WR, Golden J (1994) Bronchiolitis obliterans associated with rheumatoid arthritis: findings on HRCT and dynamic expiratory CT. J Comput Assist Tomog 18:555-558.

Arakawa H, Honma K, Shida H (2003) Computed tomography findings of Caplan syndrome. J Comput Assist Tomogr 27:758-760.

Bouros D, Hatzakis K, Labrakis H et al (2002) Association of malignancy with diseases causing interstitial pulmonary changes. Chest 121:1278-1289.

Gabbay E, Tarala R, Will R et al (1997) Interstitial lung disease in recent onset rheumatoid arthritis. Am J Respir Crit Care Med 156:528-535.

Golden MR, Katz RS, Balk RA, Golden HE (1995) The relationship of preexisting lung disease to the development of methotrexate pneumonitis in patients with rheumatoid arthritis. J Rheumatol 22:1043-1047.

Hilliquin P, Renoux M, Perrot S et al (1996) Occurrence of pulmonary complications during methotrexate therapy in rheumatoid arthritis. Br J Rheumatol 35:441-445.

Metafratzi ZM, Georgiadis AN, Ioannidou CV et al (2007) Pulmonary involvement in patients with early rheumatoid arthritis. Scand J Rheumatol 36:338-344.

Mori S, Cho I, Koga Y, Sugimoto M (2008) Comparison of pulmonary abnormalities on high-resolution computed tomography in patients with early versus longstanding rheumatoid arthritis. J Rheumatol 35:1513-1521.

Mutlu GM, Mutlu EA, Bellmeyer A, Rubinstein I (2006) Pulmonary adverse events of anti-tumor necrosis factor-alpha antibody therapy. Am J Med 119:639-646.

Perez T, Remy-Jardin M, Cortet B (1998) Airways involvement in rheumatoid arthritis: clinical, functional, and HRCT findings. Am J Respir Crit Care Med 157:1658-1665.

Remy-Jardin M, Remy J, Cortet B et al (1994) Lung changes in rheumatoid arthritis: CT findings. Radiology 193:375-382.

Tanaka N, Kim JS, Newell JD et al (2004) Rheumatoid arthritis-related lung diseases: CT findings. Radiology 232:81-91.

Systemic sclerosis

Bouros D, Wells AU, Nicholson AG et al (2002) Histopathologic subsets of fibrosing alveolitis in patients with systemic sclerosis and their relationship to outcome. Am J Respir Crit Care Med 165:1581-1586.

Fischer A, Misumi S, Curran-Everett D et al (2007) Pericardial abnormalities predict the presence of echocardiographically defined pulmonary arterial hypertension in systemic sclerosis-related interstitial lung disease. Chest 131:988-992.

Goldin JG, Lynch DA, Strollo DC et al (2008) High-resolution CT scan findings in patients with symptomatic scleroderma-related interstitial lung disease. Chest 134:358-367.

Kim DS, Yoo B, Lee JS et al (2002) The major histopathologic pattern of pulmonary fibrosis in scleroderma is nonspecific interstitial pneumonia. Sarcoidosis Vasc Diffuse Lung Dis 19:121-127.

Pearson JE, Silman AJ (2003) Risk of cancer in patients with scleroderma. Ann Rheum Dis 62:697-699.

Remy-Jardin M, Remy J, Wallaert B et al (1993) Pulmonary involvement in progressive systemic sclerosis: sequential evaluation with CT, pulmonary function tests, and bronchoalveolar lavage. Radiology 188:499-506.

Wells AU, Cullinan P, Hansell DM et al (1994) Fibrosing alveolitis associated with systemic sclerosis has a better prognosis than lone cryptogenic fibrosing alveolitis. Am J Respir Crit Care Med 149:1583-1590.

Lupus erythematosus

Bankier AA, Kiener HP, Wiesmayr MN et al (1995) Discrete lung involvement in systemic lupus erythematosus: CT assessment. Radiology 196:835-840.

Fenlon HM, Doran M, Sant SM, Breatnach E (1996) High-resolution chest CT in systemic lupus erythematosus. AJR Am J Roentgenol 166:301-307.

Swigris JJ, Fischer A, Gillis J et al (2008) Pulmonary and thrombotic manifestations of systemic lupus erythematosus. Chest 133:271-280.

Wiedemann HP, Matthay RA (1992) Pulmonary manifestations of systemic lupus erythematosus. J Thorac Imaging 7:1-18.

Dermatomyositis/Polymyostis

Arakawa H, Yamada H, Kurihara Y et al (2003) Nonspecific interstitial pneumonia associated with polymyositis and dermatomyositis: serial high-resolution CT findings and functional correlation. Chest 123:1096-1103.

Fischer A, Swigris JJ, du Bois RM et al (2009) Anti-synthetase syndrome in ANA and anti-Jo-1 negative patients presenting with idiopathic interstitial pneumonia. Respir Med 103:1719-1724.

Mino M, Noma S, Taguchi Y et al (1997) Pulmonary involvement in polymyositis and dermatomyositis: sequential evaluation with CT. AJR Am J Roentgenol 169:83-87.

Sjögren syndrome

Franquet T, Gimenez A, Monill JM et al (1997) Primary Sjogren's syndrome and associated lung disease: CT findings in 50 patients. AJR Am J Roentgenol 169:655-658.

Honda O, Johkoh T, Ichikado K et al (1999) Differential diagnosis of lymphocytic interstitial pneumonia and malignant lymphoma on high-resolution CT. AJR Am J Roentgenol 173:71-74.

Jeong YJ, Lee KS, Chung MP et al (2004) Amyloidosis and lymphoproliferative disease in Sjogren syndrome: thin-section computed tomography findings and histopathologic comparisons. J Comput Assist Tomogr 28:776-781.

Johkoh T, Müller NL, Pickford HA et al (1999) Lymphocytic interstitial pneumonia: thin-section CT findings in 22 patients. Radiology 212:567-572.

Taouli B, Brauner MW, Mourey I et al (2002) Thin-section chest CT findings of primary Sjogren's syndrome: correlation with pulmonary function. Eur Radiol 12:1504-1511.

Mixed connective tissue disease

Bodolay E, Szekanecz Z, Devenyi K et al (2005) Evaluation of interstitial lung disease in mixed connective tissue disease (MCTD). Rheumatology (Oxford) 44:656-661.

Fagan KA, Badesch DB (2002) Pulmonary hypertension associated with connective tissue disease. Prog Cardiovasc Dis 45:225-234.

Kozuka T, Johkoh T, Honda O et al (2001) Pulmonary involvement in mixed connective tissue disease: high-resolution CT findings in 41 patients. J Thorac Imaging 16:94-98.

Unclassifiable connective tissue disease, lung-dominant CTD

Fischer A, Brown KK (2014) Interstitial lung diseases in undifferentiated forms of connective tissue disease. Arthritis Care and Research doi: 10.1002/acr.22394 [Epub ahead of print].

Fischer A, du Bois R (2012) Interstitial lung diseases in connective tissue disorders. Lancet 380:689.

Vasculitis

Attali P, Begum R, Romdhane HB et al (1998) Pulmonary Wegener's granulomatosios: changes at follow up CT. Eur Radiol 8:1009-1113.

Cordier JF, Valeyre D, Guillevin L et al (1990) Pulmonary Wegener's granulomatosis. A clinical and imaging study of 77 cases. Chest 97:906-912.

Haworth SJ, Savage COS, Carr D et al (1985) Pulmonary hemorrhage complicating Wegener's granulomatosis and microscopic polyarteriitis. BMJ 290:1175.

Jennette JC, Falk RJ (2007) Nosology of primary vasculitis. Current opinion in rheumatology 19:10.

Marten K, Schnyder P, Schirg E et al (2005) Patternbased differential diagnosis in pulmonary vasculitis using volumetric CT. AJR Am J Roentgenol 184:1843.

Specks U, Deremee RA (1990) Granulomatous vasculitis. Wegener's granulomatosis and Churg Strauss syndrome. Rheum Dis Clin North Am 16: 377-397.

Susanto I, Peters JI (1997) Acute lupus pneumonitis with normal chest radiograph. Chest 111:1781.

Worthy SA, Muller NL, Hansell DM, Flower CD (1998) Churg strauss syndrome: The spectrum of pulmonary CT findings in 17 Patients. AJR Am J Roentgenol 170:297-300.

Chung MP, Yi CA, Lee HY et al (2010) Imaging of pulmonary vasculitis. Radiology 255:322-341.

Khan I, Watts RA (2013) Classification of ANCA associated vasculitis. Curr Rheumat Rep 15:383.

Castaner E, Alguersuari A, Andreu M et al (2013) Imaging findings in pulmonary vasculitis. Seminars in Ultrasound, CT and MRI 33:567-579.

Inflammatory bowel disease

Camus P, Piard F, Ashcroft T et al (1993) The lung in inflammatory bowel disease. Medicine (Baltimore) 72:151-183.

Garg K, Lynch DA, Newell JD (1993) Inflammatory airways disease in ulcerative colitis: CT and high-resolution CT features. J Thorac Imaging 8:159-163.

Kelly MG, Frizelle FA, Thornley PT et al (2006) Inflammatory bowel disease and the lung: is there a link between surgery and bronchiectasis? Int J Colorectal Dis 21:754-757.

Amyloidosis and light chain deposition disease

Bhargava P, Rushin JM, Rusnock EJ et al (2007) Pulmonary light chain deposition disease: report of five cases and review of the literature. Am J Surg Pathol 31:267-276.

Urban BA, Fishman EK, Goldman SM et al (1993) CT evaluation of amyloidosis: spectrum of disease. RadioGraphics 13: 1295-1308.

Erdheim-Chester disease

Brun A-L, Touitou-Gottenberg D, Haroche J et al (2010) Erdheim-Chester disease: CT findings of thoracic involvement. Eur Radiol 20:2579-2587.

IgG$_4$-related sclerosing disease

Ryu JH, Sekiguchi H, Yi ES (2012) Pulmonary manifestations of immunoglobulin G4-related sclerosing disease. Eur Respir J 39:180-186.

CT Evaluation of Chest Pain: Acute Coronary Syndrome and Acute Aortic Syndrome

Dominik Fleischmann[1], Udo Hoffmann[2]

[1] Department of Radiology, Stanford University School of Medicine, Stanford, CA, USA
[2] Department of Radiology, Massachusetts General Hospital, Harvard School of Medicine, Boston, MA, USA

Background

Chest pain is a common presenting symptom among patients visiting emergency departments (EDs) in the US and is responsible for over 5.5 million visits annually, second only to abdominal pain [1]. However, the number of patients ultimately diagnosed with an acute coronary syndrome (ACS), either ST-elevation myocardial infarction (MI), unstable angina, or a non-ST elevation MI, is <20% [2]. The prevalence of acute aortic chest pain is one to two orders of magnitude less than chest pain due to ACS [3]. For every 130 patients with ACS, there is only one patient with an aortic cause of chest pain.

In the evaluation of patients in the ED who present with chest pain, the goals include the rapid recognition of conditions that require emergent care, such as ACS as well as the far less common acute aortic syndromes, and risk stratification for these conditions to allow for rapid treatment and triage decisions. However, the accurate triage of individuals presenting with acute chest pain to the ED remains difficult because neither the chest pain history [1, 2], nor a single set of established biochemical markers for myocardial necrosis (troponin I, troponin T, creatine kinase, MB-type) [4, 5] nor initial 12-lead echocardiography (ECG), either alone or in combination (acute cardiac ischemia time-insensitive predictive instrument), identifies a group of patients that can be safely discharged home without further diagnostic testing [6-8]. As a result, the threshold to admit chest pain patients remains low, and over six million patients are admitted annually to US hospitals [2, 9-11]. The standard "rule out" MI protocol consists of serial ECG and cardiac biomarker measurements and usually requires a noninvasive stress test. These tests, whether exercise treadmill ECG testing (ETT), stress echocardiography (Echo), or rest or stress myocardial perfusion imaging with Tc-99m (SPECT), require the exclusion of myocardial necrosis with negative serial biomarkers and are performed to rule out the presence of a hemodynamically significant coronary stenosis. While these tests have good sensitivities (ETT: 76%, SPECT: 83%, Echo: 85%) for detecting the presence of significant coronary artery stenosis, their specificities are only moderate when compared to that of coronary angiography (ETT: 60%, SPECT: 64%, Echo: 77%) [12-14]. Moreover, these tests are time-consuming (e.g., SPECT: 2–3 h) and usually not available around the clock. Thus, the standard evaluation of patients with chest pain to rule out myocardial ischemia requires hospital admission for 24–36 h [15]. The remarkable inefficiency of current evaluation strategies is also documented by the fact that <10% of the six million patients admitted each year in the US ultimately receive a diagnosis of ACS at discharge [16, 17]. In-patient care for negative evaluations is a significant economic burden, in excess of $8 billion annually for the US healthcare system [18-20].

The rapid development and dispersion of modern computed tomography (CT) technology have resulted in the ability to acquire high-resolution three-dimensional datasets, with the elimination of cardiac motion artifacts in coronary CT and the reliable suppression of pulsation artifacts in the ascending aorta [21]. These developments have substantially changed the triage of patients presenting with acute coronary or aortic chest pain. Recent data have confirmed the ability of early coronary CT angiography (CTA) to allow the safe triage patients with suspected ACS. Our experience over more than a decade also confirms the benefits of modern ECG-gating technology in the setting of acute aortic syndromes. Here we review the clinical context and state-of-the art of ECG-gated CT in the imaging of patients presenting to the ED with acute coronary and aortic chest pain.

Acute Coronary Syndrome: Definition and Classification

The American Heart Association/American College of Cardiology (AHA/ACC) guidelines [22-24] define ACS as follows: (1) STEMI (ST-segment elevation myocardial infarction): a new finding of ST-segment elevation of >0.1 mm in at least two anatomically contiguous limb leads and/or >2 mm in at least two anatomically contiguous precordial leads in conjunction with elevated serial levels of cardiac troponin-I (>0.09 ng/ml); (2) NSTEMI (non-ST-segment elevation myocardial infarction): a new finding of ST-segment depression of >1 mm or T-wave inversion of at least 3 mm in at least two anatomically contiguous leads and elevated serial levels of troponin-I (<0.09 ng/mL); (3) UAP (unstable angina pectoris): clinical symptoms suggestive of ACS, such as typical chest discomfort or the equivalent, with an unstable pattern of chest pain (at rest, new onset, or crescendo angina), optimally with a markedly positive stress test (SPECT, Echo, or treadmill testing) and/or an invasive coronary angiogram demonstrating a >50% epicardial coronary stenosis.

Acute Aortic Syndrome: Definition and Classification

Acute aortic syndrome is a contemporary clinical term, analogous to acute coronary syndrome and referring to a spectrum of acute life-threatening abnormalities of the aorta associated with intense chest or back pain [25]. Acute aortic syndromes are much less common than acute cardiac events, with an estimated annual incidence of approximately 6 per 100,000 for acute aortic dissection [3] (the most common acute aortic condition requiring emergency operative repair) versus more than 400 per 100,000 for acute MI. While the presumptive diagnosis of acute MI is usually considered first, excluding acute thoracic aortic disease is imperative to expedite appropriate treatment, avoid deleterious thrombolysis, and circumvent unnecessary delays associated with emergency coronary angiography. The clinical picture of an acute aortic syndrome can be caused by a wide range of aortic lesions and predisposing conditions. Traditionally, acute aortic syndromes have been ascribed to three main abnormalities [25]: (1) aortic dissection, (2) intramural hematoma (IMH), and (3) penetrating atherosclerotic ulcer (PAU). Although poorly reflecting the underlying pathology and without including the full spectrum of acute aortic diseases, these categories are almost universally used in the literature [26-28]. They are also at the core of the current classifications of acute aortic diseases by the European and American Heart Associations (Table 1), with added subcategories for limited tears and iatrogenic/traumatic dissections [28, 29].

At our institution we use a conceptually different classification of acute aortic disorders that is based on the un-

Table 1. ESC Task force, and ACCF/AHA/AATS/ACR/ASA/SCA/ SCAI/SIR/STS/SVM guidelines for the diagnosis and management of aortic diseases

ESC/AHA/ACC/AATS classification	
Class 1	Aortic dissection
Class 2	Intramural hematoma
Class 3	Discrete/Subtle dissection/Limited tear
Class 4	Penetrating atherosclerotic ulcer
Class 5	Iatrogenic and traumatic dissection

ESC, European Society of Cardiology; AHA, American Heart Association; ACC, American College of Cardiology; AATS, American Association for Thoracic Surgery

Table 2. Stanford conceptual classification of acute aortic syndromes

1. Aortic dissection and dissection variants (diseased media)
   1.a Classic aortic dissection[a]
   1.b Intramural hematoma variant
   1.c Limited intimal tear (limited dissection)[a]
2. Penetrating atherosclerotic ulcer (diseased intima)[a]
3. Rupturing thoracic aortic aneurysm[a]

[a] Classic aortic dissection, limited intimal tear, penetrating atherosclerotic ulcer and rupturing aneurysm are lesions that can occur with or without associated intramural hematoma.

derlying pathology and allows for a broader spectrum of manifestations, particularly within the dissection category. We also consider symptomatic thoracic aortic aneurysms as an acute aortic syndrome, and treat IMH as a dissection variant or as an unspecific imaging finding rather than as a separate disease entity (Table 2).

ECG-Gated CT: Improved Chest Pain Triage in Patients with Acute Coronary and Acute Aortic Syndromes

Nowadays, fast scanner technology combined with heart-rate-reducing medication has made it possible to image the coronary arteries without motion artifacts in most patients. Indeed, state-of-the-art scanners acquire 64–320 cross-sections per rotation, depicting vascular details with a spatial resolution of <0.5 mm. ECG-synchronized, contrast-enhanced images of the heart and coronary arteries can be acquired in one to five heart cycles. The diagnostic performance of coronary CTA has been investigated extensively in patients with stable coronary artery disease (CAD). Using invasive angiography as a reference, coronary CTA is more sensitive (98–100%) than any other noninvasive technique [30]. Because of its high negative predictive value (99–100%), coronary CTA is recommended in patients with a low to intermediate probability of CAD and in patients with an inconclusive functional test [31]. A normal cardiac CT examination is associated with a low adverse cardiac event rate in the following years [32] The reported per-patient specificity (~85%) is lower because stenosis severity is overestimated, often due to the presence of calcifications, but it is not inferior to that of other noninvasive techniques. In addition, radiation exposure has decreased dramatically over the past years, such that doses of <5 mSv are now common practice using state-of-the-art technology; moreover, very recent innovations permit doses under 1 mSv in selected patients [33]. Given the practical limitations of functional testing in the ED setting and the relatively low prevalence of CAD in patients visiting EDs, direct coronary visualization by CTA offers an attractive diagnostic alternative for the early triage of ACS patients.

CTA of the thorax and abdomen is a well-established imaging technique for many acute abnormalities of the aorta. Even without the use of ECG gating, CTA of the aorta has high sensitivity and specificity for the detection of acute thoracic aortic diseases and it has largely replaced conventional diagnostic angiography [34]. However, over the last decade it has become clear that the spectrum of acute aortic abnormalities also includes subtle yet important aortic lesions that evade nearly all cross-sectional imaging techniques, including non-gated CTA. Conversely, using ECG-gated CTA, the aortic root, coronary arteries, and valve apparatus can be accurately assessed preoperatively. Finally, modern endovascular treatment options require much higher degrees of accuracy in the delineation of pathology and treatment planning: both the exact size and location of a primary intimal tear and the branching pattern of the aortic arch are affected by cardiac pulsation artifacts, and their suppression is highly desirable.

CT Protocols in Patients with Acute Chest Pain

The CT techniques used for the assessment of CAD are different from those used in patients with acute aortic diseases; thus, selection of the correct protocol is the first step in any CT imaging procedure and is based on clinical judgment by ED physicians.

Coronary CTA

The assessment of coronary stenosis requires coronary CTA of the highest quality. The scan range is restricted to the heart. Premedication of the patient with nitroglycerine and, above a prespecified heart rate (typically 65 bpm), with beta-blockers is necessary. The entire workflow needs to be well established, as the introduction of a coronary CTA program is not without substantial effort, even when all the technology is available. A guide on patient preparation, CT imaging protocols, CT imaging assessments, and reporting is provided below.

ECG-Gated CTA of the Aorta

In the evaluation of patients with acute aortic syndromes the goal in imaging is to eliminate or at least reduce pulsation artifacts. This can be achieved routinely even without beta-blockage. Nitroglycerine is also not required. The scan range always needs to include the entire aorta and iliofemoral access vessels as a road-map for endovascular treatment. Use of ECG-gating does not pose a major change of workflow for an established CT system operating around the clock. While routine use of ECG gating in the setting of acute aortic syndromes has several advantages, it may be an unnecessary effort outside of centers with large surgical and endovascular programs. If ECG gating is not routinely used for patients with acute aortic syndromes, a gated protocol should nevertheless be available to further evaluate indeterminate findings on a non-gated scan. Another benefit of routine ECG gating for thoracic aortic CTA is that it facilitates the imple-

mentation of ECG gating for acute coronary CTA programs.

Combined "Triple-Rule-Out" Protocol

While it is technically possible to build CT protocols that allow imaging and interpretation of the entire aorta, the coronary arteries, and the pulmonary vasculature, such studies are not performed at our institutions. A complete "triple-rule-out" protocol would require a longer injection of contrast agent (to opacify systemic and pulmonary arteries simultaneously), resulting in artifacts from the superior vena cava and the right heart. To perform a guideline-conforming work-up for aortic dissection, the scanning range would have to include not only the entire chest but also the entire abdominal aorta and iliofemoral access vessels, which implies greater radiation exposure. While it is possible to detect an aortic dissection using coronary CTA, and acute coronary abnormalities or abnormal myocardial enhancement can be identified on a gated CTA for evaluation of acute aortic syndrome, these situations tend to be rare. Some studies have suggested the limited efficacy of these protocols since they are likely to be ordered in patients with undifferentiated chest pain, who have a very low event rate for any of the syndromes [35]. Contrary to common belief, there is not a wide clinical overlap between ACS and acute aortic syndromes.

Challenges to the Implementation of a Coronary CT Program

While the potential diagnostic value of cardiac CT in the ED seems evident, there are practical obstacles that interfere with its widespread implementation. CT equipment with sufficient cardiac imaging capabilities (minimally a single-source 64-slice system), fully-trained technologists, and experienced cardiac CT readers are essential. Not all patients are eligible for cardiac CTA, including those with known CAD, cardiac arrhythmia, tachycardia, or severe obesity (typically BMI >40 kg/m^2). CTA is associated with risks due to radiation exposure, although doses have decreased substantially over the past decade. The use of iodine-containing contrast media is contraindicated in patients with renal dysfunction or related allergies. The guidelines emphasize that the choice of test, whether CT or another modality, should be based on local expertise and the individual characteristics of the patient that affect eligibility [36]. More advanced CT technology, i.e., dual-source CT systems or wider detector arrays, can improve image quality in somewhat less suitable patients. Presently, few centers have a sufficient number of experienced personnel to offer cardiac CT around the clock. Current published guidelines on the practice of cardiac CT in the ED specify the requirements for and maintenance of certification for imaging centers, interpreting physicians, and medical staff [36].

Suggested Coronary CTA Approach

The following sections provide guidance based on professional society standards and encourage the use of the recommended practices [36]. Cardiac CT should be performed and interpreted in accordance with best practice standards as delineated in the imaging guidelines of the Society of Cardiovascular Computed Tomography (SCCT), using at least 64-slice technology and interpreted by physicians at least Core Cardiology Training Symposium (COCATS) level 2 or equivalent, SCCT level 2, or certified by the Certification Board of Computed Cardiovascular Tomography (CBCCT) [29]. Below is a summary of the standards that should be considered at every institution:

Patient Preparation

Contraindications

1. Absolute: Iodinated contrast allergy not amenable to pre-treatment, pregnancy
2. Relative: Renal insufficiency, multiple myeloma/radioactive iodine therapy, untreated hyperthyroidism, inability to perform breath-hold for >15 s, cardiac rhythm (frequent ectopy/arrhythmia), unwillingness to abstain from metformin for 48 h after the CT examination.

Prior to Arrival

1. Discontinue phosphodiesterase inhibitors for 48 h before the test.
2. Consider abstaining from nonsteroidal anti-inflammatory agents.
3. Consider 48-h abstention from metformin after the CT examination.
4. Continue medications other than phosphodiesterase inhibitors/nonsteroidal anti-inflammatory drugs.
5. No solids 4 h prior to the scan, but otherwise may continue usual intake of liquids and solid foods.

In the Scanner

1. Patient positioning
   a. Heart centered within the gantry
   b. Appropriate placement of ECG leads
2. Patient preparation
   a. A test breath-hold to monitor heart rate to decide on beta-blocker requirement and usage of prospective vs. retrospective gating
   b. Use of i.v. or oral beta blockers if heart rate is >60 bpm, e.g., 5–20 mg metoprolol i.v. or 50–100 mg atenolol 1 h before (exceptions can be made for CT scanners with high temporal resolution such as dual-source or flash)
   c. Use of nitroglycerin for coronary vasodilation, e.g., 400–800 μg sublingual nitroglycerin (one to two tabs).

Important: In patients abstaining from phosphodiesterase inhibitors 48 h before the test, no nitrates should be given during CT scan acquisition.

CT Imaging Protocol

1. Iodinated contrast agent with at least 320 (or 300) mg iodine/mL.
   a. Injection rate of contrast agent: minimum of 5 ml/s and up to 8 mL/s in obese patients.
2. Determination of optimal contrast timing using either a test bolus or a bolus trigger technique
3. Amount of contrast: duration of scan but at least a 10-s injection.
4. Minimizing the radiation exposure by choosing an appropriate field of view (at the level of the carina to the dome of the diaphragm).

Steps

1. Scout: Topogram anteroposterior and/or lateral
2. Coronary calcium assessment
   a. Prospective ECG-gated/triggered, low-dose non-contrast CT scan to determine coronary artery calcification
   b. An Agatston score of >800
   c. No contrast-enhanced CTA
3. Assessment of coronary atherosclerotic plaque and stenosis: Prospective ECG-triggered or retrospective ECG-gated CT imaging using tube modulation technique
   a. Maximal temporal and spatial resolution of the equipment
   b. Candidates for prospective triggering: regular heart rate <62 bpm during breath-hold after beta-blockade, no cardiac arrhythmias or premature beats prior to or during test breath-hold and <400 AS
4. Adjusting kvp to BMI:
   a. 100 kvp if BMI <30 kg/m^2 AND body weight <220 pounds
   b. 120 kvp if BMI >30 kg/m^2
   c. For retrospective gating: use radiation safety options according to the manufacturer's guidelines (i.e., tube current modulation, width of the full tube current according to heart rate, hybrid techniques such as padding)
5. Image reconstruction
   a. ECG editing in patients with premature beats
   b. Reconstruction with approximately 50% overlap (e.g., 0.75-mm slice thickness with 0.4-mm increment or 0.6 mm slice thickness with 0.3-mm overlap)
   c. Reconstruction of the number of series necessary to eliminate motion artifacts, typically two data sets, but more if required (i.e., for the right coronary artery) in mid-diastole (65–80%) and end systole (35–45%) if retrospective technique was used.

Left Ventricular Function

1. For either prospective (extending the gate) and retrospective ECG gating, data on global and regional left ventricular function should be collected and assessed.
2. Typically 1.5- to 2-mm-thick axial images are reconstructed at 10% increments (10 phases) for single-source CT scanners or 5% increments (20 phases) for dual-source CT scanners throughout the cardiac cycle with a reduced pixel matrix of 256×256.

Full Field of View

1. If incidental findings are assessed: reconstruction of a data set of 3-mm-thick axial images, covering the portions of the thorax acquired during the cardiac CT scan
2. Reconstruction of a field of view optimized for coverage of the heart.

Documentation of Radiation Exposure

Radiation exposure should be reported as the CT dose index per volume (CTDIvol), expressed in mGy, for a given anatomic coverage (e.g., the heart) with or without the corresponding dose-length product (in mGy per cm) for each diagnostic acquisition (e.g., for the calcium score and the CT angiographic acquisition), together with a total dose length product (DLP).

CT Parameters To Be Reported

A diagnostic testing report should contain information on beta-blocker and nitrate administration, imaging sequences performed, overall contrast administration, including the contrast agent used, and the overall radiation dose.

Report on the Coronary Arteries

1. Arterial distribution (right or left dominant, co-dominant)
   a. Rate overall image quality as interpretable/uninterpretable; specify non-evaluable segments/arteries and reason
2. Presence and extent of coronary atherosclerotic plaque (none, calcified, non-calcified, both) according to American Heart Association (AHA) classification per vessel and optionally per 17 coronary segments, including presence and severity of a significant coronary stenosis (>70% luminal narrowing) per vessel and optionally per 17 coronary segments.
   a. Degree of luminal narrowing should be as follows: normal: 0%, non-significant/minor disease: 1–49%, moderate disease: 50–69% (except left main, where >50% is considered significant), significant disease: 70–99%, occluded: 100%.

Evaluation of the Left Ventricle

1. Regional left ventricular (LV) dysfunction including wall motion and wall thickening of the myocardium assessed qualitatively based on the American Heart Association, American College of Cardiology, American Society of Echocardiography (AHA/ACC/ASE) 17-segment model.
2. Whether the location of regional dysfunction matches the stenosis location.
3. Regional LV dysfunction has to be present in at least two contiguous myocardial segments or in one segment visualized in two different views to be considered a true-positive finding.
4. Each LV segment is graded as normal, hypokinetic (impaired contraction), akinetic (absent contraction), dyskinetic (paradoxical outward wall motion during systole without aneurysm formation in diastole) or aneurysmal.
5. Global LV function as normal, mildly, moderately or severely impaired.
6. Non-cardiac finding assessment should include aortic dissection, pulmonary embolism, pulmonary nodules, pneumonia, pneumothorax, pericardial effusion, hiatal hernia, rib fractures.

Coronary CTA in Patients with Suspected ACS

The absence of plaque on CTA excludes ACS (sensitivity 100%), while obstructive CAD (>50% stenosis) does not (sensitivity 77%); only half of the patients with obstructive CAD on CTA have acute coronary disease. Several randomized controlled trials have investigated the safety and economic performance of cardiac CT in acute chest pain (Table 3) [37–39]. Taken together, the three trials comprised more than 3000 patients. Follow-up analysis demonstrated that, based on the CTA results, not a single patient was discharged with a missed diagnosis of ACS. These trials demonstrated the efficiency of CTA compared to the standard of care (SOC) as evidenced by a reduction in length of stay, hospital admissions, and ED cost, while overall hospital costs remained similar to those of the SOC, driven by a higher rate of invasive angiography and revascularizations. Across the trials, patients randomized to CTA more often underwent cardiac catheterization (8.4% vs. 6.3%) and percutaneous coronary intervention (4.6% vs. 2.6%). Unfortunately, the trials were not powered to prove that higher sensitivity for the detection of obstructive CAD by CTA, with subsequently increased revascularization rates, also results in a better clinical outcome. Additionally, radiation exposure will be higher for CTA when the SOC consists of exercise tests and stress echocardiography. In summary, these trials have established cardiac CT as a viable alternative to functional testing in the triage of low-risk patients with acute chest pain. Several studies demonstrated that CTA findings of plaque, stenosis, and ventricular function

Table 3. Randomized controlled trials comparing coronary CTA with the standard of care in the evaluation of acute chest pain

Study	CT-STAT (2011)		ACRIN (2012)		ROMICAT II (2012)	
Population	699 TIMI risk score 0–4 MI 0.9%		1370 TIMI risk score 0–2 MI 1%		985 Low–intermediate risk MI 2.5%	
Randomization Control group	1:1 SPECT MPI		2:1 Usual care		1:1 Usual care	
	CTA	Controls	CTA	Controls	CTA	Controls
ACS diagnosis	1.1%	2.4%	1%	1%	9%	6%
ED discharge			*50%*	*23%*	*47%*	*12%*
ICA rate	8.0%	7.4%	5%	4%	12%	8%
Revascularization	4.3%	2.7%	3%	1%	6%	4%
Time to diagnosis (median, range)	*2.9 h*[a] *(2.1-4.0)*	*6.3 h* *(4-19)*				
Length of stay (median, range)			*18.0 h* *(8-27)*	*24.8 h* *(19-31)*	*23.2 h*[a]	*30.8 h*
1 month MACE			*0%*[a]	*0%*	0.4%	1.2%
6-month MACE	0.8%	0.4%				
Cost (US$)	*2137*[b]	*3458*			4026[c]	3874

TIMI, Thrombolysis in myocardial infarction; CTA, computed tomography angiography; ACS, acute coronary syndrome; ED, emergency department; ICA, invasive coronary angiography; MACE, major adverse cardiac event; MI, myocardial infarction.
Statistically significant results are shown in italic.
[a] Primary endpoint of the study.
[b] Represents only emergency department costs.
[c] Represents index hospitalization including angiograms and interventions.

accurately predict adverse cardiac events over the next 6 months to 2 years. While patients without CAD remain virtually event-free, those with non-obstructive CAD have a slightly increased risk, and those with obstructive CAD are at the highest risk [32].

Current Recommendations and Future Expectations

Several guideline documents discuss the role of cardiac CT in the management of acute chest pain, including the 2010 Cardiac CT Appropriateness Criteria, which included representation by the ACC, AHA, and SCCT, the 2011 ESC Non-STE-ACS management guidelines [39], and the 2014 SCCT guidelines for CCTA in acute chest pain [32, 36], suggest cardiac CT as appropriate in patients with low to intermediate risk for ACS, defined as a non-diagnostic ECG and serum biomarkers. The 2014 SCCT recommendations have been informed by the ACRIN (American College of Radiology Imaging Network) and ROMICAT (Rule Out Myocardial Ischemia/Infarction Using Computer Assisted Tomography) II results, published in 2012. It is important to emphasize that information from cardiac CT needs to be interpreted in the context of all clinical and diagnostic information available (Table 4). In the future, the diagnostic value of cardiac CT may be further strengthened by the incorporation of morphologic plaque assessment and by applications to assess the functional relevance of CAD on CTA. Additionally, high-sensitive-troponin assays may allow the safe exclusion of ACS without the need for further diagnostic testing in a proportion of patients. Hence, early triage by cardiac CT may re-focus efforts towards those patients with (conflicting) low elevations in high-sensitive-troponins.

Potential of CCTA Beyond the Coronary Lumen

Resting myocardial ischemia or MI can be identified on CTA datasets as myocardial hypo-enhancement. The presence of resting myocardial enhancement defects on CTA has a sensitivity and specificity of around 90% to identify MI patients. The hemodynamic severity of CAD can also be determined by calculation of the fractional flow reserve (FFR) from CT angiograms using computational fluid dynamics. CTA-derived FFR can confidently exclude hemodynamically significant CAD. Neither of these applications is currently the clinical standard but they add much needed information on functional testing. Moreover, they have the potential to improve the efficacy of CCTA by improving its specificity, thereby reducing unnecessary referrals to invasive angiography and other downstream testing.

Table 4. Clinical interpretation of cardiac CT in the emergency department

Immediate evaluation of life-threatening conditions		Management recommendation
Coronary arteries	>70% stenosis (myocardial hypo-enhancement)	Hospital admission, catheterization if symptoms suggestive of ACS
	Moderate stenosis (40–70%)	Observation (admission), second troponins, consider stress testing
	Atherosclerotic plaque, <40% stenosis	ACS ruled out after second negative troponins, no stress testing, (clinical) observation depending on clinical presentation, consider non-cardiac causes
	No or minimal atherosclerotic plaque	ACS ruled out, consider non-cardiac conditions
Other cardiac	Pericardial effusion, aortic valve disease, myocardial scar	As indicated
Thoracic aorta	Acute aortic syndrome (within scan range)	As indicated
Pulmonary arteries	Pulmonary emboli (as far as scan range and opacification allows)	As indicated
Extravascular	Pulmonary disease (pneumonia, pneumothorax)	Appropriate referral
Other	Relevant, but not acutely relevant, cardiac and non-cardiac abnormalities (which may be evaluated during office hours)	Appropriate referral

ACS, Acute coronary syndrome.
Simplified diagnostic algorithm, depending on local conditions and practices. Management also affected by risk profile and other findings. Cardiac CT does not exclude ACS by functional coronary artery disease (spasm).

CT Evaluation of Acute Aortic Syndromes

The sensitivity and specificity of non-gated CT for acute aortic abnormalities have been reported to approach 100%. CTA can reliably assess complications of aortic diseases and guide treatment decisions. However, there are subtle lesions of the aorta that can be missed with non-gated CT [40]. Cardiac pulsation artifacts may also mimic disease, particularly in younger individuals. While ECG gating clearly improves both assessment of the aortic root, including the coronary artery origins and the valve apparatus, and visualization of subtle aortic lesions, the superiority of gated versus non-gated CT acquisitions in acute aortic disease has yet to be assessed in a prospective trial. The possibility of reconstructing time-resolved datasets to display dynamic changes in the position of a dissection flap or the size of a true or false lumen provides intriguing insights into the hemodynamic consequences of a given pathology. The best CT protocol for the evaluation of acute aortic syndromes depends on several factors, including the scanner generation, patient population, and expected prevalence of acute aortic diseases, the comfort and training level of night- and weekend technologists, as well as the expertise of readers.

ECG-gating technologies include retrospective gating, which allows 4D reconstructions but comes with a slight radiation-dose penalty. Prospective triggering involves a lower dose of radiation but requires larger detectors if the entire thoracic aorta is to be covered. High-pitch helical scans (so-called flash mode) are an intriguing alternative, but require high-power X-ray tubes or small patient size. It is also worth mentioning that improved scanner technology reduces pulsation artifacts even without gating,

simply due to the much faster helical acquisition with short rotation times and detector bank widths of at least 4 cm.

The following guiding principles may help in the decision to implement ECG gating for acute aortic syndromes:
- Suppression of pulsation artifacts is highly desirable in the ascending aorta
- Dynamic (time resolved) visualization is intriguing but may not provide critical information beyond an artifact-free static dataset
- Assuming a prevalence of 5% of limited tears (dissection variant) that might be missed without gating and those cases in which pulsation artifacts mimic aortic lesions or do not allow their exclusion, a reasonable estimate for the proportion of patients benefitting from gating is probably in the order of 5–10%
- If ECG-gating can be achieved at no or minimal additional dose and without an unreasonably complicated workflow, it is the opinion of the authors that gating should be implemented
- If ECG-gating is not routinely used, e.g., in a setting with a low prevalence of patients with acute aortic disease, a dedicated gated protocol should still be available for problem solving (e.g., in the 5–10% of cases in which it is deemed necessary) following an inconclusive non-gated study.

Aortic Dissection and Its Variants

Our conceptual approach to acute aortic syndromes groups all the manifestations of a diseased aortic media into the dissection group. The common pathologic denominator of these diseases is the presence of an abnormal aortic medial layer, traditionally (albeit not completely accurately) described as "cystic medial necrosis." Cystic medial necrosis is the common pathologic endpoint of several underlying acquired and inherited conditions, ranging from severe hypertension and normal aging to familial aortic diseases, vasculitis, and connective tissue diseases such as Ehlers-Danlos, Loeys-Dietz, or Marfan disease.

Classic dissection (class I) is characterized by a primary intimal tear (in which blood enters the false lumen), a false channel, or a lumen within the aortic media that is separated from the true lumen by a dissection flap made of intima and a considerable portion of the media.

A common variant of aortic dissection manifests as an IMH (class II). The abnormal space within the aortic media enabled by the underlying cystic medial necrosis is filled by thrombus rather than by flowing blood. It is important to realize that elements of classic dissection and its IMH variant may coexist in the same individual. For example, it is not uncommon to find areas of intramural blood in patients who otherwise have features of classic dissection. At the same time, in most patients with IMH it is now recognized that small primary intimal tears as well as other small communications between the true lumen flow channel of the aorta and portions of the thrombosed false channel do exist [41].

A so-called limited tear of the aorta, or limited dissection (class III), is a rare lesion characterized by a partial-thickness tear of the aortic wall, extending from the intima into part or all of the media [40]. This lesion could be regarded as a very large primary intimal tear but without development of a separate flow channel in the media (false lumen) as in classic dissection. Limited tears occur more often in the ascending aorta than more distally and are associated with dilated or aneurysmal aortic diameters. The underlying pathology, typically with cystic medial degeneration, and risk profiles of patients with limited tears are similar to those with classic dissection.

Intramural Hematoma (Class II)

While the term "intramural hematoma" simply means blood in the aortic wall, it has been used misleadingly (class II lesion) to describe an entity on the same level as an aortic dissection or penetrating atherosclerotic ulcer, which has resulted in considerable confusion and inconsistent classification of aortic diseases in the literature. We do not consider IMH as a specific disease entity, but instead as an important imaging finding, because it is unspecific to the underlying pathology or etiology. Intramural blood can be seen to variable degrees in any acute aortic condition: if fresh clot fills the entirety of the dissection plane in patients with cystic medial necrosis, it is best considered a variant manifestation of aortic dissection. Intramural blood is also typically associated with PAUs: any communication between the aortic lumen and the media – be it through a primary intimal tear, a focal

penetrating ulcer, or even trauma – blood can extend into the neighboring aortic wall and result in IMH. These local hematomas typically do not extend far along the aorta or its branches when associated with a PAU, but are typically local.

While IMH can occur in underlying cystic medial necrosis as well as in PAUs, this does not make these lesions the same entity, and the notion that PAUs can become dissections and vice versa does not reflect our experience. The one patient group in which overlapping and indistinguishable features of PAU, IMH, and elements of dissection may occur in the same individual are typically older individuals with moderate atherosclerotic burden and presumed coexisting cystic medial necrosis, which is a known manifestation of normal aging as well. In this particular situation the overlapping imaging features may reflect coexisting intimal (atherosclerotic) and medial (cystic degeneration) disease in the same patient.

Penetrating Atherosclerotic Ulcer (Class IV)

The pathologic definition of a PAU is a deep ulcerated plaque that penetrates the internal elastic lamina into the medial layer of the aorta [42]. PAU is therefore a manifestation of atherosclerosis (and not of cystic medial disease). The risk profile of patients with PAU is different from that of patients with aortic dissection. Patients are typically older, with several other atherosclerotic comorbidities, including a history of stroke, peripheral vascular disease, CAD, and aortic aneurysms. CT images frequently show extensive atherosclerotic changes, often with more than one ulcer-like lesion.

Given the multiplicity of lesions and the common observation of atherosclerotic ulcers in non-symptomatic patients, it is important to try to distinguish between non-penetrating ulcers (i.e. ulcerated plaque confined to the thickened intima), chronic healed penetrating ulcers (which are re-endothelialized and not an acute threat), and those lesions that acutely penetrate the aortic wall with a high risk of complications such as perforation and rupture. The key distinguishing features of acute lesions are intramural blood and periaortic stranding, which can help identify a culprit lesion. Acute PAUs without IMH do exist, though, and in the setting of acute aortic pain a CT scan without IMH or periaortic stranding near an identifiable ulcer-like lesion does not exclude an acute aortic condition. In these cases, follow up imaging is recommended.

Iatrogenic and Traumatic Dissection (Class V)

Aortic and other arterial dissections can occur as a complication of diagnostic and interventional catheter-based procedures, as well as a complication of cardiac or vascular surgery. While patients with iatrogenic dissections may have underlying vascular diseases that predispose them to aortic dissection, even the non-diseased aortic wall can be mechanically dissected by subintimal advancement of endovascular wires and catheters.

Acute traumatic injuries of the aorta typically occur in otherwise healthy, often young patients. The presentation and underlying pathology are thus very different from the entities causing acute aortic syndromes. The spectrum of traumatic aortic lesions usually involves disruption of the intima, underlying media, and lastly the adventitia with more or less pseudoaneurysm formation. While the cross-sectional appearance of these lesions may resemble the morphology of aortic dissection on one or two transverse images, these are typically undermined, torn portions of the aortic wall and not true dissections with a separate flow channel within the medial layer of the aortic media. A normal aorta does not easily dissect. True traumatic aortic dissections may thus represent coincidences, such as in patients with underlying cystic medial necrosis who are involved in a trauma.

Rupturing Thoracic Aortic Aneurysms

Acutely expanding, unstable, and leaking aneurysms present with the prototypical symptoms that define the acute aortic syndrome [43]. It is thus most surprising that these lesions are not included in the current European and North American classification schemes. In our population, symptomatic aneurysms represent approximately 8% of acute aortic syndromes. The imaging findings in patients with symptomatic aneurysms may be limited to visualization of the aneurysmal dilatation of the aorta alone. In stable patients responding to antihypertensive and pain medication, an observational approach is often justified. CT signs of unstable aneurysms include intramural blood (within the medial layer of the aorta), intraclot hemorrhage ("crescent sign"), periaortic stranding (leaking ultrafitrate), periaortic or mediastinal hematoma (hyperdense blood), hemorrhagic pleural fluid, or frank rupture with blood beyond the confines of the aortic wall. Accurate preoperative imaging is critical for the evaluation of surgical and endovascular treatment options and specific treatment planning in surgical and endovascular candidates.

Conclusion

State-of-the art technology allows the reliable acquisition of motion-free datasets for coronary CTA as well as ECG-gated CTA of the thoracic aorta. Because this powerful technology is widely available, both methods have the potential to become widely used for diagnosing, triaging, and treatment planning in patients presenting with coronary or aortic causes of acute chest pain. Familiarity with imaging technology and interpretation, establishment of a robust workflow beyond daytime coverage, and an in-depth knowledge of the underlying pathology and current clinical triage and guidelines are all prerequisites to using this technology for the benefit of our patients.

References

1. Lee TH, Rouan GW, Weisberg MC et al (1987) Clinical characteristics and natural history of patients with acute myocardial infarction sent home from the emergency room. Am J Cardiol 60:219-224.
2. Swap CJ, Nagurney JT (2005) Value and limitations of chest pain history in the evaluation of patients with suspected acute coronary syndromes. Jama 294:2623-2629
3. Howard DP, Banerjee A, Fairhead JF et al (2013) Population-based study of incidence and outcome of acute aortic dissection and premorbid risk factor control: 10-year results from the Oxford Vascular Study. Circulation 127:2031-2037.
4. Limkakeng A, Jr., Gibler WB, Pollack C et al (2001) Combination of goldman risk and initial cardiac troponin i for emergency department chest pain patient risk stratification. Acad Emerg Med 8:696-702.
5. Zimmerman J, Fromm R, Meyer D et al (1999) Diagnostic marker cooperative study for the diagnosis of myocardial infarction. Circulation 99:1671-1677.
6. Fesmire FM, Hughes AD, Fody EP et al (2002) The Erlanger chest pain evaluation protocol: a one-year experience with serial 12-lead ECG monitoring, two-hour delta serum marker measurements, and selective nuclear stress testing to identify and exclude acute coronary syndromes. Ann Emerg Med 40:584-594.
7. Hedges JR, Young GP, Henkel GF et al (1992) Serial ECGs are less accurate than serial CK-MB results for emergency department diagnosis of myocardial infarction. Ann Emerg Med 21:1445-1450.
8. Selker HP, Beshansky JR, Griffith JL et al (1998) Use of the acute cardiac ischemia time-insensitive predictive instrument (ACI-TIPI) to assist with triage of patients with chest pain or other symptoms suggestive of acute cardiac ischemia. A multicenter, controlled clinical trial. Ann Intern Med 129:845-855.
9. Hollander JE, Sease KL, Sparano DM et al (2004) Effects of neural network feedback to physicians on admit/discharge decision for emergency department patients with chest pain. Ann Emerg Med 44:199-205.
10. McCaig LF, Burt CW (2004) National hospital ambulatory medical care survey: 2002 emergency department summary. Adv Data 1-34.
11. McCaig LF, Nawar EW (2006) National hospital ambulatory medical care survey: 2004 emergency department summary. Adv Data 1-29.
12. Fleischmann KE, Hunink MG, Kuntz KM, Douglas PS (2002) Exercise echocardiography or exercise spect imaging? A meta-analysis of diagnostic test performance. J Nucl Cardiol 9:133-134.
13. Klocke FJ, Baird MG, Lorell BH et al (2003) ACC/AHA/ASNC guidelines for the clinical use of cardiac radionuclide imaging-executive summary: a report of the American College of Cardiology/American Heart Association task force on practice guidelines (ACC/AHA/ASNC committee to revise the 1995 guidelines for the clinical use of cardiac radionuclide imaging). Circulation 108:1404-1418.
14. Cheitlin MD, Armstrong WF, Aurigemma GP et al (2003) ACC/AHA/ASE 2003 guideline update for the clinical application of echocardiography: Summary article: a report of the American College of Cardiology/American Heart Association task force on practice guidelines (ACC/AHA/ASE committee to update the 1997 guidelines for the clinical application of echocardiography). Circulation 108:1146-1162.
15. Zalenski RJ, Rydman RJ, Ting S et al (2998) A national survey of emergency department chest pain centers in the United States. Am J Cardiol 81:1305-1309.
16. Burt CW (1999) Summary statistics for acute cardiac ischemia and chest pain visits to United States eds, 1995-1996. Am J Emerg Med 17:552-559.
17. Lee TH, Goldman L (2000) Evaluation of the patient with acute chest pain. N Engl J Med 342:1187-1195.

18. Tosteson AN, Goldman L, Udvarhi IS, Lee TH (1996) Cost-effectiveness of a coronary care it versus an intermediate care unit for emergency departm patients with chest pain. Circulation 94:143-150.

19. Conti A, Paladini B, Magazzini S al (2002) Chest pain unit management of patients at low a not low-risk for coronary artery disease in the emergency artment. A 5-year experience in the Florence area. Eur J rg Med 9:31-36.

20. Solinas L, Raucci R, Terrazzino et al (2003) Prevalence, clinical characteristics, resource u zation and outcome of patients with acute chest pain in th mergency department. A multicenter, prospective, observat al study in north-eastern Italy. Ital Heart J 4:318-324.

21. Roos JE, Willmann JK, Weishaupt et al (2002) Thoracic aorta: motion artifact reduction with r ospective and prospective electrocardiography-assisted mult etector row CT. Radiology 222:271-277.

22. Braunwald E, Antman EM, Fe sley JW et al (2002) ACC/AHA guideline update for management of patients with unstable angina and non-st gment elevation myocardial infarction-2002: Summary ar le: a report of the American College of Cardiology/Amer n Heart Association task force on practice guidelines (cor ittee on the management of patients with unstable angina). rculation 106:1893-1900.

23. Luepker RV, Apple FS, Christensc RH et al (2003) Case definitions for acute coronary heart ease in epidemiology and clinical research studies: a staten t from the AHA Council on Epidemiology and Prevention; HA Statistics Committee; World Heart Federation Council o pidemiology and Prevention; The European Society of Ca ology Working Group on Epidemiology and Prevention; C ters for Disease Control and Prevention; and the National art, Lung, and Blood institute. Circulation 108:2543-254

24. Ornato JP (2003) Management of tients with unstable angina and non-st-segment elevation r cardial infarction: update ACC/AHA guidelines. Am J Eme Med 21:346-351.

25. Vilacosta I, Roman JAS (2001) A te aortic syndrome. Heart 85:365-368.

26. Erbel R, Alfonso F, Boileau C et a 001) Diagnosis and management of aortic dissection. Eur art J 22:1642-1681.

27. Evangelista A, Mukherjee D, Meh RH et al (2005) Acute intramural hematoma of the aorta: ystery in evolution. Circulation 111:1063-1070.

28. Hiratzka LF, Bakris GL, Beckma A et al (2010) 2010 ACCF/AHA/AATS/ACR/ASA/S /SCAI/SIR/STS/SVM guidelines for the diagnosis and r agement of patients with thoracic aortic disease: a report the American College of Cardiology Foundation/Americ Heart Association task force on practice guidelines, Am can Association for Thoracic Surgery, American Colleg of Radiology, American Stroke Association, Society of C liovascular Anesthesiologists, Society for Cardiovascular giography and Interventions, Society of Interventional H diology, Society of Thoracic Surgeons, and Society for ta cular Medicine. Circulation 121:e266-369.

29. Erbel RV, Aboyans V, Boileau C et (2014) 2014 ESC Guidelines on the diagnosis and treatm of aortic diseases: Document covering acute and chronic a ic diseases of the thoracic and abdominal aorta of the adult ame Task Force for the Di

30. Yang L, Zhou T, Zhang R et al (2014) Meta-analysis: diagnostic accuracy of coronary CT angiography with prospective ECG gating based on step-and-shoot, flash and volume modes for detection of coronary artery disease. European Radiology 24:2345-2352.

31. Task Force Members, Montalescot G, Sechtem U, Achenbach S et al (2013) 2013 ESC guidelines on the management of stable coronary artery disease: The task force on the management of stable coronary artery disease of the European Society of Cardiology. Eur Heart J 34:2949-3003.

32. Hulten EA, Carbonaro S, Petrillo SP et al (2011) Prognostic value of cardiac computed tomography angiography: a systematic review and meta-analysis. J Am Coll Cardiol 57:1237-1247.

33. Fuchs TA, Stehli J, Bull S et al (2014) Coronary computed tomography angiography with model-based iterative reconstruction using a radiation exposure similar to chest x-ray examination. Eur Heart J 35:1131-1136.

34. Shiga T, Wajima Z, Apfel CC et al (2006) Diagnostic accuracy of transesophageal echocardiography, helical computed tomography, and magnetic resonance imaging for suspected thoracic aortic dissection: systematic review and meta-analysis. Arch Intern Med 166:1350-1356.

35. Rogers IS, Banerji D, Siegel EL et al (2011) Usefulness of comprehensive cardiothoracic computed tomography in the evaluation of acute undifferentiated chest discomfort in the emergency department (capture). Am J Cardiol 107:643-650.

36. Raff GL, Chinnaiyan KM, Cury RC et al (2014) SCCT guidelines on the use of coronary computed tomographic angiography for patients presenting with acute chest pain to the emergency department: a report of the society of cardiovascular computed tomography guidelines committee. J Cardiovasc Comput Tomog 8:254-271.

37. Hoffmann U, Truong QA, Schoenfeld DA et al; Investigators R-I (2012) Coronary CT angiography versus standard evaluation in acute chest pain. N Engl J Med 367:299-308.

38. Litt HI, Gatsonis C, Snyder B et al (2012) CT angiography for safe discharge of patients with possible acute coronary syndromes. N Engl J Med 366:1393-1403.

39. Goldstein JA, Chinnaiyan KM, Abidov A et al; Investigators C-S (2011) The CT-STAT (coronary computed tomographic angiography for systematic triage of acute chest pain patients to treatment) trial. J Am Coll Cardiol 58:1414-1422.

40. Svensson LG, Labib SB, Eisenhauer AC, Butterly JR (1999) Intimal tear without hematoma: an important variant of aortic dissection that can elude current imaging techniques. Circulation 99:1331-1336.

41. Williams DM, Cronin P, Dasika N et al (2006) Aortic branch artery pseudoaneurysms accompanying aortic dissection. Part I. Pseudoaneurysm anatomy. J Vasc Interven Radiol JVIR 17:765-771.

42. Nathan DP, Boonn W, Lai E et al (2012) Presentation, complications, and natural history of penetrating atherosclerotic ulcer disease. J Vasc Surg 55:10-15.

43. Johansson G, Markstrom U, Swedenborg J (1995) Ruptured thoracic aortic aneurysms: a study of incidence and mortality rates. J Vasc Surg 21:985-988.

agnosis and Treatment of Aortic Diseases of the European Society of Cardiology (ESC). Eur Heart J 35:2873-2926.

Incidental Findings on Thoracic and Cardiac CT

Lynn S. Broderick[1], Shawn D. Teague[2]

[1] University of Wisconsin-Madison, Madison, WI, USA
[2] Indiana University School of Medicine, Indianapolis, IN, USA

Introduction

With the ever-increasing use of computed tomography (CT) for imaging, there is always the possibility of finding something on the exam that was not anticipated and is not related to the primary indication for obtaining the exam. These unanticipated findings have been labeled "incidentalomas" and, depending on their significance, a cascade of additional imaging exams can result. Care must be taken to limit unnecessary downstream imaging due to these unanticipated findings. In a patient with an incidental finding, the first task of the radiologist is to determine its stability. An active search of the patient's prior imaging exams in the picture archiving and communication systems is critical. Appropriate comparison exams may include prior abdominal, renal, or virtual colonoscopy CT exams, magnetic resonance (MR) or ultrasound exams of the liver or biliary tree, or a thoracic or cardiac CT in which the organs of the upper abdomen were incidentally included. For lesions of the thoracic inlet, a prior neck or cervical spine CT may be helpful. If the patient is new to your institution, comparison exams from other institutions can often be electronically transferred and thus obtained with relatively little effort, and are of great value. Obtaining prior exams can save the patient the significant cost, radiation exposure, and anxiety associated with repeat exams. If the "incidentaloma" is new or there are no comparisons to determine stability, a decision must be made regarding the overall significance of the finding, which often has yet to be fully assessed. We have included some of the incidental findings that may be encountered on routine thoracic and cardiac CT imaging, with a focus on their management.

Thoracic Inlet

Coronal reconstructed images can be helpful in detecting supraclavicular lymph nodes, which may be more difficult to differentiate from adjacent vascular structures on axial images, especially if the exam is performed without

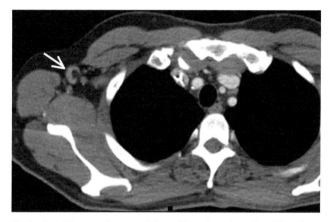

Fig. 1. Axial image shows a right axillary lymph node with a fatty hilum (*arrow*) indicating a benign lymph node

intravenous contrast. As with other incidental lymph nodes in the mediastinum and hilum, assessment for clinical significance should include a short-axis measurement as well as evaluation of the lymph node density. In general a short-axis measurement of <1.0 cm suggests a benign lymph node [1]. However, a lymph node may be enlarged secondary to reaction to local infection or to a neoplastic process. The density of the lymph node is also important since lymph nodes containing a fatty hilum (Fig. 1) are considered benign regardless of size. Diffuse, central, or peripheral eggshell calcifications also indicate a benign etiology. However, eccentric calcification should not be considered a benign feature.

The thyroid gland is usually at least partially included on a chest CT exam. Thyroid nodules are extremely common in the adult population and the vast majority are benign. Recent guidelines have been published by Hoang et al. [2] to diminish the number of unnecessary follow-up exams. (Fig. 2). For adults ≥35 years of age, a follow-up ultrasound is recommended if the nodule is ≥1.5 cm. In adults <35 years of age, a follow-up ultrasound is recommended if the nodule is ≥1 cm. In addition, any nodule in the pediatric age group or any nodule regardless of patient age that is fluorodeoxyglucose-avid on positron

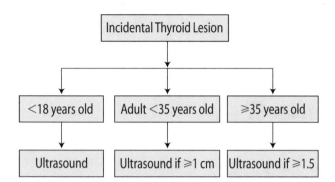

Fig. 2. The exact guideline for the evaluation of incidental thyroid nodules depends on the age of the patient and the size of the lesion

emission tomography (PET) or with evidence of invasion or adjacent lymphadenopathy should be assessed by ultrasound.

Chest Wall

Coronal and sagittal reformatted images are useful in evaluating skeletal structures. The ribs are problematic because a single rib is not visualized on a single axial image. The use of bone windows improves visualization of the lateral aspects of the ribs on sagittal images; posterior aspects are best visualized on coronal reformatted images. Rib lesions will be more obvious while scrolling through the data set than if each image is independently reviewed. Sternal fractures can be missed on axial images because of the plane of imaging but are very well depicted on sagittal views. Likewise, the vertebral column is ideally suited for review on sagittal views, where compression fractures (Fig. 3) and lytic and sclerotic lesions may be more obvious than on axial images.

CT is not ideal for breast imaging. However, assessment of breast tissue should be included in the search pattern. Breast cancer may be visible as an asymmetric soft-tissue mass that sometimes shows enhancement with the administration of intravenous contrast. Skin thickening from tumor or radiation can also be visualized, as well as evidence of prior surgery such as lymph node dissection. The presence of collateral vessels in the chest wall may alert the clinician to the presence of vascular pathology elsewhere, such as a stenosis or occlusion at the thoracic inlet.

Subcutaneous nodules such as metastases occur more commonly with lung cancer, breast cancer, or melanoma. However, soft-tissue nodules of the chest wall are more typically related to benign etiologies such as sebaceous cysts, or, when involving the anterior upper abdominal wall, injection sites from subcutaneous administration of medication. Occasionally, abnormalities such as calcifications in patients with scleroderma or neurofibromas in patients with neurofibromatosis will be present.

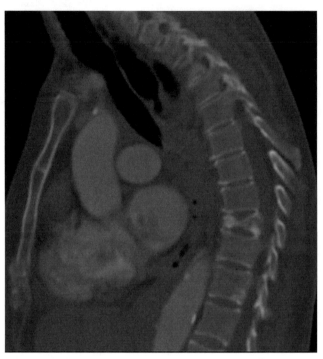

Fig. 3. Sagittal image demonstrating a compression fracture of the T9 vertebral body; the fracture was not present on the prior exam

Upper Abdomen

Liver

Although commonly encountered, most liver lesions are benign, even in patients with known malignancy. Berland et al. [3] published guidelines for the management of incidental liver findings on CT (Fig. 4). They categorized liver lesions based on the size and appearance of the lesion and the relative risk of the patient. Hepatic cysts are very common and present as sharply marginated, low-attenuation lesions of <20 Hounsfield units (HU). Typical hemangiomas show peripheral, nodular enhancement that fills in centrally on delayed images (Fig. 5). Findings that are more concerning include low-attenuation lesions with

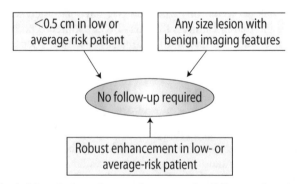

Fig. 4. Liver lesions do not always require follow-up imaging; rather, the decision depends on the imaging features and size of the lesion and the risk to the patient

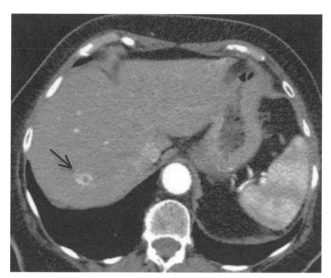

Fig. 5. Axial image demonstrates a lesion in the right lobe of the liver with peripheral contrast enhancement (*arrow*) and a central low density. The findings are consistent with the "peripheral puddling" contrast enhancement pattern seen in hemangiomas

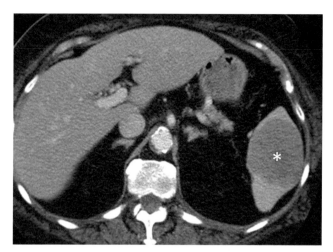

Fig. 6. Axial image shows a soft-tissue mass (*asterisk*) in the spleen, consistent with metastasis

ill-defined margins, enhancement <20 HU, and heterogeneity. These lesions will require additional imaging and/or intervention. Hyperenhancing liver lesions may be encountered – particularly on CT angiogram for the diagnosis of pulmonary embolism or evaluation of the aorta – and may represent a transient hepatic attenuation difference (THAD) flow artifact or focal nodular hyperplasia. For lesions measuring up to 1.5 cm, in patients with a low or average risk of malignancy, hyperenhancing lesions can be considered benign and no further imaging is recommended [3].

Kidneys

Renal cysts are very common. The features consistent with a cyst on unenhanced CT scans include a well-defined margin, homogeneous attenuation of 0–20 HU, absence of nodularity, septa, wall thickening, and nodular or thick calcification. Thin calcification of the wall is an acceptable benign feature of a cyst. If these features are present, no further work-up is necessary. A homogeneously dense lesion, with an intensity >70 HU and measuring <3 cm in diameter, is most likely a hyper-dense cyst. Lesions that do not demonstrate these benign imaging features will require additional work-up [3].

Spleen

Incidental splenic lesions are not as common as incidental hepatic lesions but they do occur. If the lesion is consistent with a splenic cyst, i.e., imperceptible wall, near-water attenuation (<10 HU), and lack of contrast enhancement, no further work-up is necessary. If these criteria are not met, the lesion may still be benign when it has the following imaging features: homogeneous atten-

uation of <20 HU, lack of contrast enhancement, and smooth margins. Features that should raise suspicion of a neoplasm include heterogeneous contrast enhancement, irregular margins, necrosis, and evidence of invasion (Fig. 6). When suspicious features are present, follow-up imaging or intervention is warranted [3].

Adrenal Glands

The most important parameter for incidental adrenal gland nodules is the density of the lesion. Lesions that show homogeneous macroscopic fat attenuation are consistent with myelolipoma. If the lesion does not visually appear to be a fatty lesion but has a density of ≤10 HU, it is consistent with a benign, lipid-rich adenoma. For lesions >20 HU and ≤4 cm in diameter in patients without symptoms and without a personal history of malignancy, a 1-year follow-up CT or MR study is recommended. If the lesion measures >4 cm in size, dedicated MR or CT imaging of the adrenal glands is recommended (Fig. 7) [3].

Stomach

A hiatal hernia is a common finding in routine thoracic imaging. It is important to recognize because patients with hiatal hernias may have chest pain secondary to associated reflux. At echocardiography, hiatal hernia can sometimes be misinterpreted as a mass adjacent to or involving the cardiac atria.

Incidental Cardiovascular Findings on Non-Cardiac CT

Cardiovascular structures are always included on a thoracic CT exam and should be evaluated much the same as one evaluates the mediastinum for lymph node enlargement. One of the most common incidental cardiac find-

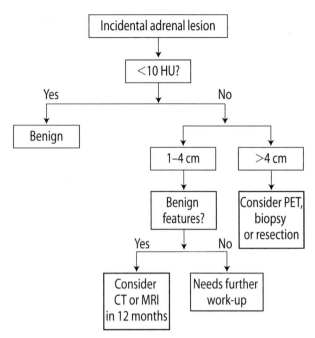

Fig. 7. The guidelines for incidental adrenal lesions depend on the density and size of the lesion

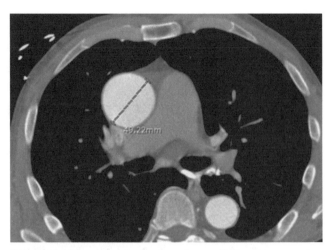

Fig. 8. Axial image shows an enlarged ascending aorta, measuring 4.9 cm at the level of the main pulmonary artery. Orthogonal measurements require double-oblique reformatted images.

ings on CT scans of the chest is coronary artery calcification, which is often seen in combination with atherosclerotic disease of the aorta. Numerous studies have shown that the more extensive the coronary artery calcification, the greater the risk of cardiac events, especially in younger patients. Whenever coronary artery calcification is detected, the association with coronary artery disease merits further attention. Subjective assessment of the amount of calcification relative to the patient's age can also be made. Calcification of the aortic valve is also commonly encountered. It is important to distinguish calcification of the aortic wall from calcification of the aortic valve leaflets. If the distinction is not obvious due to the orientation of the aortic valve plane relative to the imaging plane, oblique multiplanar reformatted images are often helpful. The significance of aortic valvular calcification depends on the amount of calcification and the patient's age. In patients <65 years of age, aortic valve calcification should raise suspicion of aortic stenosis, usually in association with a bicuspid aortic valve. As patients age, the presence of aortic valve calcification is more common and may be related to aortic valve sclerosis rather than aortic valve stenosis. In sufficiently calcified valves, the leaflets may be apparent on non-enhanced scans. The size of the great vessels should be assessed routinely, including a measurement of the ascending aorta at the level of the main pulmonary artery (Fig. 8), ensuring that an aortic aneurysm is not overlooked. There are no strict size criteria for the ascending aorta since the aortic size is related to the patient's body habitus. However, as a general rule, size should be reported if the ascending aorta measures ≥4.0 cm (measured from the external walls)

[4, 5]. Surgery is usually not contemplated until the ascending aorta measures >5 cm, unless the patient is symptomatic or has a connective-tissue disorder such as Marfan's syndrome. If the ascending aorta appears enlarged on axial images, it is important to perform double-oblique reformats to create a true transaxial image of the aorta, perpendicular to the axis of blood flow, so that an accurate measurement can be made. It is also important to evaluate the size of the pulmonary artery. If the main pulmonary artery diameter is ≥3.0 cm, then pulmonary hypertension becomes a consideration, especially if there is concomitant right ventricular hypertrophy and/or dilatation. Among the normal variant vascular anomalies are a persistent left superior vena cava (SVC), which may occur in isolation or in combination with a right SVC, and partial anomalous pulmonary venous return, most commonly with the left upper lobe pulmonary vein draining into the left innominate vein or the right upper lobe pulmonary vein draining directly into the SVC. When right heart enlargement is present, the pulmonary venous drainage pathways should be reviewed so that this diagnosis is not overlooked.

Lung Parenchyma

In the lungs, there are endemic areas where certain infections, such as histoplasmosis, coccidiodomycosis and even tuberculosis, are common and result in benign calcified pulmonary nodules. Recently, however, incidental non-calcified pulmonary nodules have received significant attention as they may indicate early stage lung cancer, which is potentially treatable. In 2005, the Fleischner Society published guidelines for the evaluation of pulmonary nodules in asymptomatic patients, with guidelines for the evaluation of subsolid pulmonary nodules published in 2013 [6, 7]. A recent review by Truong et al. summarized these guidelines and offered tips on technique and

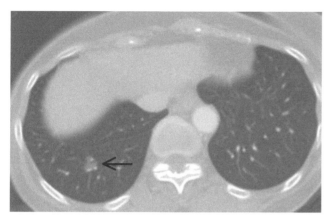

Fig. 9. Axial image shows a pure ground glass opacity nodule (*arrow*) in the right lower lobe

evaluation to ensure that patients are adequately treated [8]. The follow-up of solid nodules includes determination of their average of the length and width and of the presence of known risk factors for lung carcinoma. It should be noted that these guidelines do not apply to patients who are suspected of having, or who have, a known malignancy, patients <35 years of age, and patients with unexplained fever. The guidelines for the follow-up of subsolid (ground glass or part solid/part ground glass) nodules (Fig. 9) are based on the size of the lesion [8]. Only subsolid nodules >5 mm in diameter require follow-up. Solid nodules are followed for a period of 2 years, at which time a lack of change is considered to be evidence of a benign process; subsolid nodules require at least 3 years of surveillance, as the malignancies that demonstrate this pattern are typically slow-growing. When a lung nodule is identified, it should also be assessed on sagittal or coronal reformatted images. Nodules that appear discoid are likely benign, regardless of their conspicuity on axial images. Likewise, triangular or polygonal nodules that are intimately associated with the lung fissures most likely represent intrapulmonary lymph nodes. Emphysema is usually related to smoking and is commonly found in the same patient population undergoing CT exams for smoking-related pathologies. In emphysema, there is destruction of lung parenchymal tissue resulting in focal lucencies. It is important to distinguish emphysema from cystic lung disease, which is often managed differently. The key finding to distinguish emphysema from cystic lung disease is the ability to identify a discernible wall around the focal lucency in the lung parenchyma, which indicates the latter (i.e., pulmonary Langerhans cell histiocytosis or lymphangioleiomyomatosis) rather than

emphysema. These patients will need to be referred to pulmonology for further work-up.

Conclusion

In the routine practice of interpreting thoracic and cardiac CT exams, there will be frequent incidental findings that are not related to the patient's indication for the exam and may not be symptomatic [9]. The majority of these incidental lesions will be benign in etiology and not require additional attention. However, in patients with "incidenalomas," it is key that we, as radiologists, make efforts to compare current and prior examinations to determine the chronicity of the abnormality, in order to avoid unnecessary additional work-up. Conversely, when a new finding is significant, it is important that we recommend appropriate follow-up management, including additional imaging or specialty consultation. Appropriate management is critical for patient safety as well as for the overall resource utilization of the medical system.

References

1. Onuma Y, Tanabe K, Nakazawa G et al (2006) Noncardiac findings in cardiac imaging with multidetector computed tomography. J Am Coll Cardiol 48:402-406.
2. Hoang JK, Langer JE, Middleton WD et al (2014) Managing incidental thyroid nodules detected on imaging: white paper of the ACR incidental thyroid findings committee. J Am Coll Radiol pii: S1546-1440 (14) 00627-9 [E_pub a head to print].
3. Berland LL, Silverman SG, Gore RM et al (2010) Managing incidental findings on abdominal CT: white paper of the ACR incidental findings committee. J Am Coll Radiol 7:754-773.
4. Elefteriades JA, Farkas EA (2010) Thoracic aortic aneurysm: clinically pertinent controversies and uncertainties. J Am Coll Cardiol 55:841-857.
5. Hiratzka LF, Bakris GL, Beckman JA et al (2010) ACCF/AHA/AATS/ACR/ASA/SCA/SCAI/SIR/STS/SVM Guidelines for the diagnosis and management of patients with thoracic aortic disease. J Am Coll Cardiol 55:e27-e129.
6. MacMahon H, Austin JH, Gamsu G et al (2005) Guidelines for management of small pulmonary nodules detected on CT scans: a statement from the Fleischner Society. Radiol 237:395-400.
7. Naidich DP, Bankier AA, MacMahon H et al (2013) Recommendations for the management of subsolid pulmonary nodules detected at CT: a statement from the Fleischner Society. Radiol 266:304-317.
8. Truong MT, Ko JP, Rossi SE et al (2014) Update in the evaluation of the solitary pulmonary nodule. RadioGraph 34:1658-1679.
9. Teague SD, Rissing S, Mahenthiran J, Achenbach S (2012) Learning to interpret the extracardiac findings on coronary CT angiography examinations. J Cardiovasc Comput Tomogr 6:232-245.

Cardiac Magnetic Resonance

Didier Revel[1], David A. Bluemke[2]

[1] Department of Radiology, Université Claude Bernard Lyon 1, Bron, France
[2] Radiology and Imaging Sciences, Johns Hopkins University School of Medicine, Baltimore, MD, USA

Introduction

Magnetic resonance (MR) imaging is widely recognized for its ability to provide accurate and reliable assessments of the function and anatomy of the heart and great vessels. With the recent development of more specialized cardiovascular MR scanners, cardiac MR applications have expanded and are now utilized on a routine basis. In this chapter, the technical aspects of MR scanning of the cardiovascular system are outlined, followed by brief discussions of its applications to several diseases involving the heart in adults. A separate chapter in this volume specifically covers the use of cardiac MR for the diagnosis of coronary artery disease.

Understanding the Basic Pulse Sequences

It is extremely helpful to understand the strategy underlying the selection of a particular MR pulse sequence. This allows the user to determine the acquisition time and the corresponding imaging strategy to be employed. A fundamental characteristic of all pulse sequences is that the image is generated in the frequency domain, also referred to as k-space. Fourier reconstruction is used to generate the image. The k-space representation of the image is a pixel array generated one line at a time, typically 128–256 lines. To obtain a repetition time (TR) of 1000 (or 1 s, approximately one heart beat), each line of the image requires the duration of one heart beat for the acquisition (e.g., if 256 lines are generated, 256 heart beats at 60 beats per minute requires 256/60 = 4.3 min per image). However, new techniques incorporate fast (or turbo) imaging modes as well as parallel imaging techniques that greatly accelerate imaging times. For example, cine images of the heart are now routinely obtained in 6- to 12-s breath-holds. Real-time cine imaging is also possible. The most useful pulse sequences are discussed below.

Turbo Spin-Echo Imaging

Fast or turbo spin-echo images are a fundamental MR pulse sequence. In all parts of the body except the heart, a complete examination often consists of T1 images, which typically clearly display the anatomy, and/or T2 images, which accentuate pathologic changes, such as edema from infarction or the relationship of a tumor to the pericardium. The advantages of spin echo are the excellent signal to noise ratio and excellent contrast between the heart, epicardial fat, and adjacent structures. Fast or turbo spin-echo imaging reduces acquisition times by an acceleration factor typically ranging from 16 to 32. Parallel imaging can further accelerate speed by a factor of 2–3. Essentially all spin-echo imaging of the cardiovascular system is now done with fast/turbo spin-echo imaging, usually during a single breath-hold.

The primary disadvantage of fast/turbo spin-echo imaging is that these are very time-consuming sequences, typically one or two slices per breath-hold of 10–15 s. In so-called "black-blood" images, the blood is made to appear dark. Cine information is not routinely obtained. Despite these drawbacks, spin-echo images are important for imaging congenital anomalies and in evaluations of the pericardium, right ventricular cardiomyopathy, and cardiac tumors.

Cine MR Imaging

Cine-gradient echo images are used to evaluate motion gated to the cardiac cycle. Information from 4–12 cardiac cycles is used to obtain cine information during the entire cardiac cycle, referred to as segmented k-space cine MR imaging (MRI). Older MR scanners used so-called conventional gradient-echo pulse sequences together with gradient moment nulling, or flow compensation, to make blood bright ("bright-blood images"). In nearly all new MR scanners however, steady-state free precession (SSFP, also known as TrueFISP, Fiesta, balanced fast field echo) images are now used with a segmented

Diseases of the Chest and Heart 2015-2018,
DOI: 10.1007/978-88-470-5752-4_17 © Springer-Verlag Italia 2015

k-space acquisition. SSFP images provide very rapid imaging, with blood having very high signal intensity compared to the ventricular wall. Because there is a large amount of signal available, the SSFP technique is often combined with parallel imaging, which improves imaging speed by two- to three-fold. A single cine slice of the heart with a 40-ms temporal resolution is acquired in about 6 s on a modern MR scanner.

T1 and T2 Mapping

The detection of myocardial fibrosis using contrast-enhanced cardiac MR depends on differences in signal intensity between scarred regions and adjacent normal myocardium. However, in diffuse myocardial fibrosis these differences in signal intensity are lacking. Measurement of myocardial T1 times (T1 mapping) using non-contrast or gadolinium-enhanced inversion recovery prepared sequences has the potential to identify diffuse myocardial fibrosis that correlates well with ex vivo fibrosis content. T1 mapping calculates myocardial T1 relaxation times using image-based signal intensities and can be performed using standard cardiac MR scanners and radiology workstations. Current studies show that a myocardium with diffuse fibrosis will have greater retention of contrast and thus shorter T1 times than normal myocardium. Amyloidosis is a deposition disease in which the T1 time of the myocardium is likewise altered. These observations suggest the utility of T1 mapping in the detection of diffuse myocardial fibrosis and amyloidosis.

T2 and T2* maps of the myocardium may also be calculated. T2* maps have clinical utility in the assessment of iron content of the myocardium (e.g., hemochromatosis). T2 mapping has been used to evaluate diseases that have associated myocardial edema, such as myocarditis and acute myocardial infarction.

The different clinical and emerging applications of cardiac MRI are described below.

Assessment of Ventricular Function

MRI is a very accurate and highly reproducible technique for measuring ejection fraction and ventricular volumes noninvasively in three dimensions. For this reason, it has become the gold standard to which other modalities are compared [1]. Simpson's rule is applied to determine ejection fraction and volumes. In assessments of volumes and mass, bright-blood SSFP sequences are typically used, with 30–40 phases per cardiac cycle. Breath-holding techniques with acquisition times of 6–12 s reduce blurring of the endocardial border. Generally, for accurate measurement of volume and mass, entire coverage of the left ventricle (LV) with short-axis views from the mitral plane are recommended. Slice thickness is typically 8–10 mm, but in the evaluation of subtle changes the thickness should be reduced appropriately.

MRI is the method of choice for longitudinal follow-up in patients who are undergoing therapeutic interventions. For example, in cardiac stem cell trials MRI was the test of choice to assess changes in LV size, function, and mass [2, 3]. From a research perspective, the sample size needed to detect LV parameter changes in a clinical trial is far smaller, in the range of one order of magnitude, when MRI rather than 2D echocardiography is used, thus markedly reducing the time and cost of patient care and pharmaceutical trials [4, 5].

A unique MR technique, myocardial tagging (spatial modulation of magnetization, SPAMM technique), has been developed, in which heart muscle is labeled with a dark grid and cardiac rotation, strain, and the displacement and deformation of different myocardial layers during the cardiac cycle are analyzed in 3D (Fig. 1). SPAMM technique helps in assessing regional myocardial wall motion but it requires sophisticated software to extract local function parameters such as 2D or 3D myocardial strains [6, 7].

Assessment of Cardiomyopathies

In the visualization of left and right ventricular morphology and function, MRI is a noninvasive tool that has a high degree of accuracy and reproducibility. It is also superior to echocardiography in the determination of ventricular mass and volumes [8] and has become the gold standard for the in vivo identification of the phenotypes of cardiomyopathies [9].

Dilated Cardiomyopathy

In dilated cardiomyopathy, MRI is useful to study ventricular morphology and function (Fig. 2), by analyzing wall thickening, impaired fiber shortening, and end-systolic wall stress, which is a very sensitive parameter of a change in LV systolic function. It can also accurately assess the morphology and function of the right ventricle (RV), which is frequently affected in dilated cardiomyopathy. Late contrast-enhanced T1-weighted images are helpful in detecting the changes that occur in acute myocarditis. In this setting, increased gadolinium accumulation is thought to be due to inflammatory/hyperemia-related increased flow, slow wash-in/wash-out kinetics, and diffusion into necrotic cells [10]. There is evidence of similar changes in chronic dilated cardiomyopathy [11]. Contrast-enhanced MRI may also increase the sensitivity of endomyocardial biopsy by revealing inflamed areas, which aids in determining the appropriate biopsy site. Moreover, the presence and extent of myocardial late enhancement has been shown to predict clinical outcome [12, 13].

Hypertrophic Cardiomyopathy

Due to its high accuracy, MRI is increasingly used to assess morphology, function, tissue status, and degree of

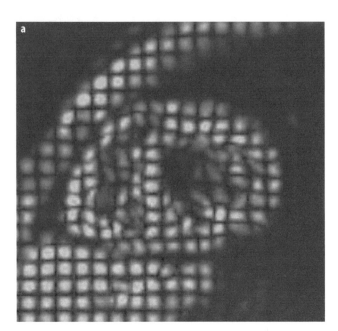
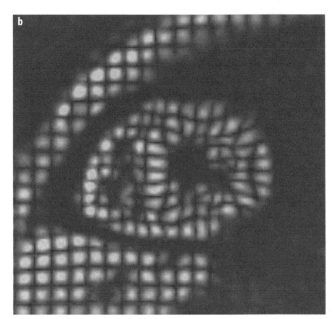

Fig. 1 a, b. Cardiac magnetic resonance (MR) tagging. Magnetic strips are placed in the heart before contraction (diastole, **a**) and then followed throughout the cardiac cycle (systole, **b**) to measure the regional contraction of different portions of the heart. Note that in the left image the tag lines are curved, representing deformation of the myocardium. Cardiac MR is considered the reference standard for the measurement of regional function of the heart compared to other imaging modalities

LV outflow tract (LVOT) obstruction in patients with hypertrophic cardiomyopathy (HCM) (Fig. 3). In addition, it is very accurate in assessing a LV mass, regional hypertrophy patterns, and the different phenotypes of HCM (e.g., apical HCM) [7]. Post-surgical changes after myomectomy can also be reliably monitored [14]. The tur-

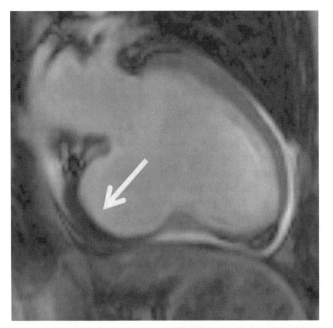

Fig. 2. Bright-blood cine image (SSMP) shows the vertical long-axis view of the left ventricle. There is an aneurysm at the base of the left ventricle; the thickened dark tissue in the aneurysm is the thrombus (*arrow*)

bulent jet during systolic LVOT obstruction is easily detected using suitable echo times (about 4 ms). MRI also detects the systolic anterior motion of the mitral valve, in a four-chamber or a short-axis view on the valvular plane [15], and can be used to document quantify mitral regurgitation. A newer technique is to measure the effective LVOT area by MR planimetry during systole, which overcomes the problem of interstudy variability of the LVOT gradient due to its independence from the hemodynamic status. There are preliminary data showing that assessment of diastolic function using MRI may be superior to the determination of conventional parameters by echocardiography. Analysis of the early untwisting motion of the myocardium could be helpful in assessing diastolic function [16]. Other functional changes that make use of myocardial tagging include a reduction in posterior rotation, reduced radial displacement of the inferoseptal myocardium, reduced 3-D myocardial shortening, and heterogeneity of regional function. With late enhancement imaging after the injection of gadolinium chelates (Fig. 4), MRI may help to detect areas of fibrosis, the prognostic value of which has been demonstrated [17, 18]. MRI also easily detects the acute and chronic changes after septal artery ablation [14, 19].

Arrhythmogenic Right Ventricular Cardiomyopathy/Dysplasia

Arrhythmogenic right ventricular cardiomyopathy/ dysplasia (ARVC/D) is a rare disorder characterized by fibrofatty replacement of the RV free wall. MRI is usually the diagnostic imaging technique of choice for ARVC/D (Fig. 5) [20, 21] as it visualizes the ventricular

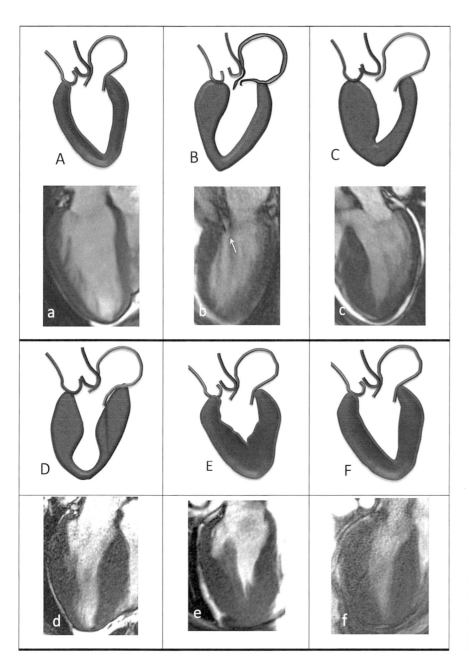

Fig. 3. Morphologic patterns in hypertrophic cardiomyopathy. **A, a** normal LV; **B, b** sigmoid septum; **C, c** reversed septal contour; **D, d** mid-ventricular hypertrophy; **E, e** apical and **F, f** symmetric hypertrophic cardiomyopathy

cavities and walls, with excellent depiction of the myocardial anatomy. Although T1-weighted spin-echo images may reveal fatty infiltration, thinned walls, and dysplastic trabecular structures, these particular findings are actually quite infrequent. Moreover, the subjective assessment of RV wall thinning, wall motion abnormalities, and fatty infiltration of the myocardium by cardiac MR may be problematic. Thus, the international Task Force proposed revised criteria for the clinical diagnosis of ARVC/D. Major and minor criteria defined by cardiac MR contribute to the final diagnosis. Regional RV dysfunction associated with an increase of RV end-diastolic volume ($>$110 mL/m^2 for males and $>$100 mL/m^2 for females) and RV ejection fraction $<$40% are considered to be major criteria for the diagnosis of ARVC/D [22].

Restrictive Cardiomyopathy

Primary infiltration of the myocardium by fibrosis or other tissues leads to the development of restrictive cardiomyopathy, which is characterized by normal LV size and systolic function, severe diastolic dysfunction, and biatrial enlargement. Restrictive cardiomyopathy needs to be differentiated from constrictive pericarditis, which is a primary disease of the pericardium rather than the myocardium. LV size and thickness are quantified using gradient-echo sequences. Atrial enlargement is assessed in a four-chamber view. Mitral regurgitation should be assessed as well. The restrictive diseases that can be effectively assessed using MRI are described below [23, 24].

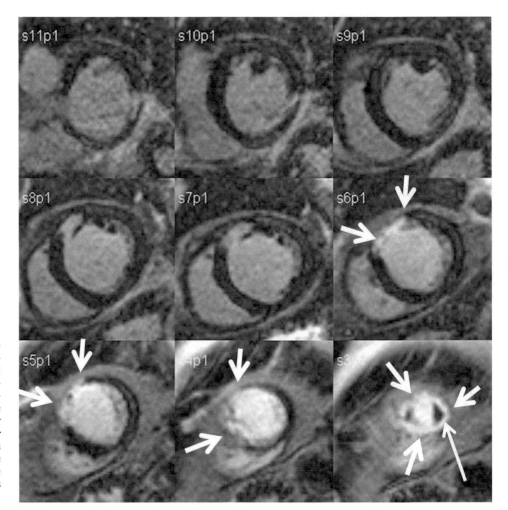

Fig. 4. Delayed gadolinium short-axis images of the heart in a patient with a history of myocardial infarction. The bright, high-signal portion of the anterior and anterolateral walls (*arrows*) of the left ventricle is the area of prior infarction. At the apex (*lower right corner*) the infarct involves the entire circumference of the heart; a small thrombus (*thin arrow*) is present at the apex as an area of dark tissue

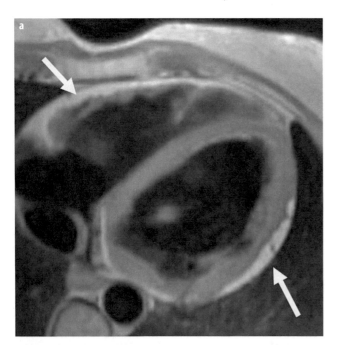
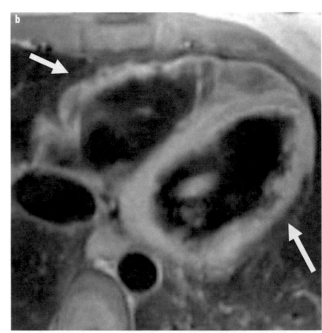

Fig. 5 a, b. Axial black-blood image of the heart. The T1 image (**a**) shows replacement of the myocardium by fat signal (*arrows*) in the left and right ventricles. The fat suppression T1-weighted image (**b**) shows dark signal at the corresponding sites of fat deposition

Sarcoidosis

Cardiac involvement in sarcoidosis produces symptoms in only 5% of patients but has been found in 20–50% of sarcoidosis patients at autopsy. During acute myocardial inflammation, sarcoid infiltrates are visible on MRI as intramyocardial, epicardial, or endocardial hyperhancement in a non-ischemic pattern with increased signal intensity on both T2-weighted and gadolinium-enhanced images [25, 26]. Occasionally, MRI may be useful in guiding endomyocardial biopsy.

Hemochromatosis, Iron Overload Conditions

Extensive iron deposits leading to wall thickening, ventricular dilatation, congestive heart failure, and death characterize cardiac hemochromatosis. Usually, the iron deposits are subepicardial; hence, endomyocardial biopsy may fail to confirm the diagnosis of hemochromatosis. MRI is able to detect the iron deposits because of the very strong paramagnetic properties of iron, which lead to extensive signal loss in native T1- and T2-weighted images. The pattern of focal signal loss in a dysfunctional myocardium associated with an abnormally "dark" liver might be sufficient to confirm the diagnosis of systemic hemochromatosis. However, iron loading in the myocardium does not always correlate with the degree of disease involvement. A particular sequence acquisition that allows T2* calculation (T2* mapping) has been established for the determination of cardiac iron concentrations. T2* values <20–25 ms indicate myocardial iron overload [27-29].

Amyloidosis

Infiltration of the heart by amyloid deposits is found in almost all cases of primary amyloidosis and in 25% of the cases of familial amyloidosis. MRI is the modality of choice for evaluating cardiac amyloidosis, by demonstrating LV wall thickening, reduced systolic function with decreased ejection fraction, and disproportionate atrial enlargement. The more specific finding, obtained on late-enhanced images, is a diffuse, heterogeneous pattern of increased signal intensity on delayed contrast-enhanced inversion recovery T1 images. During the selection of the most appropriate inversion time to null the normal myocardium signal intensity, the null point for the myocardium is often reached before the blood pool is nulled [30]. The shorter T1 of myocardium than of blood reflects the accumulation of amyloid material. This finding is of important value for the final diagnosis of cardiac amyloidosis.

Most recently, T1 mapping of the myocardium has been performed prior to gadolinium administration to determine "native" T1 times. In patients with cardiac amyloidosis, the native T1 time is longer than in normal subjects (e.g., average 1140 ms vs. 958 ms) [31].

Assessment of Pericardial Disease

MRI is ideally suited to evaluating the pericardium (Fig. 6). T1-weighted spin-echo imaging demonstrates the normal pericardium as a thin band (<2 mm) of low signal, bordered by epicardial and pericardial fat, which have a high signal. Because pericardial thickness varies at different levels, the thickness should be measured in axial images at the level of the right atrium, RV, and LV. A thickness >4 mm is considered abnormal and suggests fibrous pericarditis, either acute or chronic (due to surgery, uremia, tumor, infection or connective tissue disease) [32]. Contrast-enhanced MRI may help to better delineate the pericardium in cases of effusive-constrictive pericarditis. Breath-hold or real-time cine gradient echo

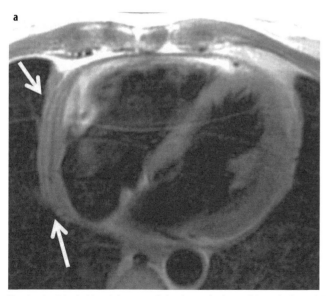
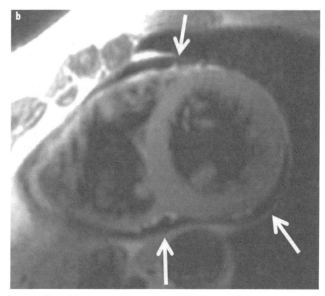

Fig. 6 a, b. Black-blood image of the heart in long (**a**) and short (**b**) axis reveals a thickened pericardium (*arrows*) and fluid (**b**, *arrows*). Pericardial effusion and thickening ⩾4 mm is abnormal

images of the ventricles and phase-velocity mapping of the cardiac valves may be helpful in assessing the significance of pericardial pathology. The same approach is useful to detect other disorders, such as congenital absence of the pericardium, pericardial cysts, or pericardial effusion undetected by other modalities.

Myocarditis

In patients in whom myocarditis is suspected, cardiac MR has become the primary tool for the noninvasive diagnosis of myocardial inflammation. Myocarditis is defined as the inflammation of myocardial tissue and is an important underlying etiology of other myocardial diseases, such as dilated cardiomyopathy. The definitive diagnosis is frequently confirmed based on the clinical history, the clinical assessment, and non-invasive test results, in which case cardiac MR is nowadays crucial. Pericardial effusion has been reported in 32–57% of patients with myocarditis although it is not specific for the diagnosis. T2-weighted or T2 mapping images sensitively detect tissue edema because of the long T2 values of edematous tissue. However, the definitive diagnosis is usually based on the observation on late enhanced images of focal signal increase typically localized to the subepicardial regions of the LV and possibly extension through the ventricular wall. Late enhancement may be multifocal or diffuse in distribution but with no coronary artery disease distribution. Consensual diagnostic criteria using cardiac MR have been proposed ("Lake Louise Consensus Criteria") for the diagnosis of acute myocarditis [33].

Evaluation of Cardiac and Paracardiac Masses

Primary cardiac tumors are rare (0.002–0.3% incidence) and the majority (75%) are benign. Metastatic tumors are 20- to 40-fold more common than primary tumors. MRI is ideal for delineating the morphologic details of a mass (including extent, origin, hemorrhage, vascularity, calcification, and effects on adjacent structures). Protocols include the combined use of axial black-blood sequences and axial bright-blood cine images. Functional MRI is useful to study the pathophysiologic consequences of a cardiac mass. Specifically, benign myxomas (the most common cardiac tumor) appear brighter than myocardium on T2 weighting; cine images may reveal the characteristic mobility of the pedunculated tumor. Lipomas (Fig. 7) appear brighter on spin-echo T1-weighted images. The diagnosis is verified by a decrease in signal intensity using a fat suppression technique [34].

Evaluation of Valvular Diseases

Echocardiography with color Doppler is usually the first-line imaging modality for diagnosing valvular diseases.

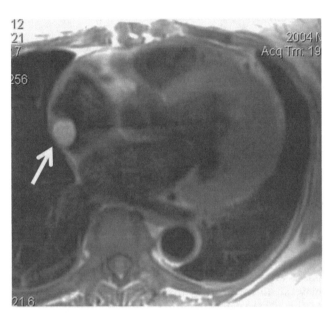

Fig. 7. Black-blood image of the heart in a long-axis view shows a mass (*arrow*) in the right atrium that was subsequently diagnosed as lipoma

MRI is generally reserved for use when other modalities fail or provide suboptimal information. Double inversion recovery sequences can show valve morphology as well as evidence of associated secondary changes (chamber dilatation, myocardial hypertrophy, post-stenotic changes in the great vessels, or thrombus in any of the chambers). Semi-quantitative assessment of valvular stenosis or regurgitation can be obtained by measuring the area of signal void on gradient-echo images. The duration or extent of the signal void correlates with the severity of the aortic stenosis, and the total area of signal loss with the severity of mitral regurgitation. This technique has a very high sensitivity (98%), specificity (95%), and accuracy (97%) for diagnosing aortic and mitral regurgitation. The signal void, however, is dependent upon certain scan parameters, such as echo time, voxel size, and image orientation relative to the flow jet. Phase-contrast MRI can be used to assess the severity of valvular stenosis (by measuring the peak jet velocity) by calculating the valve orifice area and the transvalvular pressure gradient.

Evaluation of Myocardial Perfusion and Ischemia

MRI has been validated as a reliable and useful tool in the assessment of regional left ventricular perfusion [35]. In this setting, MRI relies upon monitoring the first pass of a contrast agent. After a rapid intravenous contrast injection, there is marked signal enhancement first in the right ventricular cavity, then in the left ventricular cavity, and finally in the left ventricular myocardium. This is completed within 20–30 s. Peak signal intensity is related to the concentration of the contrast agent in the local tissue and is directly proportional to coronary blood flow. A comparison between perfusion MRI at rest and after the infusion of pharmacologic agents (adenosine, regadenoson, and persantine) and standard methods (angiography or radionuclide scintigraphy) has shown that the sensitivity of MRI is equal or superior to stress myocardial radionuclide scintigraphy, and the specificity is similar [36, 37]. Assessing wall motion further improves the performance of MRI [38].

Myocardial Viability

Viability has been defined as dysfunctional myocardium sustained by coronary artery disease with limited or absent scarring and the potential of functional recovery after revascularization. Cardiac MRI may help in predicting potential recovery based on the degree of high enhancement through the myocardium [39]. Alternatively, as in dobutamine echocardiography, inotropic stimulation of LV contraction at a low dose of dobutamine is a predictor of recovery [39, 40].

Coronary Artery Imaging

MRI of the coronary arteries has had significant progress in recent years. Whole-heart MRI technique involves axial electrocardiogram-gated SSFP acquisitions with navigator pulses to track the motion of the diaphragm [41-44]. Fat suppression is used to suppress mediastinal and pericardial fat. Acquisitions take between 5 and 15 min during free breathing. At 1.5T in particular, no contrast agent is used. The spatial resolution of whole-heart acquisitions is approximately 1 mm in the z-axis direction, which is greater than the resolution of CT scanning (0.5–0.6 mm) [43, 45]. Nevertheless, image quality is excellent for the exclusion of coronary artery anomalies. Unlike CT scanning, coronary MRI is not sensitive to highly calcified coronary artery calcification. Given the relative ease of application, coronary imaging is often added as a routine part of the protocol for young patients with unexplained chest pain. The detection rate of coronary artery stenosis in selected patient populations appears to be similar to that achieved with CT scanning, except that distal arteries less well evaluated [43, 46]. In addition, the technique has a lower technical success rate than CT scanning: non-diagnostic examinations occur in about 20% of patients.

Conclusion

MRI has emerged as a definitive examination for a wide array of complex cardiovascular problems. Its is a prominent imaging modality in multiple facets of nonischemic and ischemic cardiomyopathy. Continuing challenges are the complexity of the modality compared to CT scanning

and the wide variety of tools that the imaging physician must thoroughly understand in order to appropriately deploy them.

References

1. Hundley WG, Bluemke DA, Finn JP et al (2010) ACCF/ACR/AHA/NASCI/SCMR 2010 expert consensus document on cardiovascular magnetic resonance: a report of the American College of Cardiology Foundation Task Force on Expert Consensus Documents. J Am Coll Cardiol 55:2614-2662.
2. Makkar RR, Smith RR, Cheng K et al (2012) Intracoronary cardiosphere-derived cells for heart regeneration after myocardial infarction (CADUCEUS): a prospective, randomised phase 1 trial. Lancet 379:895-904.
3. Rokosh G, Ghafghazi S, Bolli R (2013) Mechanisms of stem cell effects: insights from MRI. Minerva Cardioangiol 61:605-616.
4. Grothues F, Smith GC, Moon JC et al (2002) Comparison of interstudy reproducibility of cardiovascular magnetic resonance with two-dimensional echocardiography in normal subjects and in patients with heart failure or left ventricular hypertrophy. Am J Cardiol 90:29-34.
5. Bellenger NG, Burgess MI, Ray SG et al (2000) Comparison of left ventricular ejection fraction and volumes in heart failure by echocardiography, radionuclide ventriculography and cardiovascular magnetic resonance; are they interchangeable? Eur Heart J 21:1387-1396.
6. Reeder SB, Du YP, Lima JA, Bluemke DA (2001) Advanced cardiac MR imaging of ischemic heart disease. Radiographics 21:1047-1074.
7. Shehata ML, Cheng S, Osman NF et al (2009) Myocardial tissue tagging with cardiovascular magnetic resonance. J Cardiovasc Magn Reson 11:55.
8. Bottini PB, Carr AA, Prisant LM et al (1995) Magnetic resonance imaging compared to echocardiography to assess left ventricular mass in the hypertensive patient. Am J Hypertens 8:221-228.
9. Hundley WG, Bluemke DA, Finn JP et al (2010) ACCF/ACR/AHA/NASCI/SCMR 2010 expert consensus document on cardiovascular magnetic resonance: a report of the American College of Cardiology Foundation Task Force on Expert Consensus Documents. Circulation 121:2462-2508.
10. Davies MJ (2000) The cardiomyopathies: an overview. Heart 83:469-474.
11. Nazarian S, Bluemke DA, Lardo AC et al (2005) Magnetic resonance assessment of the substrate for inducible ventricular tachycardia in nonischemic cardiomyopathy. Circulation 112:2821-2825.
12. Piers SR, Tao Q, van Huls van Taxis CF et al (2013) Contrast-enhanced MRI-derived scar patterns and associated ventricular tachycardias in nonischemic cardiomyopathy: implications for the ablation strategy. Circ Arrhythm Electrophysiol 6:875-883.
13. Doltra A, Amundsen BH, Gebker R (2013) Emerging concepts for myocardial late gadolinium enhancement MRI. Curr Cardiol Rev 9:185-190.
14. Wu KC (2006) Utility of cardiac MRI in the diagnosis of hypertrophic cardiomyopathy. Curr Cardiol Rep 8:41.
15. Maron MS, Olivotto I, Harrigan C et al (2011) Mitral valve abnormalities identified by cardiovascular magnetic resonance represent a primary phenotypic expression of hypertrophic cardiomyopathy. Circulation 124:40-47.
16. Ho CY, Sweitzer NK, McDonough B et al (2002) Assessment of diastolic function with Doppler tissue imaging to predict genotype in preclinical hypertrophic cardiomyopathy. Circulation 105:2992-2997.

17. Maron MS (2012) Clinical utility of cardiovascular magnetic resonance in hypertrophic cardiomyopathy. J Cardiovasc Magn Reson 14:13.
18. Noureldin RA, Liu S, Nacif MS et al (2012) The diagnosis of hypertrophic cardiomyopathy by cardiovascular magnetic resonance. J Cardiovasc Magn Reson 14:17.
19. Wu KC, Heldman AW, Brinker JA et al (2001) Microvascular obstruction after nonsurgical septal reduction for the treatment of hypertrophic cardiomyopathy. Circulation 104:1868.
20. te Riele AS, Tandri H, Bluemke DA (2014) Arrhythmogenic right ventricular cardiomyopathy (ARVC): cardiovascular magnetic resonance update. J Cardiovasc Magn Reson 16:50.
21. Jain A, Tandri H, Calkins H, Bluemke DA (2008) Role of cardiovascular magnetic resonance imaging in arrhythmogenic right ventricular dysplasia. J Cardiovasc Magn Reson 10:32.
22. Marcus FI, McKenna WJ, Sherrill D et al (2010) Diagnosis of arrhythmogenic right ventricular cardiomyopathy/dysplasia: proposed modification of the task force criteria. Circulation 121:1533-1541.
23. Friedrich MG (2000) Magnetic resonance imaging in cardiomyopathies. J Cardiovasc Magn Reson 2:67-82.
24. Schulz-Menger J, Friedrich MG (2000) Magnetic resonance imaging in patients with cardiomyopathies: when and why. Herz 25:384-391.
25. Vignaux O (2005) Cardiac sarcoidosis: spectrum of MRI features. AJR Am J Roentgenol 184:249-254.
26. Tadamura E, Yamamuro M, Kubo S et al (2005) Effectiveness of delayed enhanced MRI for identification of cardiac sarcoidosis: comparison with radionuclide imaging. AJR Am J Roentgenol 185:110-115.
27. Pennell DJ, Berdoukas V, Karagiorga M et al (2006) Randomized controlled trial of deferiprone or deferoxamine in beta-thalassemia major patients with asymptomatic myocardial siderosis. Blood 107:3738-3744.
28. Pennell DJ (2005) T2* magnetic resonance and myocardial iron in thalassemia. Ann N Y Acad Sci 1054:373-378.
29. Carpenter JP, Grasso AE, Porter JB (2013) On myocardial siderosis and left ventricular dysfunction in hemochromatosis. J Cardiovasc Magn Reson 15:24.
30. Maceira AM, Prasad SK, Hawkins PN (2008) Cardiovascular magnetic resonance and prognosis in cardiac amyloidosis. J Cardiovasc Magn Reson 10:54.
31. Karamitsos TD, Piechnik SK, Banypersad SM et al (2013) Noncontrast T1 mapping for the diagnosis of cardiac amyloidosis. JACC Cardiovasc Imaging 6:488-497.
32. Rajiah P (2011) Cardiac MRI: Part 2, pericardial diseases. AJR Am J Roentgenol 197:W621-634.
33. Friedrich MG, Sechtem U, Schulz-Menger J et al (2009) Cardiovascular magnetic resonance in myocarditis: A JACC White Paper. J Am Coll Cardiol 53:1475-1487.
34. O'Donnell DH, Abbara S, Chaithiraphan V et al (2009) Cardiac tumors: optimal cardiac MR sequences and spectrum of imaging appearances. AJR Am J Roentgenol 193:377-387.
35. Wolk MJ, Bailey SR, Doherty JU et al (2014) ACCF/AHA/ASE/ASNC/HFSA/HRS/SCAI/SCCT/SCMR/STS 2013 multimodality appropriate use criteria for the detection and risk assessment of stable ischemic heart disease: a report of the American College of Cardiology Foundation Appropriate Use Criteria Task Force, American Heart Association, American Society of Echocardiography, American Society of Nuclear Cardiology, Heart Failure Society of America, Heart Rhythm Society, Society for Cardiovascular Angiography and Interventions, Society of Cardiovascular Computed Tomography, Society for Cardiovascular Magnetic Resonance, and Society of Thoracic Surgeons. J Am Coll Cardiol 63:380-406.
36. Nandalur KR, Dwamena BA, Choudhri AF et al (2007) Diagnostic performance of stress cardiac magnetic resonance imaging in the detection of coronary artery disease: a meta-analysis. J Am Coll Cardiol 50:1343-1353.
37. Lipinski MJ, McVey CM, Berger JS et al (2013) Prognostic value of stress cardiac magnetic resonance imaging in patients with known or suspected coronary artery disease: a systematic review and meta-analysis. J Am Coll Cardiol 62:826-838.
38. Schwitter J, Wacker CM, Wilke N et al (2013) MR-IMPACT II: Magnetic Resonance Imaging for Myocardial Perfusion Assessment in Coronary artery disease Trial: perfusion-cardiac magnetic resonance vs. single-photon emission computed tomography for the detection of coronary artery disease: a comparative multicentre, multivendor trial. Eur Heart J 34:775-781.
39. Shan K, Constantine G, Sivananthan M, Flamm SD (2004) Role of cardiac magnetic resonance imaging in the assessment of myocardial viability. Circulation 109:1328-1334.
40. Gutberlet M, Frohlich M, Mehl S et al (2005) Myocardial viability assessment in patients with highly impaired left ventricular function: comparison of delayed enhancement, dobutamine stress MRI, end-diastolic wall thickness, and TI201-SPECT with functional recovery after revascularization. Eur Radiol 15:872-880.
41. Yonezawa M, Nagata M, Kitagawa K et al (2014) Quantitative analysis of 1.5-T whole-heart coronary MR angiograms obtained with 32-channel cardiac coils: a comparison with conventional quantitative coronary angiography. Radiology 271:356-364.
42. Yoon YE, Kitagawa K, Kato S et al (2012) Prognostic value of coronary magnetic resonance angiography for prediction of cardiac events in patients with suspected coronary artery disease. J Am Coll Cardiol 60:2316-2322.
43. Sakuma H (2011) Coronary CT versus MR angiography: the role of MR angiography. Radiology 258:340-349.
44. Nagata M, Kato S, Kitagawa K et al (2011) Diagnostic accuracy of 1.5-T unenhanced whole-heart coronary MR angiography performed with 32-channel cardiac coils: initial single-center experience. Radiology 259:384-392.
45. Kefer J, Coche E, Legros G et al (2005) Head-to-head comparison of three-dimensional navigator-gated magnetic resonance imaging and 16-slice computed tomography to detect coronary artery stenosis in patients. J Am Coll Cardiol 46:92-100.
46. Pouleur AC, le Polain de Waroux JB, Kefer J et al (2008) Direct comparison of whole-heart navigator-gated magnetic resonance coronary angiography and 40- and 64-slice multidetector row computed tomography to detect the coronary artery stenosis in patients scheduled for conventional coronary angiography. Circ Cardiovasc Imaging 1:114-121.

An Integrative Approach to the Imaging of Ischemic Heart Disease

Albert de Roos[1], Danilo Neglia[2]

[1] Department of Radiology, Leiden University Medical, Leiden, The Netherlands
[2] Institute of Clinical Physiology, CNR National Research Council, Pisa, Italy

Introduction

A multitude of invasive and non-invasive imaging techniques are available to evaluate coronary artery disease (CAD) and its effect on the myocardium [1]. Traditionally, invasive coronary X-ray angiography is the mainstay for diagnosing coronary artery stenosis. To a large extent, coronary computed tomography angiography (CCTA) has reached a high level of sophistication for performing coronary angiography non-invasively. CCTA is, in particular, highly successful for excluding coronary artery stenosis. Coronary magnetic resonance (MR) angiography is still hampered by a lack of robustness and consistent image quality. CT and MR techniques to image the coronary wall, even before the development of overt plaques, are still being tested. Plaque imaging is technically challenging, such that there is interest in improving the reliability and robustness of non-invasive techniques. Plaque characterization by CT largely involves the visual inspection and grading of plaques (calcified, non-calcified and partly calcified). So-called soft plaques seem to be more prone to rupture than those that are fully calcified. Other plaque characteristics that may relate to worse outcome include expansive or positive remodeling without high-grade narrowing, small or "spotty" calcifications localized in soft plaques, and adventitial high density ("ring sign"). Currently, post-processing software is available to extract the coronary tree and quantify the plaque components from CT images. However, the traditional calcium (Agatston) score is still useful for quantifying the amount of coronary calcium as a risk factor for all-cause mortality. CCTA may improve the prediction of coronary events especially when used together with the calcium score. The evaluation of comprehensive plaque burden integrates information from calcified and non-calcified components.

The limited information (i.e. vessel narrowing) provided by luminography using either invasive X-ray angiography or non-invasive CT or MR angiography has become apparent and has paved the way for functional imaging. In invasive X-ray angiography, the current method of reference, the pressure gradient across a coronary stenosis, is measured as a means to estimate the functional significance of a coronary stenosis. The fractional flow reserve, as measured by the pressure wire, indicates whether a coronary stenosis causes downstream ischemia in response to stress. This functional knowledge is crucial for the optimization and timing of revascularization therapy by stent placement or surgery. Coronary interventions guided by the fractional flow reserve have been shown to improve outcome in treated patients.

Even more relevant information on the presence of functionally significant CAD and the related risk can be gathered non invasively by stress myocardial perfusion imaging (MPI) or wall motion imaging. The preferred imaging technique varies between countries, regions, and hospitals, partly because of local expertise and customs and partly because guidelines do not specify one technique over another. Among the non-invasive tests, functionally significant CAD can be detected by assessing stress-induced changes in myocardial perfusion by MPI, as single photon computed emission tomography (SPECT), positron emission tomography (PET), or cardiac magnetic resonance (CMR), or by detecting stress-induced changes in regional myocardial function by wall motion imaging using echocardiography or CMR. Previous studies have compared the diagnostic accuracy of some of these modalities but a large multi-center study providing definitive evidence on the best imaging choice in specific patient groups has yet to be conducted.

Non Invasive Imaging in Patients with Suspected Stable CAD

Based on recent European guidelines, patients with suspected stable CAD should be managed using non-invasive cardiac imaging, to select patients for invasive coronary angiography (ICA) and to determine medical and possibly interventional treatments. Non-invasive imaging is not only used to recognize the presence of anatomically obstructive coronary disease but, more importantly, to

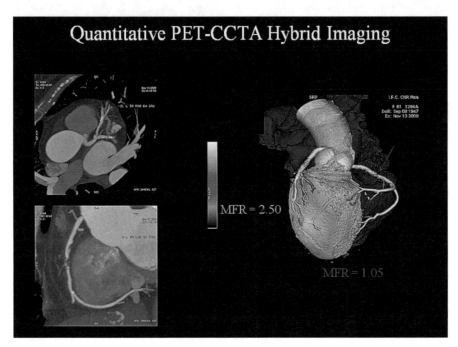

Fig. 1. Hybrid PET-CCTA imaging in a patient with stable angina. Perfusion PET images were acquired at rest and during dipyridamole stress, using 13N-ammonia as the flow tracer. Absolute myocardial blood flow (MBF) (mL/min/g) was quantified under two different conditions. Myocardial flow reserve (MFR) was computed as the ratio of dipyridamole/resting MBF. PET images show a critical downstream stenosis of the right coronary artery, documented at CCTA (*arrow*) and a large inducible perfusion defect during dipyridamole stress corresponding to a severely depressed MFR at quantitative analysis. This is an example of high-risk findings detected during imaging, which in this patient, indicated invasive coronary angiography and possible coronary revascularization

stratify future cardiovascular risk. Only patients at higher risk will be referred to interventional procedures, with the final goal of improving their outcome [2].

The management of patients with stable chest pain starts with an estimation of the pre-test probability (PTP) of CAD, based on age, sex, and type of symptoms according to an updated predictive model [3]. Patients with a PTP score <15% should not undergo further testing while in patients with a PTP >85% non invasive testing is not indicated for diagnosis but only for risk stratification [2]. According to international guidelines, patients with an intermediate PTP should preferably undergo stress MPI rather than exercise echocardiography [2, 4]. CCTA is considered a reasonable alternative in intermediate-low likelihood patients or in case of doubtful stress tests results.

Only in the presence of high-risk findings at non invasive imaging should patients be referred to invasive investigation and possible coronary intervention [2, 5]. High-risk findings are defined by the presence of left main or proximal left anterior descending arterial disease and/or three-vessel disease as determined by CTCA and/or by the documentation of significant inducible myocardial ischemia (>10% of the left ventricular myocardium) at stress testing. ICA in patients with stable CAD is not recommended as a first testing method, although in current practice as many as 30% of patients with no symptoms (including no angina) and 16% of patients without non-invasive testing, and 15% of those with prior normal non-invasive testing (resting electrocardiography, echocardiography, CT, or a stress test) undergo ICA [3]. Perhaps as a consequence, 62% of stable patients without known CAD who undergo elective coronary angiography in the USA and 42% of those in Europe have no significant stenoses [3, 6]. Conversely, non-invasive testing does not always guide clinical management since 27% of patients with high-risk imaging results do not undergo ICA [7].

Nuclear Myocardial Perfusion Imaging (MPI) and Hybrid CCTA-MPI Imaging for the Diagnosis of Stable CAD

Stress MPI by SPECT and PET is an established and widely used approach in the diagnostic and risk assessment of patients with suspected CAD. These techniques provide information on the presence, extent, and severity of myocardial perfusion abnormalities, which define the functional significance of coronary disease and are related to event risk. Since CCTA is able to depict anatomical abnormalities of the vessel wall and has a high predictive value in excluding significant coronary stenoses and in identifying high-risk coronary anatomy, a combination of functional and anatomical information, obtained either by side-by-side interpretation of stress MPI and CCTA images or by using a hybrid approach, has recently been proposed as a more accurate strategy in patients with known or suspected CAD [8] (Fig. 1).

Large observational studies have demonstrated that a normal MPI yields a favorable prognosis, with an annualized event-rate of 0.6%, while an abnormal scan implies a 3- to 7-fold increase in annual cardiac events, especially those related to the extent and severity of perfusion defects [9-11]. Additional prognostic data on left ventricular volumes and function (e.g., ejection fraction) at baseline and possible evidence of transient left ventricular dysfunction after stress are provided by the gated acquisition of SPECT data [12].

The demonstration by SPECT imaging of significant inducible myocardial ischemia not only defines a high cardiovascular risk for a specific patient but also guides treatment to modify that risk and improve outcome. Hachamovitch et al. [13] demonstrated that revascularization procedures have a beneficial impact on outcome only in the presence of ischemia involving ≥10% of the left ventricular myocardium at SPECT imaging. In a prospective nuclear substudy of the COURAGE trial, a better prognosis was related to the extent of ischemia reduction evidenced by SPECT [14]. These data justify the use of SPECT as one of the techniques recommended by the European Society of Cardiology (ESC) guidelines to diagnose CAD, stratify risk in patients with suspected disease, and guide further management and treatment of the patient to improve outcome.

In analogy to SPECT, the presence and extent of myocardial perfusion defects demonstrated by PET provide strong prognostic information [15]. PET allows measurement of absolute myocardial blood flow and flow reserve (MFR) and has incremental prognostic value compared to the evaluation of perfusion defects alone. A blunted MFR is an independent predictor of risk compared to more common prognostic indicators, such as transient regional perfusion defects, previous myocardial infarction, and left ventricular ejection fraction [16]. Interestingly, high-risk, diffuse anatomical CAD may manifest as apparently normal regional perfusion images with homogeneous tracer distribution; however, it may be recognized by global reductions of myocardial blood flow and MFR at quantitative PET imaging [17].

Improved risk stratification is obtained by combining the anatomical information of CCTA with the functional data of MPI. The likelihood of diagnosing obstructive CAD by ICA is highest when both CCTA and MPI are abnormal [18]. The hybrid approach is also useful to stratify risk in patients with doubtful results at either functional or anatomical evaluation. Accordingly, a combined anatomical and functional assessment provides complementary rather than overlapping diagnostic and prognostic information.

CT and CMR Imaging in the Diagnosis of Stable CAD

CT and MRI techniques have also been developed to evaluate myocardial perfusion. Currently, in MPI, MR is more widely used than CT. Both are performed with the patient at rest and the results are compared to perfusion under adenosine stress. MR perfusion imaging provides dynamic information on the wash-in of gadolinium-based contrast agents into the myocardium. Ischemia will be visualized during stress MR perfusion as a perfusion defect ("cold spot"). CT perfusion is more static and provides perfusion information mostly at a fixed time point in a non-dynamic manner. The difference between ischemic and normal myocardium is far greater on MR than on CT imaging.

Non Invasive Imaging of the Heart and Large Vessels

Cross-sectional CT and MR imaging are well suited to assess the gross morphology of the heart and large vessels. CT is currently routinely applied to evaluate acute chest pain (life-threatening coronary occlusion, aortic dissection, and pulmonary embolism should initially be excluded). However, it should be noted that the differential diagnosis of acute chest pain is quite extensive and many other causes may be incidentally diagnosed by CT (e.g., pneumonia, lung disease, chest wall disease, pericardial disease). In many hospitals "excluding pulmonary embolism" is a very common and sometimes misused indication for urgent CT of the chest. In the emergency setting, CT is a preferred technique due to its speed, availability, robust image quality, and ease of use in acutely ill patients who may require assisted ventilation and direct supervision. The complications of ischemic heart disease may be well shown by CT and/or MR imaging (e.g., scar, aneurysm, contained rupture, thrombus).

MR imaging is a versatile technique for evaluating many aspects of ischemic and non-ischemic heart disease. In stable patients with suspected CAD, imaging will mostly focus on the detection of coronary stenosis and defining the functional significance of the stenosis. The focus of imaging will be different in patients with suspected acute coronary syndromes (acute infarction, unstable angina pectoris). In the acute setting it will be important to use imaging tools to diagnose or exclude coronary occlusion, especially when the clinical signs and symptoms are inconclusive. CCTA is an excellent gatekeeper for excluding CAD in the emergency room setting and thereby decrease the length of stay of patients in the hospital. MR MPI has also successfully been employed as a gatekeeper in the emergency room setting for the exclusion of ischemia due to coronary artery stenosis. After coronary artery occlusion, the dependent myocardium distal from the occluded coronary artery is at risk of necrosis, thus mandating early and timely intervention. The area at risk may be visualized on T2-weighted MR sequences, which will show a region of high signal intensity due to developing edema in the area at risk. Early intervention may prevent myocardial necrosis in the area at risk ("aborted" infarction). The necrosis develops over several hours, starting as a wavefront at the endocardial site within the confines of the area at risk that, when not halted by intervention, then progresses over time and may fill the entire area at risk. There is some discussion as to whether T2-weighted techniques are reliable enough for quantification of the risk area, because of potential imaging artifacts. Nonetheless, MR-based estimates of the area at risk have been incorporated as end-points in several cardiology trials.

The wave front of progressing necrosis can be defined very accurately by late gadolinium enhancement (LGE). Combining LGE and T2-weighted MR images is an option to assess the infarct:risk ratio as an important clinical parameter. LGE has been used for over 25 years to characterize myocardial necrosis, in both the acute setting and chronic setting. T2-weighted MR techniques may be useful to distinguish acute from chronic infarcts. Acute infarcts will show LGE in conjunction with high myocardial signal (acute edema) in the area at risk, whereas chronic infarcts will show LGE in the absence (no edema present) of high signal intensity in the myocardium at risk.

CT and CMR Imaging in Patients with Heart Failure

The epidemic growth of the number of patients suffering from heart failure constitutes a diagnostic and therapeutic challenge. CT and MR imaging are playing an increasingly important role in the work-up and follow-up of patients with heart failure. The diagnostic challenge in heart failure is to identify its most likely cause. First and foremost, it is important to exclude CAD, e.g., by using CCTA to exclude coronary stenosis and plaques. However, it may also be important to evaluate the myocardium directly, to assess the presence of myocardial scar and infarction, because in a small number of patients infarction may be present after recanalization of a previously occluded coronary artery. In this respect LGE by MR imaging has a central role in the identification of ischemic myocardial scar (i.e., subendocardial LGE).

The MR protocol in the evaluation of patients with heart failure includes functional imaging (global and regional function), velocity-encoded MR to assess mitral flow, T2-weighted sequences to assess edema, T1-weighted sequences (T1 mapping with techniques such as Look-Locker technique or modified Look-Locker inversion recovery sequences) to assess diffuse fibrosis and other diffuse myocardial infiltration unseen with LGE, and LGE sequences to assess scar location, size, and distribution. The combined assessment of the location and extent of ischemic scar, the presence and severity of secondary mitral regurgitation, and precise estimates of left ventricular volumes provide a surgical road-map for planning scar resection in conjunction with mitral valve repair (e.g., Dor procedure).

These combined techniques constitute a comprehensive set of tools with which to obtain a specific diagnosis of underlying ischemic cardiomyopathy. They also offer a wide array of diagnostic features that may be helpful in differentiating ischemic from non-ischemic cardiomyopathy and in further differentiating the multitude of common and uncommon causes of non-ischemic cardiomyopathies. In the differential diagnosis of non-ischemic cardiomyopathy it may be useful to make an initial distinction between dilated (i.e., globally dilated left ventricle, thin walls) and hypertrophic (thick walls, locally or diffuse) phenotypes. The dilated phenotype is a quite common cause of heart failure and has an extensive differential diagnosis of its own. Primary (idiopathic), secondary (toxic, infiltration, etc.), and complex genetic forms of cardiomyopathy may present with the dilated phenotype. The idiopathic form of dilated cardiomyopathy is diagnosed after excluding secondary forms. Idiopathic dilated cardiomyopathy may be further characterized by LGE. Among the LGE patterns observed in dilated cardiomyopathy are the so-called midwall stripe as well as patchy, diffuse, and subepicardial enhancement. Interestingly, LGE has prognostic implications in idiopathic dilated cardiomyopathy, as the midwall stripe pattern may herald arrhythmias and sudden death. LGE patterns may be helpful for risk stratification and guiding treatment options (e.g., implantable cardioverter-defibrillator).

The differential diagnosis of hypertrophic phenotypes starts with the exclusion of arterial hypertension and aortic stenosis as the underlying causes of pressure overload on the left ventricle. It is also important to distinguish global or diffuse hypertrophy from local hypertrophy ("lumps and bumps," as seen in genetic forms of hypertrophic cardiomyopathy). The diffuse hypertrophic phenotype has a differential diagnosis that should be considered from the imaging perspective. Genetically determined hypertrophic (obstructive) cardiomyopathy may present as diffuse global hypertrophy, although localized forms are more common (e.g., classic asymmetric septal hypertrophy). Many common, but also uncommon, infiltrative myocardial diseases may present with the hypertrophic phenotype (e.g., amyloid, storage diseases, Fabry's disease, inflammatory processes such as sarcoid, medication such as amiodarone and chloroquine). Genetically determined hypertrophic cardiomyopathy has many additional morphological features that may be a clue for the correct diagnosis, such as the appearance and length of the mitral leaflets, the systolic anterior motion of the anterior leaflet of the mitral valve, secondary mitral insufficiency and atrial enlargement, crypts in the myocardial wall as an early sign of hypertrophy in a mutation carrier, and various patterns of LGE. Hypertrophic cardiomyopathy is a common cause of sudden death in athletes and apparently healthy young people, although the death rate may be lower than previously suggested. The risk of arrhythmias and sudden death may be related to the presence and extent of scar tissue as demonstrated by LGE. Typical LGE enhancement occurs at the right ventricular attachment points, although the scar can be widely distributed in various patterns. A transmural infarct-like pattern in an aneurysmatical apical scar may imply a worse prognosis.

Finally, amyloid cardiomyopathy may present as a hypertrophic phenotype. The LGE pattern may demonstrate a typical diffuse subendocardial pattern throughout the left ventricle, possibly also involving the right ventricle and atrial walls. T1 mapping techniques are currently used to characterize diffuse myocardial involvement to better advantage, such as in amyloid cardiomyopathy. T1 mapping is a promising tool for characterizing diffuse myocardial fibrosis in many forms of cardiomyopathy presenting as heart failure. The occurrence of diffuse myocardial fibrosis may be an important turning point in the natural history of aggravating heart disease, but it may also be a target for specific medical therapy.

Myocardial Perfusion Imaging in Patients with Heart Failure Who Are Candidates for Revascularization

The 2012 ESC guidelines for the diagnosis and treatment of heart failure recommend the consideration of MPI in heart failure patients with suspected CAD, to determine the extension of ischemia and the presence of viability before revascularization [19]. The assessment of myocardial viability has been an important step in therapeutic decision-making in patients with left ventricular dysfunction who are candidates for coronary revascularization. In a classical meta-analysis, patients with myocardial viability had a better outcome than those without myocardial viability [19]. However, in a sub-study of the STICH (Surgical Treatment for Ischemic Heart Failure) trial, the presence of myocardial viability in patients with ischemic severe heart failure randomized to revascularization or optimal medical therapy had no effect on all-cause mortality [20]. Conversely, in the presence of extensive viability (>10% of the myocardium), early revascularization was associated with improved survival compared with medical therapy [21]. Indeed, current heart failure guidelines recommend the consideration of noninvasive imaging for the assessment of both inducible ischemia and viable myocardium in the heart failure population.

References

1. Higgins CB, de Roos A (eds) (2014) MRI and CT of the cardiovascular system, 3rd Ed. Wolters Kluwer/Lippincott Williams & Wilkins.
2. Montalescot G, Sechtem U, Achenbach S et al (2013) ESC guidelines on the management of stable coronary artery disease: The Task Force on the management of stable coronary artery disease of the European Society of Cardiology. Eur Heart J 34:2949-3003.
3. Genders TS, Steyerberg EW, Alkadhi H et al; CAD Consortium (2011) A clinical prediction rule for the diagnosis of CAD: validation, updating, and extension. Eur Heart J 32:1316-1330.
4. American College of Cardiology Foundation Appropriate Use Criteria Task Force (2014) CCF/AHA/ASE/ASNC/ HFSA/ HRS/SCAI/SCCT/SCMR/STS 2013 multimodality appropriate use criteria for the detection and risk assessment of stable ischemic heart disease: a report of the American College of Cardiology Foundation Appropriate Use Criteria Task Force, American Heart Association, American Society of Echocardiography, American Society of Nuclear Cardiology, Heart Failure Society of America, Heart Rhythm Society, Society for Cardiovascular Angiography and Interventions, Society of Cardiovascular Computed Tomography, Society for Cardiovascular Magnetic Resonance, and Society of Thoracic Surgeons. J Am Coll Cardiol 63:380-406.
5. ACCF/SCAI/AATS/AHA/ASE/ASNC/HFSA/HRS/SCCM/ SCCT/ SCMR/STS (2012) 2012 appropriate use criteria for diagnostic catheterization: a report of the American College of Cardiology Foundation Appropriate Use Criteria Task Force, Society for Cardiovascular Angiography and Interventions, American Association for Thoracic Surgery, American Heart Association, American Society of Echocardiography, American Society of Nuclear Cardiology, Heart Failure Society of America, Heart Rhythm Society, Society of Critical Care Medicine, Society of Cardiovascular Computed Tomography, Society for Cardiovascular Magnetic Resonance, and Society of Thoracic Surgeons. J Am Coll Cardiol 59:1995-2027.
6. Patel MR, Peterson ED, Dai D et al (2010) Low diagnostic yield of elective coronary angiography. N Engl J Med 362: 886-895.
7. Hachamovitch R, Nutter B, Hlatky MA et al; SPARC Investigators (2012) Patient management after noninvasive cardiac imaging results from SPARC (Study of myocardial perfusion and coronary anatomy imaging roles in coronary artery disease). J Am Coll Cardiol 59:462-474.
8. Flotats A, Gutberlet M, Marcassa C et al; Cardiovascular Committee of the EANM, the ESCR and the ECNC, Hybrid cardiac imaging: SPECT/CT and PET/CT. A joint position statement by the European Association of Nuclear Medicine (EANM), the European Society of Cardiac Radiology (ESCR) and the European Council of Nuclear Cardiology (ECNC). Eur J Nucl Med Mol Imaging 1:201-212.
9. Shaw LJ IA (2003) Prognostic value of gated myocardial perfusion SPECT. J Nucl Cardiol 2:171-185.
10. Elhendy A, Schinkel A, Bax JJ et al (2003) Long-term prognosis after a normal exercise stress Tc-99m sestamibi SPECT study. J Nucl Cardiol 10:261-266.
11. Klocke FJ, Baird MG, Lorell BH et al (2003) ACC/AHA/ASNC guidelines for the clinical use of cardiac radionuclide imaging—executive summary: a report of the American College of Cardiology/American Heart Association Task Force on Practice Guidelines (ACC/AHA/ASNC Committee to Revise the 1995 Guidelines for the Clinical Use of Cardiac Radionuclide Imaging). Circulation 1404-1418.
12. Abidov A, Bax JJ, Hayes SW et al (2003) Transient ischemic dilation ratio of the left ventricle is a significant predictor of future cardiac events in patients with otherwise normal myocardial perfusion SPECT. J Am Coll Cardiol 42:1818-1825.
13. Hachamovitch R, Hayes S, Friedman JD et al (2003) Determinants of risk and its temporal variation in patients with normal stress myocardial perfusion scans: what is the warranty period of a normal scan? J Am Coll Cardiol 41:1329-1340.
14. Shaw LJ, Berman DS, Maron DJ et al; COURAGE Investigators (2008) Optimal medical therapy with or without percutaneous coronary intervention to reduce ischemic burden: results from the Clinical Outcomes Utilizing Revascularization and Aggressive Drug Evaluation (COURAGE) trial nuclear substudy. Circulation 117:1283-1291.
15. Murthy VL, Naya M, Foster CR et al (2011) Improved cardiac risk assessment with noninvasive measures of coronary flow reserve. Circulation 124:2215-2224.
16. Herzog BA, Husmann L, Valenta I et al (2009) Long-term prognostic value of 13N-ammonia myocardial perfusion positron emission tomography added value of coronary flow reserve. J Am Coll Cardiol 54:150-156.
17. Danad I, Raijmakers PG, Harms HJ et al (2014) Effect of cardiac hybrid 15O-water PET/CT imaging on downstream referral for invasive coronary angiography and revascularization rate. Eur Heart J Cardiovasc Imaging 15:170-179.
18. Kim H-L, Kim Y-J, Lee S-P (2014) Incremental prognostic value of sequential imaging of single-photon emission computed tomography and coronary computed tomography angiography in patients with suspected coronary artery disease. Eur Heart J Cardiovasc Imaging 15:878-885.

19. McMurray JJ, Adamopoulos S, Anker SD et al (2012) ESC Guidelines for the diagnosis and treatment of acute and chronic heart failure 2012: The Task Force for the Diagnosis and Treatment of Acute and Chronic Heart Failure 2012 of the European Society of Cardiology. Developed in collaboration with the Heart Failure Association (HFA) of the ESC. Eur Heart J 33:1787-1847.

20. Bonow RO, Maurer G, Lee KL et al (2011) Myocardial viability and survival in ischemic left ventricular dysfunction. The New England Journal of Medicine 364:1617-1625.

21. Ling LF, Marwick TH, Flores DR et al (2013) Identification of therapeutic benefit from revascularization in patients with left ventricular systolic dysfunction: inducible ischemia versus hibernating myocardium. Circ Cardiovasc Imaging 6:363-372.

Acute Aortic Syndrome: State-of-the-Art Diagnostic Imaging

Thomas Grist[1], Geoffrey D. Rubin[2]

[1] Department of Radiology, University of Wisconsin School of Medicine and Public Health, Madison, WI, USA
[2] Department of Radiology, Duke University School of Medicine, Durham, NC, USA

Introduction

The accurate detection and evaluation of acute aortic syndrome is one of the radiologist's most important and immediately impactful opportunities to improve human health. Acute aortic syndrome is often a clinical emergency and a situation that demands accurate radiologic diagnosis and intervention to provide lifesaving care. The diagnosis of acute aortic syndrome has evolved significantly over the last two decades, from an arteriographic diagnosis to a diagnosis based upon multi-detector computed tomography (CT) angiography [1] and, to a limited extent, magnetic resonance imaging (MRI). With the advent of these new techniques for diagnosis, investigators have revisited the questions and pathologies surrounding acute aortic syndromes.

Anatomic and Pathological Considerations

Acute aortic syndromes are principally diseases of the aortic wall. As a result, their categorization is aided by an understanding of the fundamental pathological features of the aortic wall.

The aorta is composed of three layers. From inner to outer, they are the intima, media, and adventitia. The intima is made up of a single layer of flattened endothelial cells with a supporting layer of elastin rich collagen, fibroblasts, and myointimal cells. As humans age, the myointimal cells tend to accumulate lipid resulting in intimal thickening which is the earliest sign of atherosclerosis. The majority of the aortic wall thickness is composed of the media, which is broad and elastic and made up of concentric fenestrated sheets of elastin, collagen, and sparsely distributed smooth muscle fibers. The predominance of elastin arrayed as elastic lamina reflects the fact that the aorta together with the pulmonary arteries are the only elastic arteries of the body. Because the aorta and the pulmonary arteries receive the entirety of the cardiac output, they undergo substantial deformation in order to accommodate the large volume changes that occur with each cardiac contraction. The remaining arteries of the body are muscular arteries, with a paucity of elastin and a predominance of smooth muscle that allows the regulation of regional blood flow throughout the body. The boundary between the intima and media is not readily defined but is recognized histologically as being formed by the internal elastic lamina, which represents the innermost of the many elastic lamellae within the aortic media. The adventitia lacks elastic lamellae and is predominantly composed of loose connective tissue and blood vessels, the so-called vasa vasorum.

Anatomically, the aorta can be divided longitudinally into five zones: the aortic root, ascending thoracic aorta, aortic arch, descending thoracic aorta, and abdominal aorta. Although acute aortic syndromes can involve any of these five anatomic zones, they only rarely originate within the abdominal aorta. An important principle in the management of acute aortic syndromes is the classification of lesions into Stanford type A or type B. Type A lesions, defined as those involving the ascending aorta or aortic root, demand urgent surgical intervention, with replacement of the diseased ascending aortic segment. The rationale for this urgent intervention is the high risk of aortic rupture, which can lead to pericardial tamponade or frank exsanguination. Type B lesions do not involve the ascending aorta and thus can occur within the aortic arch or the descending thoracic aorta. If there is evidence for active aortic rupture, then these patients should likewise be referred for urgent surgical intervention. However in the absence of active bleeding, they are typically managed with blood pressure reduction and regular monitoring to assess the evolution of aortic dimension and disease extension.

Definitions and Classifications

Collectively, acute aortic syndromes represent life-threatening conditions that are associated with a high risk of aortic rupture and sudden death. The typical presentation is the sudden onset of chest pain, which may be accompanied

Diseases of the Chest and Heart 2015-2018,
DOI: 10.1007/978-88-470-5752-4_19 © Springer-Verlag Italia 2015

by signs or symptoms of hypoperfusion or ischemia to the distal organs, extremities, or brain.

Traditionally, acute aortic syndromes have been categorized as aortic dissection, intramural hematoma, and penetrating atherosclerotic ulcer.

Aortic dissection (AD) is characterized by a separation of the aortic media, creating an intimal-medial complex that separates from the remaining aortic wall. Blood flowing between the intimal-medial complex (intimal flap), and the remaining wall is considered to be within a false lumen, whereas blood flow bounded by the intima is considered to be within a true lumen. Multiple communication points can be observed between the true and false lumens. The most proximal communication is defined as the "entry tear" and the remaining points of communication as the "exit tears," implying flow directionality from true to false lumen and from false to true lumen, respectively. The actual incidence of AD is difficult to define, since AD involving the ascending aorta is often fatal and patients frequently die prior to hospitalization. Likewise, AD is sometimes misdiagnosed on initial presentation; consequently, these patients are also at risk for death outside of the hospital. Nevertheless, various population-based studies suggest that the incidence of AD ranges from 2 to 4 case per 100,000 patients [2].

The temporal definition of acute AD is a dissection that is identified less than 2 weeks after the onset of symptoms, while sub-acute ranges from 2 to 6 weeks following an initial painful episode. Chronic AD is defined as a dissection identified >6 weeks after the onset of pain.

Intramural hematoma (IMH) is an entity that was first described approximately 25 years ago as a stagnant collection of blood within the aortic wall. The common association of IMH with pathologically detected intimal defects led to the hypothesis that most are sequelae of penetrating atherosclerotic ulcer. An alternative cause of IMH, typically invoked in the absence of an intimal defect, is rupture of the vasa vasorum. This hypothetical cause of IMH has never been definitively proven. IMH is treated similar to dissections in terms of initial diagnosis as well as clinical management. Most IMHs occur in the descending thoracic aorta and can be associated with severe pain. The imaging features vary depending on the amount of blood accumulated in the wall of the aorta, but typically the normal wall measures <7 mm in thickness. The natural history of IMH can be quite variable. Roughly one-third of them will progress to AD, one third will be stable, and one third will resolve [3]. The mortality for patients with IMH involving the ascending aorta is similar to that of patients with classic dissection; therefore these patients are treated as though they have a classic AD, with emergent surgery [4]. Patients with IMH involving the descending thoracic aorta can initially be given appropriate therapy for hypertension and then followed.

Penetrating atherosclerotic ulcer (PAU) is a condition that originates with atherosclerotic plaque involvement of the aorta, primarily the descending thoracic aorta (Fig. 1). As the plaque evolves, the ulceration "penetrates" the internal elastic lamina into the media of the aortic wall. Over time, the PAU may extend through all three layers of the aortic wall to form a false or pseudoaneurysm. A finding of PAU does not necessarily imply the existence of an acute aortic syndrome. Signs of IMH or extravasation indicate acuity.

There are two limitations to this traditional classification. The first concerns the omission of a rupturing true aortic aneurysm, as the nature of the presentation and the severity of the event are similar in PAU and the other acute aortic syndromes. The second limitation is that IMH, defined as a stagnant intramural collection of blood, can be observed in the setting of AD, PAU, and rupturing aortic aneurysm. As such, it is a feature or characteristic associated with any of the acute aortic syndromes, reflecting degradation of the aortic wall as a harbinger of impending aortic rupture.

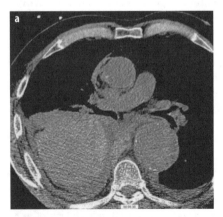 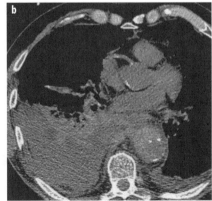 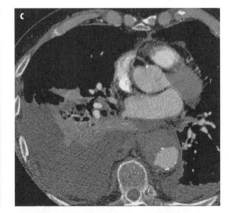

Fig. 1 a-c. Rupturing thoracic aortic aneurysm. **a** Unenhanced computed tomography (CT) demonstrates a high-attenuation hematoma in the right pleural space and middle mediastinum. There is an aneurysm of the descending aorta. **b** Unenhanced CT section 5 cm inferior to (**a**), reveals an intramural hematoma (IMH) at the inferior margin of the aneurysm, with extravasation of blood into the middle mediastinum. Note the displacement of intimal calcium along the inner wall of the IMH. **c** Following the administration of intravenous contrast material, the IMH is harder to visualize because of the wider window used to display the CT angiogram.

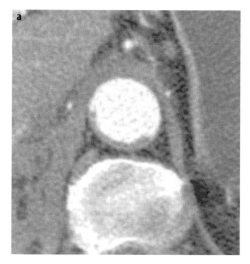
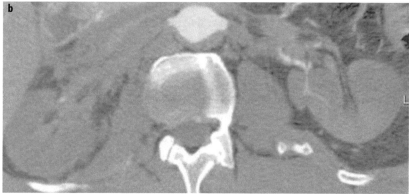

Fig. 2 a, b. Type B aortic dissection. **a** The true lumen is completely collapsed posteriorly and only the true lumen fills with contrast material. The entry tear was (not shown) in the proximal descending aorta. **b** Because of their supply from the aortic true lumen, the renal arteries do not opacity and the kidneys are not perfused

In consideration of these two points, a new classification scheme has been proposed based upon the primary location of the lesion within the aortic wall. In this new classification scheme, there are three pathological entities: AD, PAU, and rupturing aortic aneurysm [5]. These three entities are differentiated by the fact that AD principally involves the aortic media, PAU originates within the aortic intima, and aortic aneurysm is a disease of all three layers. The presence of IMH is an observation or epi-phenomenon to be applied to any of these three fundamental pathologies. In the setting of an isolated IMH without PAU, "non-communicating dissection" has been proposed as a descriptor, although the term "IMH" is more commonly associated with this lesion.

Essential Elements of Aortic Imaging Reports

In 2010, a group of medical organizations representing the disciplines of cardiology, radiology, thoracic surgery, and anesthesia published guidelines for the diagnosis and management of patients with thoracic aortic diseases. In this report, the authors identified eight essential elements that should be addressed in aortic imaging reports [2]. While these guidelines are not comprehensive, nor do they imply the necessity of reporting every element in every case, they are a useful construct from which to build any formalized description of the imaging findings of an acute aortic syndrome. They are the following.
1. The location at which the aorta is abnormal.
2. The maximum diameter of any dilation, measured from the external wall of the aorta, perpendicular to the axis of flow, and the length of the aorta that is abnormal.
3. For patients with genetic syndromes who are at risk for aortic root disease, measurements of the aortic valve, sinuses of Valsalva, the sinotubular junction, and the ascending aorta.
4. The presence of internal filling defects consistent with thrombus or atheroma.

5. The presence of IMH, PAU, or calcification.
6. Extension of the aortic abnormality to include inter-branch vessels, including dissection and aneurysm, and secondary evidence of end-organ injury (e.g., renal or bowel hypoperfusion).
7. Evidence of aortic rupture, including periaortic and mediastinal hematoma, pericardial and pleural fluid, and contrast extravasation from the aortic lumen (Fig. 2).
8. When a prior examination is available, direct image-to-image comparison to determine whether there has been any increase in lesion diameter.

CT-Based Imaging Approaches to Acute Aortic Syndromes

High-quality and comprehensive aortic and end-organ assessment is performed using multi-detector row CT with at least 16 detector rows. This scanner configuration allows for imaging from the neck through the pelvis, acquiring ≤1.5-mm-thick transverse sections during the arterial phase of enhancement from an intravenous contrast administration. It also allows for the use of electrocardiographic (ECG) gating of the scan when appropriate, as described below.

Unenhanced CT

An unenhanced scan prior to the administration of intravenous contrast can be valuable for the detection of intramural and periaortic blood, which is often subtle. It can also be useful for mapping the specific regions of the aorta that are abnormal and thus guide the mode of subsequent CT angiographic acquisition. While an associated increase in radiation exposure results from this approach, the potential value of the information almost always outweighs the risk. Using dual-energy scanning, a virtual unenhanced scan might obviate the need for a separate unenhanced acquisition. However, this approach has not been comprehensively validated in acute aortic syndromes. Moreover, it eliminates the possibility of using the preliminary unenhanced acquisition to guide the decision to gate the CT angiogram.

CT Angiography

While unenhanced imaging can reveal aortic dilation, intramural and extra-aortic hemorrhage, and in uncommon circumstances directly visualize an intimal flap, the use of intravenously administered contrast medium is required for a complete assessment in patients in whom acute aortic syndrome is suspected (Fig. 3). The volume and flow rate of the contrast material should be adjusted based on patient size. A concentrated iodine solution containing ≥350 mg of iodine/mL will assure adequate intravenous delivery of iodine with a safe and reliable flow rate of the contrast material into the peripheral vein. Typical volumes and injector flow rates for iodinated contrast range between 60 and 115 mL at flow rates between 3.5 and 6 mL/s.

To assure diagnostic aortic enhancement throughout the CT acquisition, the duration of the contrast injection should exceed the scan duration by 5–10 s, and initiation of the CT angiographic acquisition should be based on the active monitoring of the arrival of iodine within the descending thoracic aorta.

Imaging the Abdominal Aorta and Iliac Arteries

Because of the likelihood of direct extension of thoracic aortic disease into the abdominal aorta and iliac arteries,

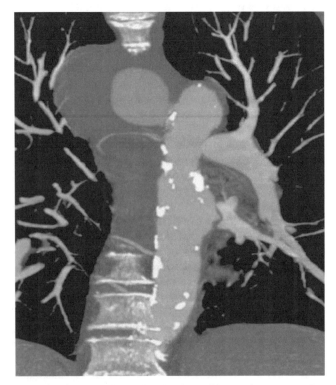

Fig. 3. Penetrating atherosclerotic ulcer with pseudoaneurysm formation in the proximal descending aorta

the presence of unrelated but important abdominal aorto-iliac pathology, the value of assessing the caliber of a transfemoral delivery route to intra-aortic repair devices, and the possibility of abdominal visceral ischemia, scan ranges that extend through the abdomen and pelvis are highly recommended as a routine approach to imaging acute aortic syndromes. By beginning the scan in the neck and extending inferiorly below the lesser trochanters of the femurs, the scan range will comfortably include several centimeters of the cervical carotid arteries through the bifurcation of the femoral artery. Scan ranges that include less anatomy risk the possibility that important observations will be missed, such that additional CT scans with further injections of iodinated contrast material may be required.

Electrocardiographic Gating

When the ascending aorta is involved by an acute aortic syndrome, electrocardiographic (ECG) gating can be valuable. ECG gating allows for clear delineation of the position of the intimal flap across the cardiac period, distinction of the involvement of the structures of the aortic root including the coronary artery ostia and the aortic annulus, elimination of pulsation-related artifacts that can blur the aortic wall, and subtle regions of extravasation. Unlike the use of ECG gating in the setting of coronary artery disease assessment, the strategy for using ECG gating in acute aortic syndromes does not rely upon the manipulation of heart rate or coronary artery dimension using β-blockers or nitrates. Regardless of the basal heart rate, the placement of ECG leads and the acquisition of a retrospectively gated CT scan (with judicious use of ECG directed X-ray tube current pulsing to minimize radiation exposure) allow for a four-dimensional assessment of the aortic root, aortic valve, coronary arteries, and ascending aorta. It is sufficient to reconstruct 10 phases every 10% of the R-R interval. Gating is only beneficial through the thoracic aorta. The abdomen and pelvis are imaged after the chest acquisitions, using a non-gated acquisition with a minimization of the delay between the two scans so that only one contrast injection is required.

MRI-Based Imaging Approaches to Acute Aortic Syndromes

Clinical Indications for MRI

While CT remains the mainstay for the initial diagnosis of patients with acute aortic syndrome, MRI does play a limited role in patients with contraindications for CT, as well as in the follow-up of patients for complications following prior AD. First, in patients who cannot tolerate iodinated contrast associated with CT, MRI may play a useful role in the diagnosis of acute AD. Investigators have demonstrated the value of cardiac-gated steady-state free precession (SSFP) MRI in detecting the intimal flap associated with dissection [6]. These scans are performed with minimal MRI table time and by using fast acquisition techniques. In patients who are stable, contrast-enhanced magnetic resonance angiography (MRA) may be used to further diagnose and characterize the configuration of the intimal flap and the involvement of branch vessels in acute AD.

In the setting of acute dissection with thrombosis lumen and intramural hematoma, SSFP MRI alone may be inadequate for detecting hemorrhage in the wall of the aorta. In this clinical scenario, T1- and T2- weighted spin-echo technique is typically necessary for diagnosis. MRI using these techniques may be useful in detecting and characterizing the age of the intramural hematoma, with typical characteristics such as a transition of the hemorrhage from deoxyhemoglobin in the early stage of IMH to extracellular methemoglobin in its late stage.

In the setting of aortic aneurysm with suspected rupture, patients typically are unstable and therefore far more complicated to image with MRI; in these cases, CT is the preferred imaging modality. MRI has been used, however, to evaluate stable patients with suspected complications of aneurysm and can be particularly helpful in patients with suspected inflammatory or infectious causes of the aneurysm, due to the exquisite sensitivity of MRI to inflammation in the tissues surrounding the aorta. In this setting, the use of gadolinium-based contrast agents, especially those with prolonged blood-pool retention, can be particularly informative.

MRI Technique

Evaluation of thoracic pathology with MRI begins with rapid SSFP imaging of the aorta and its major branches. This technique, in which high-performance gradients are applied to acquire images using a short repetition time (TR) and short echo time (TE), are especially useful for imaging aortic vascular pathology in the absence of gadolinium contrast medium (Table 1) [6]. The images are typically initially acquired in axial and oblique sagittal projections, and gated to the diastolic phase of the cardiac waveform. For a more complete characterization of intimal flap motion in the setting of AD, cine SSFP MRI can be used to further delineate the entry and exit zones of the intimal flap, as well as potential dynamic com-

pression of branch vessels, especially the coronary arteries. Likewise, cine MRI can be used to further characterize the relationship of a type A dissection flap to the aortic valve and any resultant aortic valve insufficiency. T1- and T2-weighted imaging is typically performed with fast spin-echo technique (Table 1).

Finally, gadolinium contrast-enhanced MRA is used to characterize the luminal pathology associated with acute aortic syndrome [7]. Contrast-enhanced MRA is usually acquired during the arterial phase of contrast as well as during the delayed "steady state" phase of contrast enhancement. Some authors describe the use of time-resolved 3D MRA during a small initial bolus of gadolinium-based contrast agent, thus allowing the dynamic delineation of the filling pathways of the true and false lumen and branch vessels [8]. These images are typically followed by high-resolution 3D images for more precise anatomic characterization.

Extracellular contrast agents are typically the primary diagnostic enhancement agents. Contrast agents with higher relaxivities are preferred because of their greater signal at a lower dose as well as their protein binding, which facilitates delayed imaging in the steady state. For delayed imaging, a fat-suppressed post-contrast T1-weighted gradient echo image, with spoiling of the transverse magnetization, is typically acquired. The delayed images are particularly helpful in evaluating extraluminal pathology affecting the aorta, including aortic leaks, arteritis, and infection, and in characterizing the size and extent of hematoma outside the aortic wall (Fig. 3). The arterial phase of contrast-enhanced images is used to delineate branch vessel involvement of the intimal flap, characterizing the size of aortic enlargement in dissection and/or dissecting aneurysm, and determining the nature of the intraluminal pathology associated with acute aortic syndrome, such as an intimal flap, associated thrombosis, or an atherosclerotic aortic plaque causing increased risk of distal atheroembolization.

MRI Findings in Acute Aortic Syndrome

MRI findings in classic AD are similar to those identified on CT, including a displaced intimal flap, thrombosed lumen, and demonstration of entry and exit tears [9]. One key finding on CT that is not reliable on MRI is the

Table 1. Magnetic resonance imaging techniques for the diagnosis and monitoring of acute aortic syndromes

Sequence	Plane	TR/TE (MS)	Matrix	Acceleration factor	Gating
SSFP	2D axial/sagittal	3/1.5	256×192	1–2	Yes
Time-resolved CE-MRA	3D TRICKS sagittal	3/1	192×128×32	3	
High-resolution CE-MRA	3D sagittal	3/1	320×256×128	4	No
T$_1$ fast spin echo	2D axial	~600/10	256×192	n/a	No
T$_2$ fast spin echo	2D axial	~2500/60	256×192	n/a	No
4D flow phase contrast	3D sagittal	10/4	256×128×64	6–10	Yes

TR, repetition time; TE, echo time; SSFP, steady-state free precession; CE, contrast-enhanced; MRA, magnetic resonance angiography; TRICKS, time-resolved imaging of contrast kinetics; n/a, not applicable

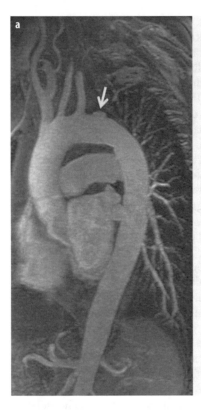
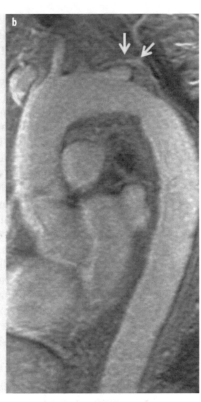

Fig. 4 a, b. a T1-weighted magnetic resonance imaging demonstrating an IMH with mixed signal intensity components, including low signal intensity corresponding to deoxyhemoglobin and high signal intensity extracellular methemoglobin, suggesting an IMH of subacute or chronic duration. **b** T2-weighted image demonstrating high signal intensity associated with extracellular methemogolobin due to chronic IMH

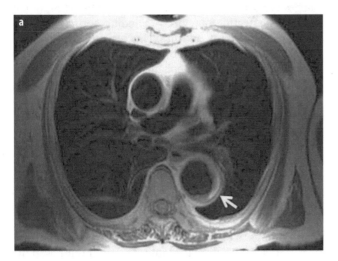
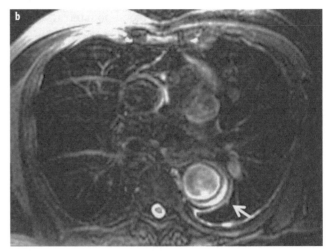

Fig. 5 a, b. Penetrating aortic ulcer. **a** Early arterial phase and **b** delayed "steady state" phase magnetic resonance angiogram (MRA) demonstrating penetrating aortic ulceration involving the superior surface of the aortic arch (*arrows*). Note the excellent delineation of the aortic adventitia on the delayed images due to contrast enhancement during the steady-state imaging phase

displaced intimal calcifications associated with a displaced intimal flap. Contrast-enhanced MRA can demonstrate filling patterns in AD and may be helpful in delineating branch-vessel and end-organ perfusion.

Spin-echo MRI may allow characterization of the age of the intramural hematoma associated with an AD or penetrating aortic ulceration. Classic features of aortic intramural hematoma include intermediate to low signal intensity in the acute phase on both T1- and T2-weighted sequences, with gradual transition to high signal intensity on

T1- and T2-weighted images in the chronic phase (Fig. 4).

The exquisite soft-tissue contrast obtained on delayed contrast-enhanced MRI may be helpful in delineating penetrating aortic ulceration. The immediate arterial-phase images on contrast-enhanced MRI may show the size and extent of ulceration, whereas delayed images enhance visualization of the aortic adventitia and the surrounding soft tissues, thus allowing a more definitive characterization of the aortic enlargement and associated structures in penetrating aortic ulceration (Fig. 5).

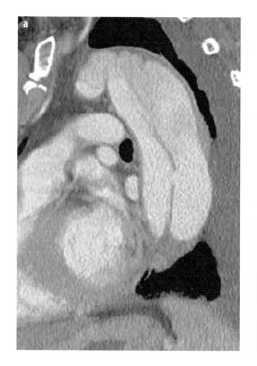
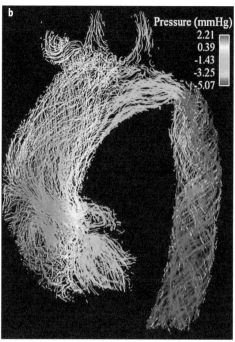

Fig. 6 a, b. CT angiography (CTA) and phase-contrast MRA in type B aortic dissection. **a** Reformatted CTA demonstrates a dissection flap with fenestration but does not reveal the cause of the patient's persistent abdominal pain and organ hypo-perfusion. **b** Pressure gradient image calculated from phase-contrast MRA 4D flow imaging demonstrates a significant pressure gradient and the dynamic obstruction of flow to the distal aorta due to compression of the true lumen by the false lumen

Finally, phase-contrast MRI typically delineates the entry and exit zone sites in classic AD and documents flow patterns in the true and false lumen (Fig. 6). In the setting of suspected branch vessel ischemia, phase-contrast MRI may demonstrate the abnormal flow waveforms associated with dissection. Future work may allow the use of computational fluid dynamics to predict the likelihood of vascular rupture in patients with dissecting aortic aneurysm or branch vessel involvement; however additional validation of the predictive power of these techniques is necessary.

Conclusion

High-resolution CT and MRI have fundamentally changed the diagnosis and treatment of acute aortic syndrome in the modern era. Multidetector CT angiography has streamlined the early diagnosis and management of these patients, and has allowed us to rethink the classification of acute aortic syndrome as a manifestation of specific pathologies involving the aortic wall. Recent improvements in understanding this entity contribute to improved patient survival, with broader treatment options for patients who are correctly diagnosed. The role of MRI is limited to the diagnosis and management of complications, follow-up studies, and in the initial diagnosis of patients who cannot undergo CT angiography. The accurate detection and evaluation of acute aortic syndrome is an opportunity for the radiologist to have an immediate impact, as a rapid and accurate diagnosis reduces the morbidity and mortality associated with this spectrum of diseases.

References

1. Rubin GD, Leipsic J, Joseph Schoepf U et al (2014) CT angiography after 20 years: a transformation in cardiovascular disease characterization continues to advance. Radiology 271:633-652.
2. Hiratzka LF, Bakris GL, Beckman JA et al (2010) ACCF/AHA/AATS/ACR/ASA/SCA/SCAI/SIR/STS/SVM guidelines for the diagnosis and management of patients with Thoracic Aortic Disease: a report of the American College of Cardiology Foundation/American Heart Association Task Force on Practice Guidelines, American Association for Thoracic Surgery, American College of Radiology, American Stroke Association, Society of Cardiovascular Anesthesiologists, Society for Cardiovascular Angiography and Interventions, Society of Interventional Radiology, Society of Thoracic Surgeons, and Society for Vascular Medicine. Circulation 121:e266-369.
3. Ganaha F, Miller DC, Sugimoto K et al (2002) Prognosis of aortic intramural hematoma with and without penetrating atherosclerotic ulcer: a clinical and radiological analysis. Circulation 106:342-348.
4. Evangelista A, Mukherjee D, Mehta RH et al (2005) Acute intramural hematoma of the aorta: a mystery in evolution. Circulation 111:1063-1070.
5. Fleischmann D, Mitchell RS, Miller DC (2008) Acute aortic syndromes: new insights from electrocardiographically gated computed tomography. Seminars in thoracic and cardiovascular surgery 20:340-347.
6. Pereles FS, McCarthy RM, Baskaran V et al (2002) Thoracic aortic dissection and aneurysm: evaluation with nonenhanced true FISP MR angiography in less than 4 minutes. Radiology 223:5.
7. Prince MR, Narasimham DL, Jacoby WT et al (1996) Three-dimensional gadolinium-enhanced MR angiography of the thoracic aorta. AJR Am J Roentgenol 166:1387-1397.

8. Finn JP, Baskaran V, Carr JC et al (2002) Thorax: Low-dose contrast-enhanced three-dimensional MR angiography with subsecond temporal resolution - Initial results. Radiology 224:896-904.

9. Gebker R, Gomaa O, Schnackenburg B et al (2007) Comparison of different MRI techniques for the assessment of thoracic aortic pathology: 3D contrast enhanced MR angiography, turbo spin echo and balanced steady state free precession. Int J Cardiovasc Imaging 23:747-756.

Interventional Techniques in the Thorax of Adults

Dierk Vorwerk

Department of Radiology, Klinikum Ingolstadt, Ingolstadt, Germany

Introduction

Interventional radiology in the thorax is somewhat ill-defined, as nonvascular interventions such as lung biopsy tend to be more common. However, many nonvascular as well as vascular interventions are performed within thoracic structures, some of which, such as radiofrequency ablation of lung tumors, are gaining in importance.

Nonvascular Interventions

Lung Biopsy

In the nonvascular field, CT-guided lung biopsies are the most well known and frequently performed intervention in this part of the body. Both fine-needle aspiration (FNA) for cytology as well as miniaturized cutting needles (not exceeding 18–20 G) for histology are used for this purpose. Automated biopsy guns have several advantages, including excellent sampling quality and the possibility to perform repeated biopsies using a single access. FNA is more often recommended if a lesion for biopsy is located close to central and vascular structures, in order to avoid major bleeding complications.

Laurent et al. [1] compared the accuracy and the complication rate of FNA and an automated biopsy device. Two consecutive series of 125 (group A) and 98 (group B) biopsies performed using 20- to 22-gauge coaxial FNA (group A) and an automated 19.5-gauge coaxial biopsy device (group B) were investigated. Among the patients in groups A and B were 100 (80%) and 77 (79%) with malignant lesions and 25 (20%) and 18 (21%) with benign lesions, respectively. The two groups did not significantly differ with respect to patient-, lesion-, and procedure-related variables. However, for a diagnosis of malignancy, the difference in sensitivity (group A: 82.7%, group B: 97.4%) between the results obtained with the automated biopsy device vs. FNA were significant. For a diagnosis of malignancy, the false-negative rate of the biopsy result was signifi-

cantly higher (p<0.005) in group A (17%) than in group B (2.6%). For a specific diagnosis of benignity, no statistically significant difference was found between the two groups (44% vs. 26%) but the automated biopsy device provided fewer indeterminate cases. There was no difference between the two groups concerning the pneumothorax rate (20% in group A and 15% in group B) or the hemoptysis rate (2.4% in group A and 4% in group B). The authors concluded that, for a diagnosis of malignancy, automated biopsy devices have a lower rate of false-negative results than FNA and a similar complication rate.

Richardson et al. [2] carried out a survey of 5444 lung biopsy in the UK. Complications included pneumothorax (20.5% of biopsies), pneumothorax requiring a chest drain (3.1%), hemoptysis (5.3%), and death (0.15%). The timing of post-procedural chest radiography was variable. Centers that performed predominantly cutting-needle biopsies had similar pneumothorax rates to those performing mainly fine-needle biopsies (18.9% vs. 18.3%). There is great variation in practice throughout the UK and most procedures are performed on an outpatient basis. Small pneumothoraces are common but infrequently require treatment. Chojniak et al. [3] carried out a retrospective study of 1,300 consecutive CT-guided biopsies performed within 6 years. Nodules or masses were suspected as the primary malignancy in 845 cases (65%) and as metastases in 455 (35%); 628 of the lesions were thoracic. For any site, sample adequacy and specific diagnosis rate were always better for cutting-needle biopsy. Among 530 lung biopsies, there were 84 cases of pneumothorax (16%) and 2 cases of hemothorax (0.3%), with thoracic drainage in 24 cases (4.9%).

Postbiopsy pneumothorax is a rather frequent complication but in most cases can be treated relatively simply. In asymptomatic patients we recommend not evacuating the pneumothorax earlier than 4 h after biopsy, in order to achieve a durable success. In symptomatic patients or those with drainage failures with a single needle approach, the use of percutaneously introduced Heimlich valves is recommended.

Diseases of the Chest and Heart 2015-2018,
DOI: 10.1007/978-88-470-5752-4_20 © Springer-Verlag Italia 2015

Minimally invasive thoracoscopic procedures have gained widespread acceptance and offer a valid alternative in patients with only a single pulmonary nodule that can be removed both for diagnostic and therapeutic reasons. In such cases, CT-guided hook marking of the nodule allows easy identification of the nodule during thoracoscopy and facilitates its removal.

Poretti et al. [4] described their experience with percutaneous CT-guided placement of hook-wires to localize nodules before video-assisted thoracoscopy (VATS). In their report, 19 patients with newly diagnosed intrapulmonary nodules underwent CT-guided hook-wire localization using a X-Reidy set, followed by a VATS resection of the lesion within a mean time of 30 min (range: 10–48 min). In all cases, resection of the nodules was successful. Eight patients developed an asymptomatic pneumothorax. In four patients, in whom the tumor was hit directly by the needle, local bleeding occurred. In one case, hemoptysis was present. There were no cases of dislocation of the hook-wire system.

Abscess Drainage

Percutaneous drainage of pleural, pulmonary, and mediastinal abscesses is a commonly employed technique that is available in almost all radiological departments. Success depends on the size of the drainage catheters, the composition of the drained material, the organization of the pseudomembrane, and the access routes, especially into mediastinal locations.

Radiofrequency Ablation of Lung Lesions

Primary and metastatic lung neoplasms with indications close to those of surgical resection can be treated by radiofrequency ablation (RFA) [5]. Thus, RFA is performed with curative intent in nonsurgical or borderline surgical candidates. Inoperability is most often due to poor respiratory function in relation to chronic obstructive pulmonary disease in patients with primary tumors, and iterative surgery in patients with metastatic disease. Because the intent is curative, a pre-ablation imaging workup must be equivalent to a pre-surgical workup. In addition, the size and number of the tumors matter not only for the oncologic indication but also for the technical possibilities. It is generally agreed that the number of tumors per hemithorax should not be more than 5, and the largest diameter should be <5 cm, ideally <3.5 cm.

Local Efficacy

In a review of 17 recent publications, the median reported rate of complete ablation was 90%, although there was high variability between publications, as ranges between 38% and 97% were reported [5]. Tumors <2 cm in size can be ablated in 78–96% of cases, according to several reports of CT-guided RFA in which there was a lengthy imaging follow-up of treated patients.

Survival

Survival data for patients treated with RFA are scarce and still preliminary, with few series achieving survival beyond 3 years [5]. Accordingly, there are as yet no comparative studies of RFA and surgery, either for small (stage I) non-small-cell carcinomas (NSCLCs) or for lung metastases. There are also no studies comparing RFA and other local ablative therapies. Although in early reports survival rates after RFA have been close to the rates after surgery, the data are preliminary. Ideally, comparative randomized studies are needed in patients treated with curative intent.

Gillams et al. [6] recently published survival data for 122 patients with 256 procedures and metastatic disease. The initial number of metastases ablated was 2.3 (range 1–8); the total number was 3.3 (range 1–15). The maximum tumor diameter was 1.7 (range 0.5–4) cm, and the number of procedures was 2 (range 1–10). The major complication rate was 3.9 %. Overall median and 3-year survival rates were 41 months and 57%. Survival was better in patients with smaller tumors: a median of 51 months, with a 3-year survival of 64% for patients with tumors ≤2 cm vs. 31 months and 44% for those with tumors 2.1–4 cm (p=0.08). The authors concluded that, among patients with inoperable colorectal lung metastases, a 3-year survival of 57% is better than would be expected with chemotherapy alone.

Schlijper et al. [7] performed a systematic review comparing surgery, RFA, and stereotactic body radiation (SBRT) as treatment options for metastases from colorectal cancer. The review included 27 studies matched according to the a priori selection criteria, the most important being >50 patients and a follow-up period of >24 months. Since there were no eligible SBRT studies, the review was conducted on four RFA series and 23 surgical series. Four of the surgical studies were prospective, all others were retrospective. There were no randomized trials. The reporting of data differed between the studies, which led to difficulties in the analyses. Treatment-related mortality rates for RFA and surgery were 0% and 1.4–2.4%, respectively, whereas morbidity rates were reported inconsistently but seemed to be lowest for surgery.

According to the authors [7] "due to the lack of phase III trials, no firm conclusions can be drawn, although most evidence supports surgery as the most effective treatment option. High-quality trials comparing currently used treatment modalities such as SBRT, RFA and surgery are needed to inform treatment decisions."

In a microsimulation model, Tramontano et al. [8] calculated a survival gain of 2.02 years for patients with stage I inoperable NSCLC undergoing RFA for peripheral tumors and SBRT for central tumors, compared to universal radiation.

Technical Considerations

The delivery of RFA therapy must be adapted to tumor location because impedance before ablation is significantly different among tumors, depending on whether >50% or <50% of the tumor abuts the pleura, or whether the tumor does not abut the pleura at all. A tumor surrounded by lung parenchyma is highly electrically and thermally insulated by the air-filled lung parenchyma compared to a tumor with pleural contact and will require less energy deposition.

Vascular Interventions

Vascular interventions can be divided into arterial and venous interventions. Among the former are balloon angioplasty of the supra-aortic arteries, such as the subclavian artery, implantation of thoracic endografts, and embolization of bronchial arteries. Rarely performed interventions include transarterial techniques for tumor treatment, such as chemoperfusion of the lateral thoracic, mammarian, and bronchial arteries in the treatment of bronchial or breast cancer. Vascular interventions involving the pulmonary artery include the occlusion of arterioportal fistulas, particularly in patients with hereditary hemorrhagic telangiectasia. Local thrombolysis or thrombodestruction of pulmonary emboli is another rare intervention but it is a promising alternative in emergency cases involving pulmonary embolism (PE).

Venous interventions in the thorax include central venous stents, either to treat malignancies or to recanalize central venous stenoses in order to allow successful drainage in dialysis patients, the placement and maintenance of central venous catheters, fibrin sheath stripping, and the removal of foreign bodies.

Only some of these interventions merit further discussion in the following. However, embolization of the bronchial arteries and treatment of malignant venous stenoses, while uncommon, might be helpful in treating patients with acute symptoms and are considered below.

Arterial Interventions

Stent Graft Implantation

The routine commercial availability of stent grafts for the thoracic aorta has drastically changed the treatment of traumatic or iatrogenic pseudoaneurysms, true aneurysms, intramural hematomas, and symptomatic type B aortic dissections. There has been a change of strategy for some types of thoracoabdominal aneurysms but they still present a challenging but luckily small group of cases. There is currently no good endoluminal alternative for type A aortic dissections or other aneurysms of the ascending thoracic aorta.

Technically, stent graft implantation into the thoracic aorta is straightforward, as it involves the insertion of a simple tube graft or several tube grafts. Important landmarks are the left subclavian artery, which can be usually covered by a stent graft in case the right vertebral artery is patent; sometimes the left common carotid artery, which should not be covered without performing a carotid-carotid bypass; and the celiac trunk. Elongation of the aortic arch can make an exact and easy placement of the stent graft difficult. Paraplegia is a rare but serious side effect in case the descending aorta is treated but is a less common occurrence than in open surgery.

Matsumura et al. [9] evaluated the safety and effectiveness of thoracic endovascular aortic repair (TEVAR) with a contemporary endograft system compared with open surgical repair of descending thoracic aortic aneurysms and large ulcers. They included 230 patients and compared 16 TEVAR subjects treated with a single type of stent graft with 70 patients undergoing open surgery. The 30-day survival rate was non-inferior (p<0.01) for the TEVAR group compared with the open group (98.1% vs. 94.3%). Cumulative major morbidity scores were significantly lower at 30 days in the TEVAR group than in the open group (1.3 ± 3.0 vs. $2.\pm3.6$, p<0.01). TEVAR patients had fewer cardiovascular, pulmonary, and vascular adverse events. No ruptures or conversions occurred in the first year after the procedure. Reintervention rates were similar in both groups. At 12 months, aneurysm growth was identified in 7.1% (8/112), endoleak in 3.9% (4/103), and migration (>10 mm) in 2.8% (3/107); other device-related problems were infrequent. At 1 year of follow-up, they concluded that thoracic endovascular aortic repair with the Zenith TX2 endovascular graft (William Cook Europe, ApS, Bjaeverskov, Denmark) is a safe and effective alternative to open surgical repair for the treatment of anatomically suitable aneurysms and ulcers of the descending thoracic aorta.

In a prospective trial, Nienaber et al. [10] investigated 140 patients with stable type B aortic dissection who were randomly assigned to elective stent-graft placement in addition to optimal medical therapy (n=72) or to optimal medical therapy (n=68) with surveillance. There was no difference in all-cause mortality: cumulative survival was $97.0\%\pm3.4\%$ with optimal medical therapy vs. $91.3\%\pm2.1\%$ with thoracic endovascular aortic repair (p=0.16). Aorta-related mortality was not different (p=0.42), and the risk for the combined end point of aorta-related death (rupture) and progression (including conversion or additional endovascular or open surgical intervention) was similar (p=0.86). Three neurologic adverse events occurred in the thoracic endovascular aortic repair group (one case each of paraplegia, stroke, and transient paraparesis) vs. one episode of paraparesis with medical treatment. It was concluded that in survivors of uncomplicated type B aortic dissection, elective stent-graft placement does not improve 1-year survival and adverse events.

The same group recently published their long-term results [11], reporting that patients with best medical treatment but no TEVAR had an aortic-related mortality of 3.6% while those with TEVAR did not show late aortic events between 2 and 5 years. This difference was significant although the overall mortality was not different between the two treatment approaches. However, the authors did find stabilization of the dissection in patients with TEVAR beyond 1 year of follow-up, while patients with optimal medical therapy had a constant progression over time. Paraplegia after TEVAR is a significant risk, requiring immediate treatment with corticosteroid and spinal drainage.

Percutaneous Transluminal Angioplasty of Supra-aortic Vessel Origins

Supra-aortic percutaneous transluminal angioplasty (PTA) is mainly performed on the left subclavian artery, but in some cases on the brachiocephalic trunk, the proximal carotid arteries, and the right subclavian artery. Stenosis or occlusions may be caused mainly by atherosclerosis and less by inflammatory processes such as Takayasu arteritis. Indications for interventions are embolic events, neurological symptoms due to steal or malperfusion, or brachial claudication. Dilatation of the left subclavian artery is relatively safe, with a low rate of vertebral embolization. However stent placement is frequently necessary due to an insufficient post-PTA result.

Sixt el al. [12] retrospectively analyzed 108 interventions of atherosclerotic lesions in subclavian arteries or the brachiocephalic trunk, representing 92% of the patients treated for subclavian artery obstructive disease during a 10-year period. The primary success rate was 97%: 100% for stenoses (78/78) and 87% for total occlusions (26/30). Treatment modalities included PTA alone (13%; n=14) or stenting (87%; n=90) with balloon-expandable (n=61) or self-expanding (n=17) devices, or both (n=12). The 1-year primary patency rate of the 97 patients eligible for follow-up was 88%: 79% for the PTA subgroup and 89% for the stenting subgroup (p=0.2).

Babic et al. [13] reported a reasonably high technical success of 82% and a complication rate of 7% in 56 patients treated for chronic total occlusions of the subclavian artery. Patency after 3 years was 83%.

Van Hattum et al. [14] evaluated the results of PTA and stent placement in isolated brachiocephalic trunk lesions in 30 patients with isolated clinically significant stenoses (n=25) or occlusions (n=5) of the brachiocephalic artery. The initial technical success rate was 83% (occlusions, 60%; stenoses, 88%), and the clinical success rate 81%. Two patients had major complications, and four experienced minor complications. At a median follow-up of 24 months (4 weeks to 92 months), the primary clinical patency rate was 79% (95% confidence interval (CI): 57%, 104%), with 83% (95% CI: 60%, 105%) for arteries with stents and 67% (95% CI: 13%, 120%) for those without stents (p=0.11). The primary technical patency rate was 50% (95% CI: 24%, 76%).

AbuRahma et al. [15] compared the results of a large series of PTA/stenting procedures in the subclavian artery with the results of a series of carotid-subclavian bypass grafts (CSBG). Subclavian artery PTA/stenting was performed in 121 patients, who were compared with a group of 51 patients with isolated subclavian artery occlusive disease treated with CSBG using polytetrafluoroethylene grafts. The mean follow-up for the PTA/stent group was 3.4 years vs. 7.7 years for the CSBG group. The technical success rate for the CSBG group was 100% vs. 98% (119/121) for the PTA/stent group. The overall perioperative complication rate in the stent group was 15.1% (18/119: 11 minor and 7 major complications) vs. 5.9% (3/51: 2 phrenic nerve palsies and 1 myocardial infarction) in the bypass group (p=0.093). There was no perioperative stroke or mortality in the CSBG group. The major perioperative complications in the stent group included four thromboembolic events, one case of congestive heart failure, one case of reperfusion arm edema, and one of pseudoaneurysm. The 30-day patency rate was 100% for the bypass group and 97% (118/121) for the PTA/stent group. The primary patency rates at 1, 3, and 5 years were 100%, 98%, and 96% for the CSBG group vs. 93%, 78%, and 70% for the stent group, respectively (p<0.0001). Freedom from symptom recurrence was also statistically superior in the bypass group vs. the stent group (p<0.0001). The authors concluded that PTA/stenting of the subclavian artery should be the procedure of choice for high-risk patients, but CSBG should be offered to good-risk surgical candidates who may be seeking a more durable procedure.

Bronchial Artery Embolization

Bronchial artery embolization (BAE) is not a simple intervention for several reasons. First, the anatomy of the bronchial artery is variable and the arteries are frequently very small, which often makes their cannulation difficult. Feeders to bronchial artery bleeding sources – mainly arteriopulmonary fistulae due to tumoral or inflammatory changes – may originate not only from the bronchial artery but also from many other arteries in the thorax, such as the subclavian artery, the thyrocervical trunk, or the mammarian or costal arteries. Moreover, there is variation in collaterals in the region, including the spinal arteries.

Particles, glue and coils are used as embolization materials but a golden rule requires that the artery is sealed as close as possible to the bleeding source, to avoid recurrence via collateral feeders shortly thereafter.

Benign reasons for bronchial bleeding include bronchiectasis, chronic bronchitis, aspergillosis, tuberculosis, pneumonia, and abscesses. Malignant sources are predominantly bronchial cancers.

The results of percutaneous intervention are relatively good. Kato et al. [16] treated 101 patients and achieved a technical success of 100%, a 1-year success of 77.7%, and a 5-year success of 62.5%. A better outcome was observed in patients with tuberculosis and bronchitis and a less favorable one in those with pneumonia and abscesses.

Lee et al. [17] described their experience with BAE in 54 patients that were treated for massive hemoptysis in a 5-year period. The underlying pathologies included bronchiectasis (n=31), active tuberculosis (n=9), pneumoconiosis (n=3), lung cancer (n=2), and pulmonary angiodysplasia (n=1). Surgery was considered if the patient had acceptable pulmonary reserve and a bleeding source was clearly identified. If the patient was not considered fit for surgery, BAE was attempted. Hemoptysis ceased with conservative management only in seven patients (13%). In the 27 (50%) patients who underwent surgical resection, the procedures included lobectomy (n=21), bilobectomy (n=4), and pneumonectomy (n=2). In-hospital mortality after surgery was 15%. Postoperative morbidity occurred in eight patients, including prolonged ventilatory support, bronchopleural fistulae, empyema, and myocardial infarction. BAE was also used in 21 patients not eligible for surgery. The procedure was successful in 17 patients, without any complications.

Woo et al. [18] retrospectively compared BAE with particles vs. bucrylate glue. In a considerably large cohort (293 procedures with particles, 113 with glue), they achieved a technical success of 94% vs. 97%. The complication rate was similar but freedom from rebleeding was better: at 1, 3, and 5 years, 88%, 85%, and 83% with glue vs. with 77%, 68%, and 66% particles.

Witt et al. [19] performed BAE using platinum coils with Dacron fibers in 30 consecutive patients with bleeding from bronchial carcinoma. The aim of that study was to compare immediate results with respect to bleeding cessation as well as recurrence, and survival rates with BAE vs. conservative management. Active bleeding stopped immediately in all patients. A comparison of the BAE group with the controls showed that the cessation of first-time hemoptysis was 100% in the BAE group vs. 93% in the non-BAE group. The rates of bleeding recurrence were similar in the two groups (BAE 50% vs. non-BAE 47%). In case of recurrent bleeding, repeated BAE led to a definite cessation of pulmonary hemorrhage in every case. By contrast, all patients with recurrent hemoptysis without a repeated BAE (8 patients, 27%) and all patients with bleeding recurrence who were in the non-BAE group died from pulmonary hemorrhage (8 patients, 53%). The mean survival time of the BAE group was significantly longer than that of the non-BAE group. The authors therefore concluded that BAE was beneficial in patients tumoral pulmonary bleeding.

Venous Interventions

Pulmonary Artery Embolization

Pulmonary artery embolization is an infrequently used tool to treat traumatic damage to the pulmonary artery induced by catheters or trauma and to treat pulmonary artery-vein shunts. In single institutions it has been modified as chemoembolization and used in the palliative treatment of patients with lung cancer [20]. There are no clinical randomized data on pulmonary artery embolization, only an experimental study in rats [21] that showed a significant reduction of tumor size compared to intravenous chemotherapy.

Recently, an Italian group described a a single cohort study in which a combination of segmental pulmonary artery embolization and RFA was used in 17 patients with 20 nodules. The technical success rate was good and a clinical complete response was achieved in 65% [22].

Pulmonary Artery Embolectomy

Treatment of acute symptomatic PE by catheter-directed methods has long been a goal of interventional radiologists but its realization has been hampered by two problems in particular. First, massive PE may lead to relatively mild symptoms not necessitating aggressive treatment. Second, intravenous thrombolysis is usually effective in most patients. Moreover, those patients who are candidates for a percutaneous approach die early or are in very poor clinical condition, as most are hemodynamically unstable and require emergency treatment but are not transportable. This logistical aspect has prevented the widespread use of catheter-based interventions. Nonetheless, among the small cohorts of patients treated with this approach, the results have been encouraging.

Kuo et al. [23] retrospectively analyzed 70 consecutive patients over a 10-year period with suspected acute PE who had been referred for pulmonary angiography and/or intervention. The criteria for study inclusion were patients who received catheter directed intervention (CDI) due to angiographically confirmed massive pulmonary embolism and hemodynamic shock (shock index $\geqslant 0.9$). CDI involved suction embolectomy and fragmentation with or without catheter thrombolysis. Twelve patients were treated with CDI. Seven patients (58%) were referred for CDI after failing to respond to systemic infusion with 100 mg of tissue plasminogen activator, and five patients (42%) had contraindications to systemic thrombolysis. Catheter-directed fragmentation and embolectomy were performed in all patients (100%) and catheter-guided thrombolysis in eight patients (67%). Technical success was achieved in all 12 cases (100%). There were no major procedural complications. Significant hemodynamic improvement (shock index: <0.9) was reported in 10 of the 12 patients (83%). The remaining two patients (17%) died secondary to cardiac arrest within 24 h. The authors concluded that CDI is potentially a life-saving treatment for patients who have not responded to or cannot tolerate systemic thrombolysis.

Lin et al. [24] evaluated the treatment outcome in patients with massive PE who were treated with either ultrasound-accelerated thrombolysis using the EkoSonic Endovascular System (EKOS; EKOS; Bothell, WA) or catheter-directed thrombolysis (CDT). Twenty-five patients underwent 33 CDI for massive pulmonary embolism during the study period. Among them, EKOS was performed in 15 (45%) and CDT in 18 (55%). In the EKOS group, complete thrombus removal was achieved in 100% cases. In the CDT cohort, complete or partial thrombus removal was accomplished in 7 (50%) and 2 (14%) cases, respectively. Comparing treatment success based on thrombus removal, EKOS resulted in an improved treatment outcome compared with the CDT group (p<0.02). The mean time of thrombolysis was 17.4 ± 5.23 h and 25.3 ± 7.35 h in the EKOS and CDT groups, respectively (p=0.03). The mortality rate was 9.1% and 14.2% (not significant). Treatment-related hemorrhagic complication rates in the EKOS and CDT group were 0% and 21.4%, respectively (p=0.02). A significant reduction in Miller scores was noted in both groups following catheter-based interventions.

Malignant Venous Obstruction (Superior Vena Cava Syndrome)

Another percutaneous procedure that has become increasingly popular is the placement of metallic stents to treat superior vena cava syndrome (SVCS). Unlike emergency radiation, stenting gives rapid relief of symptoms within a few hours or even immediately. The technique is relatively simple and can be achieved from either a brachial or a transfemoral approach. If the obstruction is associated with thrombus, stenting can be combined with thrombolysis.

Lanciego et al. [25] used stent placement as the first-choice treatment for the relief of symptoms in 52 cancer patients who were diagnosed with SVCS confirmed by cavography or phlebography. Wallstent prostheses (n=73) were inserted in all patients. A single stent was sufficient in 37 patients, two stents were required in 11, three stents in 2, and four stents in another 2 patients. Contraindications for the procedure were severe cardiopathy or coagulopathy. Resolution of symptoms was achieved in all patients within 72 h. At follow-up, six obstructions, one partial migration to the right atrium, two incorrect placements, and four stent "shortenings" were noted. All were successfully resolved by repeat stenting. Symptom-free survival ranged from 2 days to 17 months (mean: 6.4 months). The authors concluded that the Wallstent vascular endoprosthesis is an effective initial treatment in patients with SVCS of neoplastic origin.

Nagata et al. [26] retrospectively investigated the utility of metallic stent placement, mainly the spiral Z-stent (S-Z-stent), for the treatment of malignant obstruction of the SVC in 71 patients with SVCS. The 71 patients who underwent stent placement were followed until death. The technical success rate was 100%, the initial clinical success rate was 87% (62/71), the primary clinical patency rate was 88% (57/65), and the secondary clinical patency rate was 95% (62/65). Stent obstruction occurred at a rate of 12% (8/65), requiring secondary stenting. The survival times of the 57 patients in whom there was no SVCS recurrence ranged from 1 week to 29 months (mean: 5.4 months). The S-Z-stent was considered to be suitable for the treatment of malignant obstruction of the SVC. Unilateral stent placement was effective for relief of SVCS in patients with bilateral brachiocephalic vein obstruction.

Benign Venous Stenoses and Occlusions

Partial venous obstruction usually does not become clinically evident as long as there is a collateral network. In patients with dialysis fistulas, however, high venous flow may result in severe venous congestions in case the ipsilateral venous outflow is obstructed. These obstructions are frequently sequelae of an earlier placement of venous dialysis catheters into the subclavian vein. However, since over time the policy has changed to a jugular access for those catheters, there are fewer central venous outflow problems.

Treatment of benign venous stenoses is not simple, as balloon angioplasty usually fails to gain long-term improvement. Stent placement yields excellent short-term results but is burdened by a high rate of recurrent stenoses due to massive neointimal tissue growth within the stents, thus requiring frequent reinterventions. Polymer-covered stent grafts may be more promising in preventing recurrent stenoses but the results of larger studies are still pending.

Haage et al. [27] analyzed the effectiveness of stent placement as the primary treatment for central venous obstruction in 50 patients undergoing hemodialysis. Stent deployment (n=57, Wallstent stents) was successful in all patients, with early rethrombosis (within 1 week) noted in only one patient (2%). Among the 73 episodes of re-obstruction, 54 (74%) were treated percutaneously with angioplasty alone and 19 (26%) necessitated additional stent placement. The 3-, 6-, 12-, and 24-month primary patency rates were 92%, 84%, 56%, and 28%, respectively. Cumulative overall stent patency was 97% after 6 and 12 months, 89% after 24 months, and 81% after 36 and 48 months.

Bakken et al. [28] compared the outcomes of primary angioplasty (PTA) vs. primary stenting (PTS) in a dialysis access population. PTS was used to treat 26 patients (26 stenoses) and PTA in 47 patients with 49 central venous stenoses. The PTS group underwent 71 percutaneous interventions (average, 2.7 ± 2.4 interventions per stenosis), and the PTA group 98 interventions (average, 2.0 ± 1.6 interventions per stenosis). Primary patency was equivalent between the two groups by Kaplan-Meier analysis, with 30-day rates of 76% for both and 12-month rates of 29% for the PTA group and 21% for the PTS group (p=0.48). Assisted primary patency was also equivalent (p=0.08), with a 30-day patency rate of 81% and a 12-month rate of 73% for the PTA group, vs. 84% at 30 days and 46% at 12 months in the PTS group. Ipsilateral hemodialysis access survival was equivalent in the two groups. The authors concluded that PTS does not improve the patency rates compared to PTA and does not add to the longevity of ipsilateral hemodialysis access sites.

Jones et al. [29] used a stent graft (Viabahn) to treat 30 patients with central venous stenosis. Surveillance was carried out at 3, 6, 9, 12, 18, and 24 months using diagnostic fistulography. The technical success rate was 100%. Primary patency rates were 97%, 81%, 67%, and 45%;

primary assisted patency rates were 100%, 100%, 80%, and 75% at 3, 6, 12, and 24 months, respectively. Twelve patients required further stent-grafts to maintain patency.

Ferguson et al. [30] used stents in six patients with fibrosing mediastinitis with venous obstruction. Four patients were treated with intravascular stents placed percutaneously. One patient underwent surgical intravascular stent placement and one patient declined surgical therapy. The right pulmonary artery was treated in three patients, the SVC in one patient, and three pulmonary veins in the fifth patient. Each intervention resulted in hemodynamic improvement with subsequent clinical improvement. Reintervention was required within 12 months in two of the four percutaneously treated patients. The authors concluded that stents are an effective option in improving short-term vascular patency. In-stent stenosis was a frequent complication in patients with fibrosing mediastinitis.

Riley et al. [31] investigated the treatment of SVCS as a complication of pacemaker implantation, carrying out a Pubmed search to identify cases of symptomatic SVCS that developed following the implantation of permanent pacemakers or implantable cardioverter defibrillators. Patients in the study had been treated with one of five different modalities: anticoagulation, thrombolysis, venoplasty, stenting, and surgical reconstruction. The literature search identified 74 publications reporting 104 eligible cases in which SVCS presented at a median of 48 months after device implantation. Anticoagulation, thrombolysis, and venoplasty alone were all associated with high recurrence rates. Surgery and stenting were more successful, with recurrence rates of 12% and 5% over a median follow-up of 16 (range: 2–179) and 9.5 (range: 2–60) months, respectively. Based on our own observations, over the last 40 years conservative treatments have been replaced by surgical reconstruction, and most recently by stenting, as the most common therapeutic modality employed.

There is some evidence [32] that covered stents with an expanded polytetrafluoroethylene coating are more effective in preventing restenosis than PTA alone, but bare stents have yet to be compared with stent grafts. Limitations in size and diameter and the problem of overriding collateral veins restrict the wide-spread use of stent grafts in the thoracic venous circulation.

Conclusion

The great variation of vascular and nonvascular procedures in the thorax offers a vast opportunity for the use of many different therapeutic techniques, some rarely performed or restricted to just a few centers, and others with a relevance and general importance for many patients.

References

1. Laurent F, Latrabe V, Vergier B, Michel P (2000) Percutaneous CT-guided biopsy of the lung: comparison between aspiration and automated cutting needles using a coaxial technique. Cardiovasc Intervent Radiol 23:266-272.
2. Richardson CM, Pointon KS, Manhire AR, Macfarlane JT (2002) Percutaneous lung biopsies: a survey of UK practice based on 5444 biopsies. Br. J Radiol 75:731-735.
3. Chojniak R, Isberner RK, Viana LM et al (2006) Computed tomography guided needle biopsy: experience from 1,300 procedures. Sao Paulo Med J 124:10-14
4. Poretti FP, Brunner E, Vorwerk D (2002) Simple localization of peripheral pulmonary nodules - CT-guided percutaneous hook-wire localization. Rofo Fortschr Geb Rontgenstr Neuen Bildgeb Verfahr 174:202-207.
5. de Baère T., Farouil G, Deschamps F (2013) Lung Cancer Ablation: What is the evidence? Semin Intervent Radiol 30: 151-156.
6. Gillams A, Khan Z, Osborn P, Lees W (2013) Survival after radiofrequency ablation in 122 patients with inoperable colorectal lung metastases. Cardiovasc Intervent Radiol 36: 724-730.
7. Schlijper RC, Grutters JP, Houben R et al (2014) What to choose as radical local treatment for lung metastases from colo-rectal cancer surgery or radiofrequency ablation? Cancer Treat Rev 40:60-67.
8. Tramontano AC, Cipriano LE, Kong CY (2013) Microsimulation model predicts survival benefit of radiofrequency ablation and stereotactic body radiotherapy vs. radiotherapy for treating inoperable stage I non-small cell lung cancer. AJR Am J Roentgenol 200:1020-1027.
9. Matsumura JS, Cambria RP, Dake MD; TX2 Clinical Trial Investigators (2008) International controlled clinical trial of thoracic endovascular aneurysm repair with the Zenith TX2 endovascular graft: 1-year results. J Vasc Surg 47:247-257.
10. Nienaber CA, Kische S, Akin I et al (2010) Strategies for subacute/chronic type B aortic dissection: the Investigation Of Stent Grafts in Patients with type B Aortic Dissection (INSTEAD) trial 1-year outcome. J Thorac Cardiovasc Surg 140(6 Suppl):S101-108.
11. Nienaber CA, Kische S, Rousseau H et al; INSTEAD-XL trial (2013) Endovascular repair of type B aortic dissection: long-term results of the randomized investigation of stent grafts in aortic dissection trial. Circ Cardiovasc Interv 6:407-416.
12. Sixt S, Rastan A, Schwarzwälder U et al (2009) Results after balloon angioplasty or stenting of atherosclerotic subclavian artery obstruction. Catheter Cardiovasc Interv 73:395-403.
13. Babic S, Sagic D, Radak D et al (2012) Initial and long-term results of endovascular therapy for chronic total occlusion of the subclavian artery. Cardiovasc Intervent Radiol 35: 255-262.
14. van Hattum ES, de Vries JP, Lalezari F et al (2007) Angioplasty with or without stent placement in the brachiocephalic artery: feasible and durable? A retrospective cohort study. J Vasc Interv Radiol 18:1088-1093.
15. AbuRahma AF, Bates MC, Stone PA et al (2007) Angioplasty and stenting vs. carotid-subclavian bypass for the treatment of isolated subclavian artery disease. J Endovasc Ther 14: 698-704.
16. Kato A, Kudo S, Matsumoto K et al (2000) Bronchial artery embolization for hemoptysis due to benign diseases: immediate and long-term results. Cardiovasc Intervent Radiol 23: 351-357.
17. Lee TW, Wan S, Choy DK (2000) Management of massive hemoptysis: a single institution experience. Ann Thorac Cardiovasc Surg 6:232-235.
18. Woo S, Yoon CJ, Chung JW et al (2013) Bronchial artery embolization to control hemoptysis: comparison of N-butyl-2-cyanoacrylate and polyvinyl alcohol particles. Radiology 269:594-602.
19. Witt Ch, Schmidt B, Geisler A et al (2000) Value of bronchial artery embolisation with platinum coils in tumorous pulmonary bleeding. Eur J Cancer 36:1949-1954.

20. Vogl TJ, Wetter A, Lindemayr S, Zangos S (2005) Treatment of unresectable lung metastases with transpulmonary chemoembolization: preliminary experience. Radiology 234:917-922.

21. Schneider P, Kampfer S, Loddenkemper C et al (2002) Chemoembolization of the lung improves tumor control in a rat model. Clin Cancer Res 8:2463-2468.

22. Gadaleta CD, Solbiati L, Mattioli V et al (2013) Unresectable lung malignancy: combination therapy with segmental pulmonary arterial chemoembolization with drug-eluting microspheres and radiofrequency ablation in 17 patients. Radiology 267:627-637.

23. Kuo WT, van den Bosch MA, Hofmann LV et al (2008) Catheter-directed embolectomy, fragmentation, and thrombolysis for the treatment of massive pulmonary embolism after failure of systemic thrombolysis. Chest 134:250-254.

24. Lin PH, Annambhotla S, Bechara CF et al (2009) Comparison of percutaneous ultrasound-accelerated thrombolysis vs. catheter-directed thrombolysis in patients with acute massive pulmonary embolism. Vascular 17 Suppl 3:S137-147.

25. Lanciego C, Chacon JL, Julian A et al (2001) Stenting as first option for endovascular treatment of malignant superior vena Cavasyndrome. AJR Am J Roentgenol 177:585-593.

26. Nagata T, Makutani S, Uchida H et al (2007) Follow-up results of 71 patients undergoing metallic stent placement for the treatment of a malignant obstruction of the superior vena cava. Cardiovasc Intervent Radiol 30:959-967.

27. Haage P, Vorwerk D, Piroth W et al (1999) Treatment of hemodialysis-related central venous stenosis or occlusion: results of primary Wallstent placement and follow-up in 50 patients. Radiology 212:175-180.

28. Bakken AM, Protack CD, Saad WE et al (2007) Long-term outcomes of primary angioplasty and primary stenting of central venous stenosis in hemodialysis patients. J Vasc Surg 45:776-783.

29. Jones RG, Willis AP, Jones C et al (2011) Long-term results of stent-graft placement to treat central venous stenosis and occlusion in hemodialysis patients with arteriovenous fistulas. J Vasc Interv Radiol 22:1240-1245.

30. Ferguson ME, Cabalka AK, Cetta F, Hagler DJ (2010) Results of intravascular stent placement for fibrosing mediastinitis. Congenit Heart Dis 5:124-133.

31. Riley RF, Petersen SE, Ferguson JD, Bashir Y (2010) Managing superior vena cava syndrome as a complication of pacemaker implantation: a pooled analysis of clinical practice. Pacing Clin Electrophysiol 33:420-425.

32. Haskal ZJ, Trerotola S, Dolmatch B (2010) Stent graft vs. balloon angioplasty for failing dialysis-access grafts. N Engl J Med 362:494-503.

Nonvascular Interventional Radiology of the Thorax

Albert A. Nemcek, Jr.

Department of Radiology, Northwestern Memorial Hospital, Chicago, IL, USA

Percutaneous Transthoracic Needle Biopsy

Transthoracic biopsy of pulmonary and mediastinal lesions is a commonly performed diagnostic procedure. It is used to confirm malignancy in anticipation of appropriate therapy or to spare patients with benign disease from unnecessary surgery. In the following, space limitations prohibit a detailed discussion of techniques and complications; instead, the reader is referred to several reviews of this topic for details [1-5]. Current areas of interest include the use of alternate image-guidance methods, such as real-time ultrasound for peripheral lung lesions and cone-beam computed tomography (CT) [6, 7]; integrated navigational systems for guidance [8]; methods to decrease the rate of post-procedural pneumothorax [9]: and the procurement of tissue for genomic analysis [10].

Lung Tumor Localization

Pulmonary nodule localization may be requested in patients scheduled for thoracoscopic resection of small, peripheral pulmonary nodules, in order to confidently localize these lesions [11]. Several methods of localization have been described, including hook-wire localization, image-guided dye injection, the placement of fiducials or clips, intraoperative ultrasound of the deflated lung, and radionuclide injection. A method using microcoil deployment through the nodule and trailing to the pleural surface has been described that appears to have several advantages compared to previously described methods [12].

Drainage of Thoracic Fluid Collections

Thoracentesis

One of the most common image-guided interventions in the thorax is thoracentesis. Thoracentesis is performed for two main, sometimes overlapping indications: In diagnostic thoracentesis, an aliquot of collected fluid is sent to laboratory analysis to try to more specifically identify the cause of pleural fluid accumulation. In therapeutic thoracentesis, fluid is withdrawn to relieve symptoms such as dyspnea (most often) or hemodynamic compromise.

The benefits of real-time ultrasonography in improving the success and safety of thoracentesis (as well as chest tube placement) have been clearly documented, such that its use is now strongly recommended [13, 14]. Ultrasound evaluation confirms the presence and location of fluid, improves the characterization of fluid collections, and helps to avoid puncture of the lungs or other organs during the procedure.

Hemorrhagic complications may occur as a result of thoracentesis, although the degree of risk relative to various coagulation parameters is controversial [13]. Since the intercostal neurovascular bundle is typically on the undersurface of the rib, it is prudent to try to enter the pleural space above the rib. However, there is considerable variability in the position of the intercostal artery and its branches based on age and relative thoracic position. The British Thoracic Society therefore recommends that unless fluid is loculated posteriorly, thoracentesis should be performed in the "triangle of safety," bordered anteriorly by the lateral edge of the pectoralis major muscle, laterally by the lateral edge of the latissimus dorsi, inferiorly by the fifth intercostal space, and superiorly by the base of the axilla [14].

Pneumothorax may also develop during thoracentesis, with lower rates generally associated with the use of ultrasound guidance. In pneumothorax resulting simply from the leakage of air via the needle or catheter there is no clinical significance. However, pneumothorax may also develop due to direct injury to the visceral pleural surface, although this should be largely avoidable with good technique and imaging guidance. Finally, air may leak into the lung as an ex-vacuo phenomenon in cases of trapped lung. In these instances, as fluid is aspirated the lung fails to expand, and air may leak from the lung as the intrapleural pressures decrease. This has been reported as the primary cause of pneumothorax following

Diseases of the Chest and Heart 2015-2018,
DOI: 10.1007/978-88-470-5752-4_21 © Springer-Verlag Italia 2015

therapeutic thoracentesis [15], but patients with these types of pneumothorax rarely require therapy.

Another potential complication of therapeutic thoracentesis is re-expansion pulmonary edema. This complication is rare, generally mild, and responds to conservative measures including oxygen administration and diuresis. It seems more common in younger patients, those with more chronic effusions, and those in whom large amounts of fluid are removed [16]. The latter consideration has led to recommendations of maximal fluid amounts during thoracentesis (usually 1000–1500 mL). However, it has also been argued that larger volumes of pleural fluid can be safely withdrawn as long as the patient does not develop vague chest discomfort or excessively negative (<-20 cm H_2O) intrapleural pressures, as measured by pleural manometry [17].

Malignant Pleural Effusions

Malignant pleural effusions are the second most common cause of exudative pleural effusions and the most common cause of such effusions in patients over 60 years of age. While malignant pleural effusions can occur with virtually any primary tumor, they are most often the result of lung cancer, breast cancer, or lymphoma. Patients tend to present with dyspnea (over 50% of patients), chest pain (usually dull in nature), cough, and generalized systemic symptoms that reflect advanced metastatic disease. There are many techniques for the management of malignant effusions [18-20], depending on the type and stage of malignancy. In advanced malignancy, the goal is palliative and is directed primarily toward relieving the dyspnea, with the exception of the pharmacologic management of pain. Indeed, opiate therapy, in combination with oxygen, is often underutilized in patients with a short life expectancy but may be quite helpful in relieving dyspnea. Therapeutic thoracentesis is a first step in more definitive therapy as it is important to determine whether fluid removal does, in fact, result in improvement in dyspnea. However, thoracentesis rarely provided lasting control of dyspnea, with fluid reaccumulating in 98–100% of patients within 30 days.

Indwelling tunneled catheters, placed with imaging guidance, are another management option in patients with malignant pleural effusions. These catheters are well-accepted by patients, provide good palliation of dyspnea, and result in "auto-pleurodesis" in over 50% and as high as 70% of patients, thus allowing eventual catheter removal.

Tube thoracostomy can be combined with chemical pleurodesis, with the aim of causing inflammation and the adherence of the visceral and parietal pleural surfaces. Talc is a commonly used agent, although its optimal dosage and formulation remain uncertain; in addition, patients may require prolonged hospitalization during this form of therapy. Pleurodesis can also be performed thoracoscopically; while more invasive, this approach can provide excellent distribution of the sclerosing agents and be combined with mechanical abrasion.

Pleuroperitoneal shunts, placed surgically or percutaneously, allow patients to actively treat their dyspnea on their own. The disadvantages include obstruction or infection of the device and the need to pump the device multiple times per day.

Another option, unavailable as a percutaneous technique, is surgical stripping of the pleura. Although very effective, this method carries high morbidity and an approximately 10% mortality rate.

Empyema and Parapneumonic Effusion

Pleural effusions associated with infection (parapneumonic effusion and empyema) tend to evolve in stages. In the initial, exudative stage, the fluid is thin and sterile and associated with a low white blood cell (WBC) count. In the fibropurulent stage, bacteria invade the pleural space, the WBC count increases (an empyema is defined as grossly purulent fluid), and fibrin begins to be deposited on pleural surfaces and as septae within the fluid. Finally, in the organization stage, a thick peel of fibrous tissue encapsulates the pleural space. Chest-tube drainage is most effective in the earlier stages but ineffective in the organization stage. Intuition would suggest that elimination of the fibrin while fluid is being drained would facilitate drainage. Indeed, encouraging studies in this regard appeared as early as the 1940s [21] although interest waned partly due to allergic reactions to streptokinase, the primary fibrinolytic agent used at that time. A recent multicenter trial [22] compared patients with pleural infection (purulent pleural fluid, pleural fluid with pH <7.2, and signs of infection, or proven bacterial infection of the pleural space) in a double-blind trial. The 454 patients were randomly assigned to treatment with intrapleural streptokinase or placebo. There were no significant differences between the groups with regard to endpoints of death or requirement for surgery. More recent studies have also looked at deoxyribonucleases in combination with fibrinolytic agents [23]. In one such study, 210 patients with pleural infection were randomly assigned to receive one of four treatments: (1) double placebo; (2) intrapleural tissue plasminogen activator (t-PA) and a DNase; (3) t-PA and placebo; (4) DNase and placebo. The combined treatment group was associated with improved fluid drainage, reduced frequency of surgical referral, and a shorter hospital stay compared to the placebo group. The use of either agent alone did not differ significantly from placebo. Thus, the efficacy of these agents remains controversial [22-24].

Thoracic Ablation Procedures

While surgical resection remains the standard of care for early-stage lung cancer, a variety of ablative techniques have shown promise in the treatment of select primary and metastatic pulmonary malignancies [25, 26]. The largest reported experience is with radiofrequency ablation, although experience with microwave ablation, cryoablation, and other techniques is accumulating as well. Lesions most amenable to successful ablation are small (<3 cm), solitary, and remote from critical structures. Complications are similar to, although greater in frequency than, percutaneous lung biopsy. Few studies have, as yet, compared either the various ablative techniques or ablation with surgery vs. stereotactic radiation therapy.

References

1. Winer-Muram HT (2006) The solitary pulmonary nodule. Radiology 239:34-49.
2. Manhire A, Charig M, Clelland C et al (2003) Guidelines for radiologically guided lung biopsy. Thorax 58:920-936.
3. Ahrar K, Wallace M, Javadi S, Gupta S (2008) Mediastinal, hilar, and pleural image-guided biopsy: current practice and techniques. Semin Respir Crit Care Med 29:350-360.
4. Moore EH (2008) Percutaneous lung biopsy: an ordering clinician's guide to current practice. Semin Respir Crit Care Med 29:323-334.
5. Wu CC, Maher MM, Shepard JA (2011) Complications of CT-guided percutaneous needle biopsy of the chest: prevention and management. AJR Am J Roentgenol 196: W678-682.
6. Moreira BL, Guimaraes MD, de Oliveira AD et al (2014) Value of ultrasound in the imaging-guided transthoracic biopsy of lung lesions. Ann Thorac Surg 97:1795-1797.
7. Lee SM, Park CM, Lee KH et al (2014) C-arm cone-beam CT-guided percutaneous transthoracic needle biopsy of lung nodules: clinical experience in 1108 patients. Radiology 271:291-300.
8. Grasso RF, Faiella E, Luppi G et al (2013) Percutaneous lung biopsy: comparison between an augmented reality CT navigation system and standard CT-guided technique. In J Comput Assist Radiol & Surg 8:837-848.
9. Zaetta JM, Licht MO, Fisher JS et al (2010). A lung biopsy tract plug for reduction of postbiopsy pneumothorax and other complications: results of a prospective, multicenter, randomized, controlled clinical study. J Vasc Interv Radiol 21:1235-1243.
10. Marshall D, LaBerge JM, Firetag B et al (2013) The changing face of percutaneous image-guided biopsy: molecular profiling and genomic analysis in current practice. J Vasc Interv Radiol 24:1094-1103.
11. Tamara M, Oda M, Fujimori H et al (2010) New indication for preoperative marking of small peripheral pulmonary nodules in thoracoscopic surgery. Interact Cardiovasc Thorac Surg 11:590-593.
12. Mayo JR, Clifton JC, Powell TI et al (2009) Lung nodules: CT-guided placement of microcoils to direct video-assisted thoracoscopic surgical resection. Radiology 250:576-578.
13. Sachdeva A, Shepherd RW, Lee HJ (2013) Thoracentesis and thoracic ultrasound: state of the art. Clin Chest Med 34: 1-9.
14. Havelock T, Teoh R, Laws D et al (2010) Pleural procedures and thoracic ultrasound: British Thoracic Society pleural disease guideline 2010. Thorax 66:828-829.
15. Heidecker J, Huggins JT, Sahn SA, Doelken P (2006) Pathophysiology of pneumothorax following ultrasound-guided thoracentesis. Chest 130:1173-1184.
16. Echevarria C, Thowmey D, Dunning J, Chanda B (2008) Does re-expansion pulmonary oedema exist? Interact Cardiovasc Thorac Surg 7:485-489.
17. Feller-Kopman D, Berkowitz D, Boiselle P, Ernst A (2007) Large-volume thoracentesis and the risk of reexpansion pulmonary edema. Ann Thorac Surg 8:1656-1661.
18. Thomas JM, Musani AI (2013). Malignant pleural effusions: a review. Clin Chest Med 34:459-471.
19. Davies HE, Lee YCG (2013) Management of malignant pleural effusions: questions that need answers. Curr Opin Pulm Med 19:374-379.
20. Kastelik JA (2013) Management of malignant pleural effusion. Lung 191:165-175.
21. Tillett WS, Sherry S (1949) The effect in patients with streptococcal fibrinolysis (streptokinase) and streptococcal desoxyribonuclease on fibrinous, purulent, and sanguinous pleural exudations. J Clin Invest 28:173-190.
22. Maskell NA, Davies CWH, Nunn AJ et al (2005) U.K. controlled trial of intrapleural streptokinase for pleural infection. N Engl J Med 352:865-874.
23. Rahman NM, Maskell NA, West A et al (2011) Intrapleural use of tissue plasminogen activator and Dnase in pleural infection. N Engl J Med 365:518-526.
24. Rahman NM (2012) Intrapleural agents for pleural infection: fibrinolytics and beyond. Curr Opin Pulm Med 18:326-332
25. De Baere T (2011) Lung tumor radiofrequency ablation: where do we stand? Cardovasc Intervent Radiol 34:241-251.
26. Charmarthy MR, Gupta M, Hughes TW et al (2014) Image-guided percutaneous ablation of lung malignancies: a minimally invasive alternative for nonsurgical patients or unresectable tumors. J Bronchol Intervent Pulmonol 21:68-81.

Dose-Lowering Strategies in Computed Tomography Imaging of the Lung and Heart

André Euler[1], Zsolt Szucs-Farkas[2], John R. Mayo[3], Sebastian T. Schindera[1]

[1] Clinic of Radiology and Nuclear Medicine, University of Basel Hospital, Basel, Switzerland
[2] Institute of Radiology, Hospital Centre of Biel, Biel, Switzerland
[3] Department of Radiology, Vancouver General Hospital, Vancouver, BC, Canada

Introduction

Since its first introduction by Hounsfield and Cormack in 1972, computed tomography (CT) has become one of the most important imaging modalities in diagnostic imaging, because of its strong impact on patient outcome. As a result, CT utilization has risen 10% per year during the last 15 years in the USA [1] and 142% between 1998 and 2008 in Switzerland [2]. In 2008, CT was responsible for 68% of the yearly Swiss medical radiation exposure while accounting for only 6% of the ionizing radiation examinations [2]. Current knowledge on the attributable risk of cancer induction by low level medical imaging radiation exposure (<100 submillisievert, mSv) is largely based on longitudinal studies of atomic bomb survivors [3]. These data were recently augmented by two large, retrospective, epidemiologic cohort studies that showed a correlation between CT radiation exposure and a slightly increased cancer risk in children and young adults [4, 5]. However, the disease status of these patients represents a confounding factor in the interpretation of these data.

Given the rapid rise in CT frequency and the potential risk of cancer induction, it is the responsibility of the radiologic community (radiologists, technologists, medical physicists, CT manufacturers) to optimize radiation dose. In addition to ensuring CT examination justification, supervising radiologists are responsible for using the lowest diagnostic CT radiation dose, in accordance with the ALARA (as low as reasonable achievable) principle. In chest examinations, the reasons for rigorous dose optimization include highly radiosensitive organs (breast tissue, bone marrow, lung) within the scanned volume and the frequent scanning of radiosensitive young adults (e.g., to query pulmonary embolism).

The radiation dose in a chest CT can be reduced without degradation of the diagnostic accuracy by taking advantage of the large differences in attenuation between air and soft tissue. The intrinsic high subject contrast allows the acceptance of higher image noise. In addition, CT technical advances have facilitated dose reduction while maintaining image quality. This chapter summarizes the currently available methods for dose reduction/optimization in cardiothoracic CT.

Practical Methods for Dose Reduction

Practical methods for dose reduction are independent of the CT scanner and are controlled by the operator.

Limitation of the Enhancement Phases

A first and simple step in dose reduction is the limitation of the number of acquisition phases dependent on the clinical question. An additional pre-contrast phase in a chest CT is indicated only in a few clinical situations; e.g., to assess an intramural aortic hematoma or an aortic stent graft endoleak. Two-phase scanning for these indications may be eliminated by the use of dual-energy CT, which derives a virtual non-contrast image from a contrast-enhanced dual energy acquisition [6]. However, to realize a reduction in the radiation dose, the dual-energy CT protocol needs to be optimized.

Reduction of Scan Length

In general, the scanned volume should be adapted to the clinical question. For example, in suspected pulmonary embolism, the radiation dose in CT pulmonary angiography can be reduced by up to 30% by only scanning to the level of the subsegmental pulmonary arteries and excluding the lung apex and base [7] (Fig. 1), which harbor distal vessels that will not impact clinical treatment in most cases. The negative impact of this dose reduction strategy is the potential to miss a clinically significant alternative diagnosis, such as a malignant lung nodule.

Diseases of the Chest and Heart 2015-2018,
DOI: 10.1007/978-88-470-5752-4_22 © Springer-Verlag Italia 2015

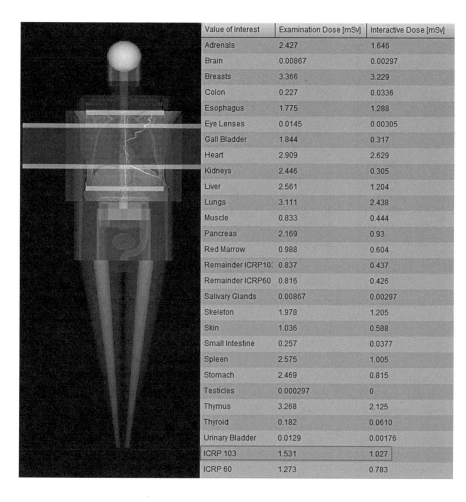

Value of Interest	Examination Dose [mSv]	Interactive Dose [mSv]
Adrenals	2.427	1.646
Brain	0.00867	0.00297
Breasts	3.366	3.229
Colon	0.227	0.0336
Esophagus	1.775	1.288
Eye Lenses	0.0145	0.00305
Gall Bladder	1.844	0.317
Heart	2.909	2.629
Kidneys	2.446	0.305
Liver	2.561	1.204
Lungs	3.111	2.438
Muscle	0.833	0.444
Pancreas	2.169	0.93
Red Marrow	0.988	0.604
Remainder ICRP10:	0.837	0.437
Remainder ICRP60	0.816	0.426
Salivary Glands	0.00867	0.00297
Skeleton	1.978	1.205
Skin	1.036	0.588
Small Intestine	0.257	0.0377
Spleen	2.575	1.005
Stomach	2.469	0.815
Testicles	0.000297	0
Thymus	3.268	2.125
Thyroid	0.182	0.0610
Urinary Bladder	0.0129	0.00176
ICRP 103	1.531	1.027
ICRP 60	1.273	0.783

Fig. 1. Simulation of reduced scan length and estimated organ doses in pulmonary CT angiography to rule out pulmonary embolism, in which the lung apex and base are excluded. A reduction of the effective dose by about one third compared with the original scan volume is estimated by the dose management software (Radimetrics, Bayer, Germany)

Positioning of the Arms

In thoracic CT, the patient's arms should be raised over his or her head to achieve a dose-efficient thoracic CT scan with acceptable image quality. The increased attenuation by the arms in the x-axis forces the automatic tube current modulation to increase the radiation dose to maintain constant image quality, thus increasing the radiation dose to most organs. Furthermore, with the arms next to the thorax, beam-hardening artifacts are increased, degrading image quality (Fig. 2). Compared to arm-down positioning, placing the arms above the head increases subjective and objective image quality [8] and leads to a dose reduction of up to 45% in CT of the thorax and abdomen [9]. If a patient is unable to lift one arm, the technician should still position the other arm above the head.

Patient Positioning in the Isocenter of the CT Scanner

The detrimental radiation dose effect of mis-centering patients within the scanner gantry is often not appreciated by technicians and radiologists. The increased radiation dose associated with mis-centering arises from the pre-patient X-ray beam bowtie filters installed in all modern CT scan-

ners. These filters modify beam strength by strongly attenuating the peripheral projections and weakly attenuating central ones. This evens the X-ray fluence at the detector and reduces the radiation dose to less-attenuating peripheral structures. Incorrect centering defeats the purpose of the bowtie filter, leading to an increased radiation dose to peripheral structures and a decreased image quality [10]. Clinical studies have found that up to 95% of patients receiving a thoracic or abdominal CT scan are not centered properly in the vertical plane [10], with an average error of 2.6 cm. Li et al. quantified this effect, thereby demonstrating that a vertical mis-centering of 3 cm results in an increase in the peripheral radiation dose of up to 18%, with a 6% increase in image noise [10]. Thus, technicians should be trained to meticulously center patients such that the bowtie filters are utilized optimally.

Technical Advances for Dose Reduction

In the last 10 years, CT manufacturers have introduced a number of effective tools that reduce the radiation dose while maintaining or improving image quality. The clinical consequence of impaired image quality associated with dose reduction has been demonstrated in experimental

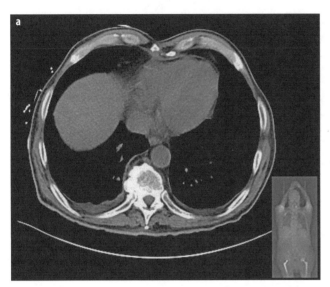
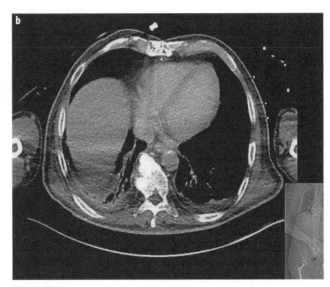

Fig. 2 a, b. Localizer radiograph and transverse CT slice of the lung base in a patient who underwent two CT examinations, one in which the arms were raised over the head (**a**) and the other with the arms placed next to the thorax due to immobility (**b**). The second CT scan resulted in an increase of beam hardening artifacts and reduced image quality in the lung bases

studies using computer-simulated low-dose scans [11]. In the experimental design, intra-observer agreement was lower when noisy, low-dose rather than higher dose exams were interpreted [12]. The authors concluded that optimal dose reduction should be achieved without sacrificing image quality. Since CT manufacturers use diverse technical approaches for dose reduction, there are some differences in the technical implementations and their resultant effectiveness.

Automatic Tube Current Modulation

Since radiation dose is linearly related to tube current at constant kVp, a decrease in the tube current results in dose reduction. Although image noise is impacted by dose reduction, there is no impact on the CT numbers (Hounsfield units) of the body tissues scanned. The aim of automatic tube current modulation (ATCM) is to maintain operator-selected image quality throughout the scan while reducing the radiation dose to the patient. State-of-the-art ATCM modulates the tube current in three dimensions (x-, y-, and z-axes) for every slice of the scan, based on the X-ray attenuation within the slice. Tube current modulation is implemented based on either:

1. attenuation measurements obtained from the topogram or scout views: This approach is used by all manufacturers for z-axis (longitudinal) ATCM modulation, but is used by GE and Toshiba for the x- and y-axes (transverse or angular) [13, 14];
2. tube current adjustment "on the fly" using the measured attenuation of the previous one-half gantry rotation: This approach is used by Siemens for x, y (transverse or angular) ATCM modulation [15].

The noise level or desired image quality is user-programmable and typically adjusted according to the clini-

cal task specified on the clinical requisition. Therefore, the effectiveness of ATCM dose reduction is dependent on the radiologist. Each manufacturer uses a proprietary method to define the desired image quality (e.g., reference mA by Siemens, noise index by GE, standard deviation by Toshiba, reference images by Philips). In chest CT, a dose reduction of 20–26% can be achieved in average-size patients using ATCM rather than fixed tube current [16]. However, in very large patients, ATCM can result in increased radiation doses [17] because the system attempts to maintain uniform image quality almost independently of body size. Thus, the operator needs to be aware of this important caveat and to adjust the image quality level in obese patients.

A few years ago, organ-based tube current modulation was introduced by one manufacturer with the goal of reducing the tube current (x–y plane) when the X-ray tube was positioned over radiosensitive organs, including the female breast, the thyroid gland, and the lens of the eye. Long term follow-up data from the Life Span Study have shown that the radiation sensitivity of female breast tissue is higher than previously thought. Consequently, in the 2007 ICRP (International Commission on Radiological Protection) publication [18], the tissue weighting factor of the female breast was increased. Because in chest CT the breasts are included in the scan range but are not the target organ of the imaging procedure, it is important to decrease the radiation dose to these radiosensitive tissues. Organ-based tube current modulation reduces the tube current in the anterior 120° arc of the rotation by up to 25% of the tube current, while increasing the tube current to 125% over the remaining 240° of the rotation to maintain constant image quality in the center of the patient [19] (Fig. 3). In phantom studies, an average reduction of the breast dose up to 37% was achieved [20].

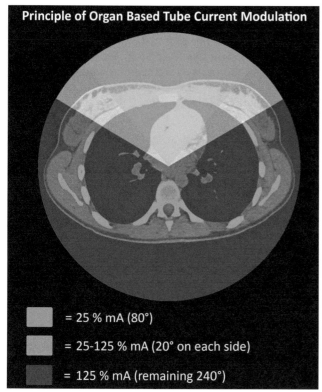

Fig. 3. Principle of organ-based tube current modulation: to protect radiosensitive organs such as the female breasts, the tube current is reduced during the anterior 120° of the gantry rotation. To maintain image quality in the center of the image, the tube current is augmented for the remaining 240° of rotation

Nevertheless, recent clinical studies showed that in a majority of women (up to 99%) parts of the glandular breast tissue are located outside the dose-reduced sector and therefore might be at increased risk of overexposure when organ-based tube current modulation is used [20, 21].

Further refinement of this technique will be required to better protect radiosensitive breast tissue.

Adjustment of the Tube Voltage for Pulmonary CT Angiography

Increasing attention is being paid to the use of lower tube voltages (80–100 kVp) in contrast-enhanced CT. In the chest, pulmonary CT angiography to rule out an embolism is well suited for a low tube voltage technique for two reasons (Fig. 4): while the radiation dose decreases at a more than linear rate, the iodine contrast enhancement increases substantially (by a factor of 2, for example, when the tube voltage is decreased from 140 to 80 kVp). The increased attenuation of contrast medium at reduced kVp (70–100) is secondary to the enhanced photoelectric effect at a lower kVp. Two publications demonstrated that image quality did not decrease when the peak tube voltage for pulmonary CT angiography was lowered to 100 kVp, while resulting in a dose reduction of up to 50% [22, 23]. Furthermore, Schueller-Weidekamm et al. reported an increase in analyzable segmental pulmonary arteries at 100 kVp compared to 140 kVp [23]. The first large-scale prospectively randomized study (REDOPED) investigating the accuracy of low-dose pulmonary CT angiography provided clear evidence that, in patients up to 100 kg body weight, an 80-kVp protocol yields very similar accuracy, diagnostic confidence, and image quality but with a dose that is 30% lower than in a 100-kVp protocol [24]. The estimated effective dose was only 2.25 mSv at 80 kVp. The study also suggested the potential for further dose reduction since it employed a dated CT technology using slow scan times and no iterative reconstruction.

Reduced tube voltage can be implemented either manually or using an automated technique. We employ a manual technique based on clinical observation and

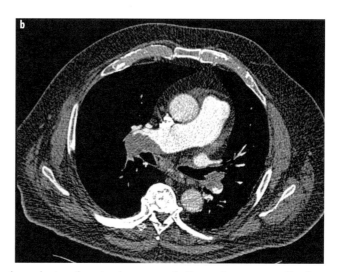

Fig. 4 a, b. Examples of lowering the tube voltage in pulmonary CT angiography to rule out pulmonary embolism. **a** A transverse slice in a male patient (95 kg body weight) who was scanned with 80 kVp [150 mA; volume CT dose index (CTDIvol) of 4.2 mGy]. **b** An obese male patient (150 kg body weight) scanned with 100 kVp (100 mA, CTDIvol of 9.3 mGy). Both images were acquired on a 16-slice MDCT scanner and reconstructed with filtered back projection. The images clearly demonstrate that, even with dated CT technology, lowering of the tube voltage in pulmonary angiography is possible without impairing diagnostic accuracy

measurements; specifically, an 80-kVp protocol is applied for patients with a body weight up to 100 kg and a 100-kVp protocol for patients with a body weight >100 kg (Fig. 4). At least two manufacturers offer automatic tube voltage selection, which selects an optimal tube voltage based on patient size, selected CT protocol, and operator-defined image quality [25]. In a prospective study, Niemann et al. demonstrated a dose reduction of 39% in pulmonary CT angiography using automatic tube voltage selection [25]. Instead of the standard tube voltage of 120 kVp, in 28% of the cases a tube voltage of 100 kVp and in 69% of the cases a tube voltage of 80 kVp were automatically selected.

Iterative Reconstruction Technique

While the commonly used filtered back-projection image reconstruction technique is computationally efficient, it suffers from noise and artifact limitations. Despite their availability over 20 years ago, iterative reconstruction (IR) techniques never gained acceptance due to their computational intensity and slow image reconstruction speed. The advent of faster computer platforms and the demand for a reduction of the radiation dose without an increase in image noise has spurred research into IR. The nomenclature of IR techniques is not yet standard. Manufacturers have developed a number of proprietary techniques involving different strengths and varying in reconstruction speed, spatial resolution, and image noise. In general, in IR an initial image is formed that is then used to generate simulated raw scan data, which are compared to the acquired scan data. A new image is then generated based on the difference. This process is repeated, or iterated, to further improve the image. IR can operate either with image and raw scan data space (Adaptive Statistical Iterative Reconstruction, ASIR, GE Healthcare; Adaptive Iterative Dose Reduction 3D, AIDR 3D, Toshiba, Sinogram Affirmed Iterative Reconstruction, SAFIRE, Siemens Healthcare; and iDose, Philips Healthcare) or raw scan data space alone (MBIR or Veo, GE Healthcare; Advanced Modeled Iterative Reconstruction, ADMIRE, Siemens Healthcare). IR is a powerful tool to either improve image quality in large patients or to maintain diagnostically adequate noise while decreasing radiation dose in small or intermediate sized patients.

There are numerous reports of substantial dose reductions using IR rather than standard filtered back projection while maintaining image quality [26, 27]. However, radiologist applying IR techniques have to be aware of the fact that images thus reconstructed tend have a blotchier and more pixilated appearance, impacting the evaluation of normal anatomic lung structure such as the interlobular fissures, subsegmental bronchial walls, and small peripheral blood vessels [27]. This occurs particularly with very aggressive noise reduction in order to achieve sub-mSv chest CT scans. Moreover, the image quality of sub-mSv chest CT is suboptimal for diagnosing mediastinal structures such as lymph nodes [27]. In the use of IR techniques for dose reduction in general, radiologists are advised to pay extra attention to the diagnostic accuracy with respect to the detection of small pulmonary nodules on the IR images. This advice is given against the background of the substantially decreased image noise achieved with IR but no impact of improved lesion detectability [28].

Special Indications

Pulmonary CT Angiography in Pregnancy

Low-dose pulmonary CT angiography is a valuable alternative for a ventilation/perfusion scan to exclude pulmonary embolism in a pregnant woman with elevated D-dimer level and negative compression sonography of the veins of the lower extremities. The use of tube voltages of 80 or 100 kVp and limiting the scan range from the aortic arch to the diaphragm will effectively reduce the radiation dose. The increased radiosensitivity of the glandular breast tissue during pregnancy deserves particular attention. Although the impact of using breast shields in preventing higher absorbed breast dose is controversial [29, 30], a reduction of tube current in the anterior part of the thorax with organ-based tube current modulation might offer a partial solution, as mentioned earlier.

Lung Cancer Screening

Recent US and Japanese lung cancer screening trial data have shown a statistically significant ($p < 0.05$) reduction in lung cancer mortality when lung cancers are diagnosed at an early stage [31, 32]. Ultra low dose lung cancer screening is possible because the large contrast differences between the pulmonary nodules and surrounding air-filled lung allows the use of images with very high noise levels; however, mediastinal images will have reduced diagnostic accuracy with these techniques. The image quality and diagnostic accuracy for the lung parenchyma using low mA values have been investigated [12, 33]. Results from phantom studies showed that 80 or 100 kVp can be combined with 25 mA with no deterioration in the detection of small lung nodules [33]. A recent phantom study achieved high image quality and sensitivity in pulmonary nodule detection at an effective dose of 0.06 mSv using a novel IR technique and tin filtration for spectral shaping [34].

Cardiac CT Dose Reduction

In cardiac CT, the requirement for scan acquisition to be synchronized to the phase of the cardiac cycle leads to specialized dose reduction strategies [35]. The initial approach to cardiac gating was retrospectively gated helical acquisitions that used low pitch values (approximately 0.2–0.5 depending on heart rate and single vs. dual tube gantry configuration) to provide raw scan data at all spatial locations in all phases of the cardiac cycle. Initial retrospective helical acquisition allowed the reconstruction of low-noise images at multiple cardiac phases. The images were typically reconstructed at 5 or 10% increments of the R to R interval. These image sets provided visualization of the coronary arteries and the motion of the ventricular walls and valves but at the cost of a high radiation dose (9–32 mSv). Moreover, this acquisition technique was radiation dose wasteful for pure coronary artery imaging, as the arteries are only motion free at 60–80% of the R to R interval for heart rates below 80 beats per minute.

The dose efficiency of retrospective helical acquisition was improved by >50% with the implementation of EKG tube current modulation, which reduces tube current by 50–90% during high-motion portions of the cardiac cycle. This provides low-noise coronary artery images in diastole and noisier wall and valve motion images at selected increments through the remaining cardiac cycle. The use of tube current modulation is recommended for all retrospective cardiac-gated acquisitions.

Prospective cardiac gating provides further dose reductions for coronary artery imaging by acquiring raw scan data only at 60–80% of the cardiac cycle. This scan acquisition mode is a modification of "step and shoot," with the scanner table stationary while a full detector width (e.g., 40 mm) of raw scan data are acquired. The scan table is then moved (e.g., 35 mm) and raw data are acquired at another position of the heart during the next heart beat. Thus, the detector steps through the entire cardiac volume, while the 5-mm overlap ensures there are no gaps in the coronary artery anatomy due to minor variations in heart positions between acquisitions. This results in a pitch factor of 0.875. Depending on the size of the heart and the width of the detector, three to five table steps are used. The result is a 77% dose reduction compared to retrospective helical acquisition without tube current modulation. Wide-area detectors capable of covering the entire z-axis length of the heart (e.g., 16 cm) can perform this acquisition without table movement. This allows a pitch factor of 1 but requires cone beam corrections in the image reconstruction.

A further modification of prospective gating is provided in dual tube CT scanners operating in helical mode. This technique is known as high-pitch or flash imaging. Using two CT tubes, complete raw scan data sets can be obtained using a pitch factor of 3.2. The high table speed allows coverage of the entire heart during diastole in patients with a heart rate below 65 beats per minute. This mode is not useful secondary to motion artifact in patients with higher heart rates.

In all prospective acquisitions, transient elevation in heart rate or arrhythmias can seriously degrade image quality. With the exception of high-pitch acquisitions, this source of image degradation can be partially mitigated by acquiring redundant projections. This modification is referred to as padding and allows movement of the acquisition window within the diastolic interval to search for the most motion-free time point for the coronary arteries. In some cases, motion-free visualization of different parts of the vessels (e.g., proximal vs. distal portion of the right coronary artery) occurs at different time points. However, these additional projections are associated with an increased radiation dose such that some authors recommend against the routine use of padding [36].

Conclusion

This review has outlined a number of practical methods for dose reduction that are independent of the CT scanner make and model. Other very effective scanner-specific technical innovations are also available on current-generation scanners. They require that radiologists are aware of the benefits and limitations of their use. When all current dose reduction strategies are utilized, sub-mSv cardiothoracic CT is achievable in non-obese patients.

References

1. Mettler FA, Jr., Bhargavan M, Faulkner K et al (2009) Radiologic and nuclear medicine studies in the United States and worldwide: frequency, radiation dose, and comparison with other radiation sources 1950-2007. Radiology 253:520-531.
2. Aroua A, Samara ET, Bochud FO et al (2013) Exposure of the Swiss population to computed tomography. BMC Medical Imaging 13:22.
3. Preston DL, Ron E, Tokuoka S et al (2007) Solid cancer incidence in atomic bomb survivors: 1958-1998. Radiation Res 168:1-64.
4. Pearce MS, Salotti JA, Little MP et al (2012) Radiation exposure from CT scans in childhood and subsequent risk of leukaemia and brain tumours: a retrospective cohort study. Lancet 380:499-505.
5. Mathews JD, Forsythe AV, Brady Z et al (2013) Cancer risk in 680,000 people exposed to computed tomography scans in childhood or adolescence: data linkage study of 11 million Australians. BMJ 346:f2360.
6. Flors L, Leiva-Salinas C, Norton PT et al (2013) Endoleak detection after endovascular repair of thoracic aortic aneurysm using dual-source dual-energy CT: suitable scanning protocols and potential radiation dose reduction. AJR Am J Roentgenol 200:451-460.
7. Prokop M (2008) [Radiation dose in computed tomography. Risks and challenges]. Der Radiologe 48:229-242.
8. Karlo C, Gnannt R, Frauenfelder T et al (2011) Whole-body CT in polytrauma patients: effect of arm positioning on thoracic and abdominal image quality. Emerg Radiol 18:285-293.
9. Brink M, de Lange F, Oostveen LJ et al (2008) Arm raising at exposure-controlled multidetector trauma CT of thoracoabdominal region: higher image quality, lower radiation dose. Radiology 249:661-670.
10. Li J, Udayasankar UK, Toth TL et al (2007) Automatic patient centering for MDCT: effect on radiation dose. AJR Am J Roentgenol 188:547-552.
11. Mayo JR, Whittall KP, Leung AN et al (1997) Simulated dose reduction in conventional chest CT: validation study. Radiology 202:453-457.
12. Mayo JR, Kim KI, MacDonald SL et al (2004) Reduced radiation dose helical chest CT: effect on reader evaluation of structures and lung findings. Radiology 232:749-756.
13. Kalra MK, Maher MM, Toth TL (2004) Comparison of Z-axis automatic tube current modulation technique with fixed tube

current CT scanning of abdomen and pelvis. Radiology 232:347-353.

14. Kalra MK, Maher MM, Kamath RS et al (2004) Sixteen-detector row CT of abdomen and pelvis: study for optimization of Z-axis modulation technique performed in 153 patients. Radiology 233:241-249.

15. Greess H, Lutze J, Nomayr A et al (2004) Dose reduction in subsecond multislice spiral CT examination of children by online tube current modulation. Eur Radiol 14:995-999.

16. Kalra MK, Rizzo S, Maher MM et al (2005) Chest CT performed with z-axis modulation: scanning protocol and radiation dose. Radiology 237:303-308.

17. Schindera ST, Nelson RC, Toth TL et al (2008) Effect of patient size on radiation dose for abdominal MDCT with automatic tube current modulation: phantom study. AJR Am J Roentgenol 190:W100-W105.

18. The 2007 Recommendations of the International Commission on Radiological Protection (2007) ICRP publication 103. Annals of the ICRP 37:1-332.

19. Duan X, Wang J, Christner JA et al (2011) Dose reduction to anterior surfaces with organ-based tube-current modulation: evaluation of performance in a phantom study. AJR Am J Roentgenol 197:689-695.

20. Lungren MP, Yoshizumi TT, Brady SM et al (2012) Radiation dose estimations to the thorax using organ-based dose modulation. AJR Am J Roentgenol 199:W65-73.

21. Taylor S, Litmanovich DE, Shahrzad M (2014) Organ-based tube current modulation: are women's breasts positioned in the reduced-dose zone? Radiology 140694 [Epub ahead of print].

22. Heyer CM, Mohr PS, Lemburg SP et al (2007) Image quality and radiation exposure at pulmonary CT angiography with 100- or 120-kVp protocol: prospective randomized study. Radiology 245:577-583.

23. Schueller-Weidekamm C, Schaefer-Prokop CM, Weber M et al (2006) CT angiography of pulmonary arteries to detect pulmonary embolism: improvement of vascular enhancement with low kilovoltage settings. Radiology 241:899-907.

24. Szucs-Farkas Z, Christe A, Megyeri B et al (2014) Diagnostic accuracy of computed tomography pulmonary angiography with reduced radiation and contrast material dose: a prospective randomized clinical trial. Invest Radiol 49:201-208.

25. Niemann T, Henry S, Faivre JB et al (2013) Clinical evaluation of automatic tube voltage selection in chest CT angiography. Eur Radiol 23:2643-2651.

26. Kalra MK, Woisetschlager M, Dahlstrom N et al (2013) Sinogram-affirmed iterative reconstruction of low-dose chest CT: effect on image quality and radiation dose. AJR Am J Roentgenol 201:W235-244.

27. Padole A, Singh S, Ackman JB et al (2014) Submillisievert chest CT with filtered back projection and iterative reconstruction techniques. AJR Am J Roentgenol 203:772-781.

28. Schindera ST, Odedra D, Raza SA et al (2013) Iterative reconstruction algorithm for CT: can radiation dose be decreased while low-contrast detectability is preserved? Radiology 269:511-518.

29. Vollmar SV, Kalender WA (2008) Reduction of dose to the female breast in thoracic CT: a comparison of standard-protocol, bismuth-shielded, partial and tube-current-modulated CT examinations. Eur Radiol 18:1674-1682.

30. Hurwitz LM, Yoshizumi TT, Goodman PC et al (2009) Radiation dose savings for adult pulmonary embolus 64-MDCT using bismuth breast shields, lower peak kilovoltage, and automatic tube current modulation. AJR Am J Roentgenol 192:244-253.

31. Aberle DR, DeMello S, Berg CD et al (2013) Results of the two incidence screenings in the National Lung Screening Trial. New England J Med 369:920-931.

32. Nawa T, Nakagawa T, Mizoue T et al (2012) A decrease in lung cancer mortality following the introduction of low-dose chest CT screening in Hitachi, Japan. Lung Cancer 78:225-228.

33. Christe A, Charimo-Torrente J, Roychoudhury K et al (2013) Accuracy of low-dose computed tomography (CT) for detecting and characterizing the most common CT-patterns of pulmonary disease. Eur J Radiol 82:e142-150.

34. Gordic S, Morsbach F, Schmidt B et al (2014) Ultralow-dose chest computed tomography for pulmonary nodule detection: first performance evaluation of single energy scanning with spectral shaping. Invest Radiol 49:465-473.

35. Mayo JR, Leipsic JA (2009) Radiation dose in cardiac CT. AJR Am J Roentgenol 192:646-653.

36. Leipsic J, LaBounty TM, Ajlan AM et al (2013) A prospective randomized trial comparing image quality, study interpretability, and radiation dose of narrow acquisition window with widened acquisition window protocols in prospectively ECG-triggered coronary computed tomography angiography. J Cardiovasc Comput Tomogr 7:18-24.

NUCLEAR MEDICINE SATELLITE COURSE "DIAMOND"

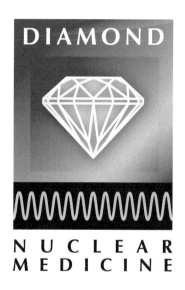

DIAMOND

NUCLEAR
MEDICINE

FDG-PET Imaging for Advanced Radiotherapy Treatment of Non-Small-Cell Lung Cancer

Matthias Guckenberger, Leonie Rudofsky, Nicolaus Andratschke

Department of Radiation Oncology, University Hospital Zürich (USZ), Switzerland

Introduction

Radiation oncology has benefited from the enormous progress that followed rapid technical developments over the last few decades. Until the 1980s, large volumes were unnecessarily irradiated during radiotherapy, due to the lack of imaging techniques to identify tumor extension, the lack of technologies to accurately conform the radiotherapy dose with the tumor, and the inability to accurately deliver radiotherapy over a prolonged fractionated course of treatment. Consequently, in many solid tumors, the radiation tolerance of the surrounding normal tissue limited the maximum irradiation dose that could be delivered safely.

In non-small-cell lung cancer (NSCLC) for example, radiation-induced pneumonitis limited the irradiation dose in many patients to a maximum of 60–66 Gy, which achieved local tumor control in fewer than 50% of the cases [1]. Simultaneously, studies had shown that substantially higher irradiation doses (>80 Gy) were necessary to locally control locally advanced NSCLC [2] and that higher irradiation doses with improved local tumor control also translated into increased overall survival (OS) [3]. In prostate cancer, irradiation doses were limited to a similar dose of 60–66 Gy because of the proximity of the prostate to the rectum, and therefore a risk of radiation-induced proctitis [4].

Research in radiation oncology thus focused on the development of technologies aiming at accurately confining the irradiation dose to the tumor while simultaneously minimizing the exposure of adjacent normal tissue. By broadening the therapeutic ratio, escalated irradiation doses could be delivered without the risk of increased toxicity.

The first major step was the integration of computed tomography (CT) into target-volume definition and treatment planning, thus enabling a patient-tailored assessment of tumor location and tumor size. The development of powerful computers allowed for three-dimensional conformal radiotherapy (3D-CRT) while multi-leaf collimators enabled the faster delivery of these multiple-field treatment plans. Randomized controlled trials have demonstrated the clinical benefit of 3D-CRT compared to conventional radiotherapy, e.g., in the treatment of prostate cancer [5].

In the last 10 years, intensity-modulated radiotherapy (IMRT) has become broadly available. IMRT has improved radiotherapy of complex-shaped target volumes. Imaging technologies (electronic portal imaging, X-ray, cone-beam CT, magnetic resonance) have been integrated into radiation treatment delivery machines to accurately visualize and target the tumor on a daily basis. Additionally, imaging and treatment-delivery technologies have been expanded to the fourth dimension, meaning that intra-treatment motion, e.g., breathing-induced, of the tumor can be compensated in real time. Irradiation with particles, for example, protons and carbon ions, instead of photons, has further improved the physics of radiotherapy. Together, these technologies allow the precise targeting of virtually every tumor within the brain or body of the patient, with nearly sub-millimeter accuracy.

As a result of these technological advances, the process of target-volume definition, that is, what to treat with which irradiation dose, has become the limiting factor in the overall accuracy of radiotherapy. Soft-tissue contrast is limited, especially in CT, and the value of magnetic resonance imaging (MRI) is limited, especially in the thoracic region. Nodal and distant staging are suboptimal using CT and MRI only. Response assessment during and after radio(chemo)therapy is restricted to an evaluation of volume and not of function and biology.

Therefore, functional imaging using positron emission tomography (PET) is now the standard of care in radiation oncology. This chapter summarizes the current applications of PET imaging in radiation oncology and provides an outlook on its future applications. It focuses first on the use of 18F-fluorodeoxyglucose (FDG)-PET for lung cancer and then briefly discusses novel tracers.

Diseases of the Chest and Heart 2015-2018,
DOI: 10.1007/978-88-470-5752-4_23 © Springer-Verlag Italia 2015

FDG-PET Imaging in NSCLC

FDG-PET for Staging in NSCLC

Selection of the appropriate patients for radical local treatment, whether surgery, radiotherapy, or multimodal treatment, is essential. Today, FDG-PET for the staging of nodal and distant metastases is the standard of care, based on international guidelines. In a prospective study of NSCLC patients with mostly locally advanced disease, initial staging was performed using CT and with FDG-PET thereafter. FDG-PET led to a change from curative to palliative therapy by upstaging the disease extent in 25% of the patients [6]. A similar study was performed in a patient cohort referred for radical radiotherapy based on CT staging [7]. The 76 patients were mostly cN+. After FDG-PET staging, radical radiochemotherapy was performed in only 66% of the patients, with palliative treatment in the remaining 34% mostly because of the detection by FDG-PET imaging of distant metastases or of more extensive nodal disease considered too extensive for successful radical radiochemotherapy. At 4 years after treatment with curative and palliative intent, OS was 35.6% and 4.1%, respectively, thus confirming the accurate selection of a high-risk population using FDG-PET staging.

The timely performance of FDG-PET staging, before the start of radical treatment, is crucial. If the interval between staging and the start of radical treatment is too long, FDG-PET needs to be repeated. Everitt et al. evaluated two sequential FDG-PET/CT images acquired from 82 patients with a median interval of 24 days prior to the start of treatment [8]. Interscan disease progression (TNM stage) was detected in 11 (39%) patients. Treatment intent changed from curative to palliative in 8 (29%) because of the detection of newly developed distant metastases in the second FDG-PET/CT; in 7 of these patients the change in treatment was based on the PET image component. The average standardized uptake value (SUV) increased by 16%.

In patients with NSCLC, FDG-PET is especially useful for nodal staging, which is of fundamental importance in therapeutic decision-making (curative vs. palliative; surgical vs. non-surgical; conventionally fractionated radiotherapy vs. stereotactic body radiotherapy) and for target-volume definition in radical radiotherapy. It is well documented that nodal staging using CT imaging is of low sensitivity and specificity. This is especially true in patients with cN0 disease. D'Cunha et al. reported the results of the CALGB 9761 study of 502 patients with clinical stage I disease as determined by CT staging [9]. After surgical resection and mediastinal lymph node dissection, 14% of the patients were shown to have had pathologic stage II disease and another 13.5% stage III disease.

Two studies evaluated the value of FDG-PET staging in patients with clinical stage IA disease based on CT staging. Park et al. reported a retrospective study of 147 patients who had clinical stage IA disease according to

FDG-PET staging [10]. After systematic lymph node dissection in the majority of the patients, 14.3% had occult nodal (N1 or N2) metastasis. Total N1 and N2 involvement was detected in 9.5% and 4.8%, respectively. Multivariate analysis demonstrated that a primary tumor with a SUV$_{max}$ >7.3 was an independent predictor of occult nodal metastasis. In the retrospective study by Stiles et al. of 266 patients with stage IA disease according to CT- and FDG-PET-based staging, mediastinal lymph node dissection detected N1 and N2 disease in 6.8% and 4.9% of the patients, respectively [11]. Tumor size >2 cm and FDG-PET positivity were risk factors for understaging by FDG-PET.

Overall mediastinal staging accuracy was evaluated in a meta-analysis. For CT staging, the median sensitivity and specificity of mediastinal staging were 61% and 79%, respectively. For FDG-PET, the corresponding values were 85% and 90. However, the specificity of FDG-PET staging was lower when CT showed enlarged lymph nodes [12]. Consequently, all positive nodal findings in FDG-PET need to be confirmed pathologically, using endobronchial ultrasound or mediastinoscopy.

Consequences of Improved Staging Accuracy Using FDG-PET

In patients with stage I NSCLC based on FDG-PET staging, stereotactic body radiotherapy (SBRT) of the primary tumor only, without elective treatment of the hilar or mediastinal lymph node regions, is the guideline-recommended standard of care in all patients who are medically inoperable [13]. The omission of elective nodal irradiation combined with other high-precision technologies (respiration correlated imaging, image guidance, intrafractional motion management) allows for irradiation with escalated irradiation doses, which are delivered in a hypo-fractionated manner: biological equivalent doses (BED) >100 Gy are delivered in 1–8 fractions.

Local tumor control in SBRT is significantly improved compared to conventionally fractionated radiotherapy and reaches >90% in the majority of studies. This improved local control translates into significantly improved OS [14], which is mainly limited by the comorbidities of the patients as well as systemic progression of the disease. Regional failures are rare after FDG-PET staging. Senthi et al. reported a 7.8% regional failure rate at 2 years in a large cohort of 676 patients [15].

In locally advanced NSCLC, involved-field irradiation without elective nodal irradiation is currently practiced in most studies and centers, if FDG-PET had been performed for staging purposes. Involved-field irradiation reduces the irradiated volume substantially, thus allowing either a reduction of toxicity or iso-toxic escalation of the irradiation dose [16]. Early studies confirmed low rates of isolated regional failures in un-irradiated hilar and mediastinal regions [17], with only 1 out of 44 patients treated with involved-field irradiation developing an isolated nodal failure. The value of involved-field irradiation after FDG-PET staging is currently being evaluated in a prospective randomized multi-center trial (PET-Plan, NCT00697333).

FDG-PET as a Prognostic Marker in NSCLC

The correlation of pre-treatment, intra-treatment, or early post-treatment FDG-PET characteristics with outcome could be used for patient stratification and subsequent treatment adaptation. However, whether FDG-uptake is a prognostic maker in NSCLC is discussed controversially in the literature. The uncertainty is at least partially explained by differences in the methodology of outcome modeling. Firstly, different endpoints have been used to determine a correlation with FDG-PET characteristics: local tumor control, progression-free survival, and OS. Secondly, different metrics of FDG-PET images have been used for outcome correlation: SUV_{max}, metabolic tumor volume, and, more recently, texture characteristics such as coarseness, contrast, and busyness. Additionally, tumor volume is a well known independent prognostic marker, which could confound analysis using FDG-PET as a prognostic marker [18]. Another matter of controversy is whether or to what extent inflammatory reactions during or shortly after radio(chemo)therapy influence the value of FDG-PET for outcome modeling.

The prognostic value of pre-treatment FDG-PET was evaluated in a meta-analysis of 21 studies by Paesmans et al. [19]. The endpoint was OS. Data from individual data patients were not available; instead, the median SUV value of each study was used as a threshold. The study detected a poor prognosis for patients with a high vs. a low SUV, with an overall combined hazard ratio of 2.08. However, it did not find an optimal SUV threshold but only that higher SUVs resulted in worse outcome. This may have been a consequence of the limitations of the meta-analysis or that rather than two groups of patients there was a continuous increase in the hazard with increasing SUV.

Matchay et al. reported one of the largest prospective studies, in which the pre- and post-treatment FDG-PET characteristics of 250 patients with locally advanced NSCLC treated with conventional concurrent platinum-based radiochemotherapy without surgery were analyzed [20]. The 2-year survival rate for the entire population was 42.5%. Neither pre-treatment SUV_{peak} nor SUV_{max} correlated with OS, which is in contrast to the meta-analysis described above. In contrast, SUV_{peak} and SUV_{max} in FDG-PET images acquired approximately 14 weeks after treatment correlated with OS. Patients with higher residual FDG-PET uptake had a significantly worse OS.

In a further analysis, Aerts et al. analyzed the spatial correlation between pre- and post-treatment SUV in 55 patients treated with chemoradiation for locally advanced NSCLC [21]. Pre- and post-treatment FDG-PET images were acquired about 2 weeks and 12 weeks prior to and after radiotherapy, respectively. The authors reported that patients with residual metabolic-active areas within the tumor had a significantly worse survival than patients with a complete metabolic response. Most importantly, the location of residual metabolic-active areas within the primary tumor after therapy correlated with the initially high FDG uptake areas determined pre-radiotherapy. Consequently, pre-treatment FDG-PET imaging could be used to identify subvolumes of the primary tumor at risk for incomplete response after definitive radiotherapy.

A similar study was performed by a group from the University of Michigan [22]. In 15 stage I–III NSCLC patients treated with a definitive dose of fractionated radiotherapy, pre-treatment (2 weeks), intra-treatment (after approximately 45 Gy), and post-treatment (3–4 months) FDG-PET/CT images were acquired. A significant correlation between metabolic tumor response during radiotherapy and metabolic tumor response 3 months post-radiotherapy was determined.

Consequences of FDG-PET as a Prognostic Marker

If either the pre-treatment or the intra-treatment FDG-PET characteristics of the tumor correlate with local tumor control and/or survival, the appropriate strategy would then be to adapt radiotherapy to these tumor-individual functional and biological characteristics. This concept of adaptive radiotherapy was first proposed more than 10 years ago [23] and is currently under clinical investigation.

Key questions in adaptive radiotherapy remain unanswered, which has prevented its board adaptation. A discussion of these issues in detail is beyond the scope of this chapter but the questions include: Which functional imaging modality, PET tracer, and image characteristics are most appropriate for tumor characterization? What are the relevant time points for image acquisition and subsequent treatment adaptation? What are the dynamics of functional and biological tumor characteristics and is multiple-step adaptation required? Are biological characteristics representative for one patient and one tumor as a whole, or can tumors be subdivided into areas of different biology and function? How can biology, treatment, and outcome be correlated with one another? How can biological information be translated into a robust radiotherapy plan? How can the outcome of adaptive radiotherapy be evaluated? And how can functional and biological markers other than imaging, e.g., genomic markers and RNA expression, be integrated into treatment?

Despite these uncertainties, the most advanced studies on adaptive radiotherapy for locally advanced NSCLC are summarized below.

The University of Michigan group reported a pilot study in which radiotherapy was adapted after the delivery of 40–50 Gy based on FDG-PET/CT [24]. Among the 14 patients with stages I–III NSCLC, the mid-treatment FDT-PET/CT showed a metabolic complete response in two and increased FDG uptake in the adjacent lung tissue in another two. In the remaining 10 patients, CT-morphological and FDG-PET metabolic volumes decreased by 26% (range, +15% to −75%) and 44% (range, +10% to −100%), respectively. Re-planning of radiotherapy based on a reduced metabolic volume was then performed in six patients and allowed a substantial intensification of radiotherapy of 30–102 Gy (mean 58 Gy) without an increased risk of toxicity compared to a scenario without mid-treatment plan adaptation (iso-toxic dose escalation approach). Even this small study by Feng et al. [24] clearly demonstrated that: (1) adaptive radiotherapy is not feasible in all patients; (2) not all patients will benefit from adaptive radiotherapy; but that (3) the potential benefit of normal tissue sparing or treatment intensification is considerable in some patients. This concept of adaptive radiotherapy using mid-treatment FDG-PET/CT is currently being investigated in a randomized phase II trial (NCT01507428).

Another study based on the experiences of Aerts et al. [21] is underway. In this randomized phase II study of patients with inoperable stage IB to stage III NSCLC (NCT01024829) [25], patients are randomized to conventional radiotherapy with a total dose of 66 Gy given in 24 fractions of 2.75 Gy with an integrated boost to the primary tumor as a whole (Arm A) or with an integrated boost to the 50% SUV_{max} area of the primary tumor (from the pre-treatment FDG-PET scan) (Arm B). The primary endpoint of this study is progression-free survival. No results have been published so far.

Normal Tissue Characterization Using FDG-PET Imaging

FDG uptake in inflammatory processes may negatively influence tumor imaging and characterization but at the same time may help in the visualization, quantification, or prediction of inflammatory radiation-induced toxicity. Pneumonitis is the most relevant toxicity in patients undergoing radiotherapy for lung cancer. Its development correlates with the radiotherapy dose, i.e., the mean lung dose and the volume of the lung exposed to 20 Gy, but the correlation is rather weak.

A group from Melbourne correlated post-treatment (median 70 days) FDG uptake in the lungs with the development of radiation-induced pneumonitis [26]. The authors reported a significant association between the worst Radiation Therapy Oncology Group (RTOG) grade of pneumonitis occurring at any time after radiotherapy and the severity of FDG uptake in the lung. No associated between FDG uptake and the duration of pneumonitis was found. The authors concluded that FDG-PET may be useful in the prediction, diagnosis, and therapeutic monitoring of radiation pneumonitis.

However, the post-treatment prediction of pneumonitis or lung toxicity has no value in terms of modifying radiotherapy to reduce the risk of pneumonitis, e.g., by redistribution of the radiotherapy dose or dose de-escalation. Petit et al. [27] reported promising results from a study in which pre-treatment FDG uptake in the lungs was shown to correlate with the post-radiotherapy development of radiation-induced lung toxicity. The hypothe-

sis was that pre-treatment inflammation in the lungs makes pulmonary tissue more susceptible to radiation damage. The authors reported that the 95th percentile of FDG uptake in the lungs, excluding clinical tumor volume, correlated significantly with the risk of developing radiation-induced pneumonitis. Pre-treatment FDG-PET could therefore be used for risk stratification and in the selection of patients for closer follow-up. Even more important from a radiotherapy perspective is the finding that the fraction of the 5%, 10%, and 20% highest SUV voxels that received irradiation doses >2–5Gy improved the correlation with radiation-induced lung toxicity. Sparing these lung areas from low-dose irradiation could therefore decrease the risk of lung toxicity.

Gross Tumor Definition Using FDG-PET Imaging

Target-volume definition of peripheral early-stage NSCLC is associated with small inter- and intra-observer variability. However, the accurate analysis of breathing-induced tumor motion and its integration into target-volume definition are essential steps in the treatment process. Respiration-correlated 4D-CT is the current method of choice, despite its limitations due to residual motion artifacts and the short image acquisition time. FDG-PET imaging, with its long image acquisition time, may provide a tool similar to slow CT scanning to evaluate tumor motion. Although this concept appears straightforward, studies have shown only a poor correlation between PET and the gold-standard of 4D-CT [28]. FDG-PET for the assessment of tumor-motion amplitude and motion patterns is therefore not recommended.

Several 4D technologies have been developed to acquire and/or reconstruct respiration-correlated 4D PET images [29]. Using these technologies should allow for more precise tumor characterization and delineation even in the presence of large tumor motion.

Definition of the target volume is associated with substantial uncertainties especially in locally advanced-stage NSCLC. These uncertainties have been quantified in several studies that evaluated inter-observer variability in target-volume definition and the variability in the target contours between multiple experts in lung cancer treatment. In the study of Steenbackers et al. based on 22 patients with early and locally advanced stage NSCLC [30], 11 experts delineated the gross tumor volume using CT images only and then, 1 year later, on matched FDG-PET/CT images. The variability between the experts was reduced from 1 cm (one standard deviation) to 0.4 cm, clearly showing the added value of the FDG-PET imaging component. Two clinical situations have been identified in which FDG-PET makes a relevant difference compared to CT imaging only: The difficulties of nodal staging were described above, and FDG-PET is essential for defining the nodal target volume, especially in cases of involved-node irradiation. The other situation in which FDG-PET can reduce uncertainties in target-volume definition is the differentiation between macroscopic tumor and atelectasis.

Automatic segmentation of the gross tumor volume has been analyzed for many years and multiple segmentation algorithms and FDG uptake cut-off values have been evaluated [31]. However, none have proven to be robust and reliable enough to replace manual segmentation in CT images.

Follow-up Response Assessment Using FDG-PET

Evaluation of treatment response at follow-up is especially difficult after high-dose radiotherapy. The majority of patients treated with SBRT for stage I NSCLC will develop radiation-induced pneumonitis grade I with fibrotic changes in the high-dose region. The fibrotic changes are known to change in size and morphology for many years after treatment. These long-term changes make it difficult to distinguish a normal tissue response from local recurrence. The use of invasive procedures to verify or exclude local recurrence should be practiced with caution in the usually fragile patient population with few salvage options.

FDG-PET has been recommended as a crucial tool in the differentiation between fibrotic changes and local tumor recurrence [32]. However, the value of FDG-PET is very limited early after SBRT, since active inflammatory changes are frequently seen in the first few months following treatment. Inflammatory processes last for approximately 3–6 months, such that FDG-PET should only be used after this time interval. Thereafter, SUV-max >5 or above the pre-treatment value has been suggested as highly suspicious for local recurrence.

Novel PET Tracers and Their Application in Lung Cancer

As discussed in detail above, FDG-PET imaging in NSCLC is associated with several limitations. Novel radiotracers may allow some of these to be overcome. For example, hypoxia is a well-established biomarker for increased radioresistance. Several tracers are currently under evaluation (e.g., FMISO, FAZA, HX4, Cu-ATSM) to quantity hypoxia. The information on radioresistance that they provide can be integrated into radiotherapy, either by modifying the radiotherapy component or by hypoxia-sensitizing systemic treatments.

Summary

FDG-PET has become mandatory in radiotherapy planning and in the treatment of NSCLC, influencing and improving all steps of the treatment chain: staging, target-volume definition, tumor and normal tissue characterization, and response assessment. Novel PET tracers may someday overcome the limitations of FDG and allow for even better individualization of radiotherapy for patients with early and locally advanced stage NSCLC.

References

1. Perez CA, Pajak TF, Rubin Pet al (1987) Long-term observations of the patterns of failure in patients with unresectable non-oat cell carcinoma of the lung treated with definitive radiotherapy. Report by the Radiation Therapy Oncology Group. Cancer 59:1874-1881.
2. Partridge M, Ramos M, Sardaro A et al (2011) Dose escalation for non-small cell lung cancer: analysis and modelling of published literature. Radiother Oncol 99:6-11.
3. Auperin A, Le Pechoux C, Rolland E et al (2010) Meta-analysis of concomitant versus sequential radiochemotherapy in locally advanced non-small-cell lung cancer. J Clin Oncol 28:2181-2190.
4. Lyons JA, Kupelian PA, Mohan DS et al (2000) Importance of high radiation doses (72 Gy or greater) in the treatment of stage T1-T3 adenocarcinoma of the prostate. Urology 55: 85-90.
5. Dearnaley DP, Khoo VS, Norman AR et al (1999) Comparison of radiation side-effects of conformal and conventional radiotherapy in prostate cancer: a randomised trial. Lancet 353:267-272.
6. Kalff V, Hicks RJ, MacManus MP et al (2001) Clinical impact of (18)F fluorodeoxyglucose positron emission tomography in patients with non-small-cell lung cancer: a prospective study. J Clin Oncol 19:111-118.
7. Mac Manus MP, Everitt S, Bayne M et al (2013) The use of fused PET/CT images for patient selection and radical radiotherapy target volume definition in patients with non-small cell lung cancer: Results of a prospective study with mature survival data. Radiother Oncol 106:292-298.
8. Everitt S, Herschtal A, Callahan J et al (2010) High rates of tumor growth and disease progression detected on serial pretreatment fluorodeoxyglucose-positron emission tomography/computed tomography scans in radical radiotherapy candidates with nonsmall cell lung cancer. Cancer 116:5030-5037.
9. D'Cunha J, Herndon JE 2nd, Herzan DL et al (2005) Poor correspondence between clinical and pathologic staging in stage 1 non-small cell lung cancer: results from CALGB 9761, a prospective trial. Lung Cancer 48:241-246.
10. Park HK, Jeon K, Koh WJ et al (2010): Occult nodal metastasis in patients with non-small cell lung cancer at clinical stage IA by PET/CT. Respirology 15:1179-1184.
11. Stiles BM, Servais EL, Lee PC et al (2009) Point: Clinical stage IA non-small cell lung cancer determined by computed tomography and positron emission tomography is frequently not pathologic IA non-small cell lung cancer: the problem of understaging. J Thorac Cardiovasc Surg 137:13-19.
12. Gould MK, Kuschner WG, Rydzak CE et al (2003) Test performance of positron emission tomography and computed tomography for mediastinal staging in patients with non-small-cell lung cancer: a meta-analysis. Ann Intern Med 139:879-892.
13. Vansteenkiste J, De Ruysscher D, Eberhardt WEE et al (2013) Early and locally advanced non-small-cell lung cancer (NSCLC): ESMO Clinical Practice Guidelines for diagnosis, treatment and follow-up. Annals of Oncology 24(suppl 6):vi89-vi98.
14. Shirvani SM, Jiang J, Chang JY et al (2012) Comparative effectiveness of 5 treatment strategies for early-stage non-small cell lung cancer in the elderly. Int J Radiat Oncol Biol Phys 84:1060-1070.
15. Senthi S, Lagerwaard FJ, Haasbeek CJ et al (2012) Patterns of disease recurrence after stereotactic ablative radiotherapy for early stage non-small-cell lung cancer: a retrospective analysis. Lancet Oncol 13:802-809.
16. Belderbos JS, Kepka L, Spring Kong FM et al (2008) Report from the International Atomic Energy Agency (IAEA) consultants' meeting on elective nodal irradiation in lung cancer: non-small-Cell lung cancer (NSCLC). Int J Radiat Oncol Biol Phys 72:335-342.

17. De Ruysscher D, Wanders S, van Haren E et al (2005) Selective mediastinal node irradiation based on FDG-PET scan data in patients with non-small-cell lung cancer: a prospective clinical study. Int J Radiat Oncol Biol Phys 62:988-994.

18. Reymen B, Van Loon J, van Baardwijk A et al (2013) Total gross tumor volume is an independent prognostic factor in patients treated with selective nodal irradiation for stage I to III small cell lung cancer. Int J Radiat Oncol Biol Phys 85:1319-1324.

19. Paesmans M, Berghmans T, Dusart M et al (2010) Primary tumor standardized uptake value measured on fluorodeoxyglucose positron emission tomography is of prognostic value for survival in non-small cell lung cancer: update of a systematic review and meta-analysis by the European Lung Cancer Working Party for the International Association for the Study of Lung Cancer Staging Project. J Thorac Oncol 5:612-619.

20. Machtay M, Duan F, Siegel BA et al (2013) Prediction of survival by [18F]fluorodeoxyglucose positron emission tomography in patients with locally advanced non-small-cell lung cancer undergoing definitive chemoradiation therapy: Results of the ACRIN 6668/RTOG 0235 Trial. J Clin Oncol 31:3823-3830.

21. Aerts HJ, van Baardwijk AA, Petit SF et al (2009) Identification of residual metabolic-active areas within individual NSCLC tumours using a pre-radiotherapy (18)Fluorodeoxyglucose-PET-CT scan. Radiother Oncol 91:386-392.

22. Kong FM, Frey KA, Quint LE (2007) A pilot study of [18F]fluorodeoxyglucose positron emission tomography scans during and after radiation-based therapy in patients with non small-cell lung cancer. J Clin Oncol 25:3116-3123.

23. Ling CC, Humm J, Larson S et al (2000) Towards multidimensional radiotherapy (MD-CRT): biological imaging and biological conformality. Int J Radiat Oncol Biol Phys 47:551-560.

24. Feng M, Kong FM, Gross M et al (2009) Using fluorodeoxyglucose positron emission tomography to assess tumor volume during radiotherapy for non-small-cell lung cancer and its potential impact on adaptive dose escalation and normal tissue sparing. Int J Radiat Oncol Biol Phys 73:1228-1234.

25. van Elmpt W, De Ruysscher D, van der Salm A et al (2012) The PET-boost randomised phase II dose-escalation trial in non-small cell lung cancer. Radiother Oncol 104:67-71.

26. Mac Manus MP, Ding Z, Hogg A et al (2011) Association between pulmonary uptake of fluorodeoxyglucose detected by positron emission tomography scanning after radiation therapy for non-small-cell lung cancer and radiation pneumonitis. Int J Radiat Oncol Biol Phys 80:1365-1371.

27. Petit SF, van Elmpt WJ, Oberije CJ et al (2011) [(1)(8)F]fluorodeoxyglucose uptake patterns in lung before radiotherapy identify areas more susceptible to radiation-induced lung toxicity in non-small-cell lung cancer patients. Int J Radiat Oncol Biol Phys 81:698-705.

28. Hanna GG, van Sornsen de Koste JR, Dahele MR et al (2012) Defining target volumes for stereotactic ablative radiotherapy of early-stage lung tumours: a comparison of three-dimensional 18F-fluorodeoxyglucose positron emission tomography and four-dimensional computed tomography. Clinical oncology (Royal College of Radiologists (Great Britain)) 24:e71-80.

29. Kruis MF, van de Kamer JB, Houweling AC et al (2013) PET motion compensation for radiation therapy using a CT-based mid-position motion model: methodology and clinical evaluation. Int J Radiat Oncol Biol Phys 87:394-400.

30. Steenbakkers RJ, Duppen JC, Fitton I et al (2006) Reduction of observer variation using matched CT-PET for lung cancer delineation: a three-dimensional analysis. Int J Radiat Oncol Biol Phys 64:435-448.

31. Sridhar P, Mercier G, Tan J et al (2014) FDG PET metabolic tumor volume segmentation and pathologic volume of primary human solid tumors. AJR Am J Roentgenol 202:1114-1119.

32. Huang K, Senthi S, Palma DA (2013) High-risk CT features for detection of local recurrence after stereotactic ablative radiotherapy for lung cancer. Radiother Oncol 109:51-57.

Staging, Restaging and Response Evaluation of Non-Small-Cell Lung Cancer

Lars Husmann, Paul Stolzmann

Division of Nuclear Medicine, Department of Medical Radiology, University Hospital of Zurich, Switzerland

Introduction

Lung cancer is the most common cancer in terms of incidence and it is associated with the highest mortality worldwide. The 5-year survival rate of all lung cancer patients is only 15%. However, progress has been made in the last years, especially regarding screening, minimally invasive techniques for diagnosis, treatment, and targeted therapies.

Treatment approaches for non-small cell lung cancer (NSCLC) include surgery, radiation therapy, and chemotherapy. They are used as stand-alone treatments or in combined therapies depending not only on the stage of disease but also on individual patient characteristics such as patient performance status. Treatment concepts are considered as being either curative or palliative. In advanced tumor stages, treatment may be shifted from standardized to personalized strategies, as targets for specific molecular tumor characteristics have been identified and can be used for new and effective treatment.

Appropriate staging of lung cancer is critical prior to treatment. Computed tomography (CT) and positron emission tomography/computed tomography with 18F-fluorodeoxyglucose (FDG-PET/CT) are the key imaging modalities in the staging of disease. CT has significant limitations in differentiating between normal or malignant tissue regarding both organ and lymph node status. FDG-PET/CT has been shown to be superior to CT in lung cancer staging, despite the known limitation of FDG-PET/CT as being non-specific for malignant tissue. Thus, false-positive findings may occur in inflammatory processes. Generally, all imaging findings and patient factors should be evaluated by a multidisciplinary team prior to initializing therapy in a patient with lung cancer.

Classification

The WHO divides lung cancer into two major classes: NSCLC (85%) and small cell lung cancer, based on pathobiology, therapy, and prognosis. The former includes squamous carcinomas and non-squamous carcinomas, such as adenocarcinomas and large cell carcinomas, as the major histopathological subtypes.

Squamous cell carcinoma is associated with smoking. It has the best prognosis, due to a slow growth rate and a low incidence of distant metastases. Squamous cell carcinomas tend to become large tumors, often with a central necrosis; regional lymph nodes metastases are common. They are the most common cause of Pancoast tumors.

Large-cell carcinomas are also associated with smoking, tend to grow rapidly, metastasize early, and are thus associated with a poor prognosis.

Adenocarcinoma is the most common type of lung cancer in nonsmokers and its incidence is rising [1]. The subclassification of pulmonary adenocarcinoma has recently been revised. This is important for the daily work of radiologists and nuclear medicine physicians as use of the term bronchioloalveolar cell carcinoma (BAC) is no longer recommended. New histological subtypes comprise adenocarcinoma in situ, lepidic predominant invasive adenocarcinoma, or invasive mucinous adenocarcinoma [2]. However, some radiologists continue to use the old terminology in their reports, referring to lesions as "formerly called BAC;" others have decided to call these lesions "adenocarcinomas with lepidic growth," or simply "adenocarcinomas." Adenocarcinomas may be difficult to diagnose by imaging alone, as they may appear as a pneumonia-like consolidation, as a solitary pulmonary nodule, or as multiple nodules throughout the lung. These adenocarcinomas may or may not be metabolically active in FDG-PET/CT. Additionally, not only is the imaging diagnosis difficult but now also the terminology. All adenocarcinomas should be tested for the epidermal growth factor receptor (EGFR) mutation and for anaplastic lymphoma kinase (ALK) rearrangements for further classification, as new targeted tumor therapies exist for these tumors (such as EGFR kinase inhibitors gefitinib/erlotinib and ALK kinase inhibitor crizotinib) [3].

Diseases of the Chest and Heart 2015-2018,
DOI: 10.1007/978-88-470-5752-4_24 © Springer-Verlag Italia 2015

Staging

Lung cancer staging guides patient management and provides prognostic information. The TNM staging system is used to classify NSCLC and is based on the characteristics of the primary tumor (T), the degree of lymph node involvement (N), and the presence or absence of metastasis (M) (Table 1). In detail, the addition of a "c" to the term cTNM means clinical staging and includes all imaging findings whereas pTNM describes the pathological staging. The combination of T, N, and M descriptors are used to identify the overall stage group (Table 2).

The 7th revision of the TNM system for lung cancer staging was published in 2010 [4] (Table 1). Significant changes from the 6th edition aim to provide a stronger correlation between the TNM stage and survival data.

Table 1. Definition of T, N, and M (TNM staging)

T	Primary Tumor
T1	Tumor ≤3 cm in greatest dimension, surrounded by lung or visceral pleura, without bronchoscopic evidence of invasion more proximal than a lobar bronchus (i.e., not in the main bronchus)
	T1a Tumor ≤2 cm in greatest dimension
	T1b Tumor >2 cm but ≤3 cm in greatest dimension
T2	Tumor >3 cm but ≤7 cm or tumor with any of the following features:
	Involves main bronchus, ≥2 cm distal to the carina
	Involves visceral pleura
	Associated with atelectasis or obstructive pneumonitis that extends to the hilar region but does not involve the entire lung
	T2a Tumor >3 cm but ≤5 in greatest dimension
	T2b Tumor >5 cm but ≤7 cm in greatest dimension
T3	Tumor >7 cm that directly invades any of the following: chest wall (including superior sulcus tumors), diaphragm, phrenic nerve, mediastinal pleura, parietal pericardium, or tumor in the main bronchus <2 cm distal to the carina but without involvement of the carina or associated atelectasis or obstructive pneumonitis of the entire lung or separate tumor nodule(s) in the same lobe
T4	Tumor of any size that invades any of the following: mediastinum, heart, great vessels, trachea, recurrent laryngeal nerve, esophagus, vertebral body, carina, separate tumor nodule(s) in a different, ipsilateral lobe
N	Regional Lymph Nodes
N0	No regional lymph node metastasis
N1	Metastasis to ipsilateral peribronchial and/or ipsilateral hilar lymph nodes, and intrapulmonary nodes including involvement by direct extension
N2	Metastasis in ipsilateral mediastinal and/or subcarinal lymph node(s)
N3	Metastasis in contralateral mediastinal, contralateral hilar, ipsilateral or contralateral scalene, or supraclavicular lymph node(s)
M	Distant Metastasis
M0	No distant metastasis
M1	Distant metastasis
	M1a Separate tumor nodule(s) in a contralateral lobe, tumor with pleural
	Nodule(s) or malignant pleural (or pericardial) effusion
	M1b Distant metastasis

The T descriptor has been reclassified according to size of the primary tumor (Table 1):
- T1 (<3 cm) is now split into T1a (<2 cm) and T1b (2–3 cm).
- T2 is split into T2a (3–5 cm) and T2b (5–7 cm).
- T3 includes tumors >7 cm.

Additional pulmonary nodules are reclassified as either
- T3, with location in the same lobe
- T4, with nodules in another lobe on the same side
- M1a, with nodules in the contralateral lung.

The N descriptor remains unchanged [5] (Tables 1 and 3):
- N1 disease refers to peribronchial and ipsilateral hilar metastases, including direct extension. All N1 nodes lie distal to the mediastinal pleural reflection and within the visceral pleura [5].
- N2 disease refers to ipsilateral paratracheal and/or subcarinal lymph node metastases.
- N3 disease refers to contralateral mediastinal, contralateral hilar, and ipsilateral or scalene or supraclavicular nodal metastases.

Notably, for paratracheal lymph nodes, the left lateral border of the trachea and not the midline differentiates left from right. Thus, a pretracheal lymph node metastases may be N2 disease in lung cancer of the right lung,

Table 2. Resultant stage groupings (TNM staging)

Stage grouping	TNM			
Stage IA	T1a,b	N0	M0	
Stage IB	T2a	N0	M0	
Stage IIA	T2b		N0	M0
	T1a,b	N1	M0	
	T2a		N1	M0
Stage IIB	T2b		N1	M0
	T3		N0	M0
Stage IIIA	T1-2a,b	N2	M0	
	T3		N1-2	M0
	T4		N0-1	M0
Stage IIIB	T4		N2	M0
	any T	N3	M0	
Stage IV	any T	any N	M1	

Table 3. Lymph node map: Definitions of nodal stations

N2 nodes - all N2 nodes lie within the mediastinal pleural envelope

1	Highest mediastinal nodes
2	Upper paratracheal nodes
3	Prevascular and retrotracheal nodes
4	Lower paratracheal nodes
5	Subaortic nodes (aorto-pulmonary window)
6	Para-aortic nodes (ascending aorta or phrenic)
7	Subcarinal nodes
8	Paraesophageal nodes (below carina)
9	Pulmonary ligament nodes

N1 nodes - all N1 nodes lie distal to the mediastinal pleural reflection and within the visceral pleura

10	Hilar nodes
11	Interlobular nodes
12	Lobar nodes
13	Segmental nodes
14	Subsegmental nodes

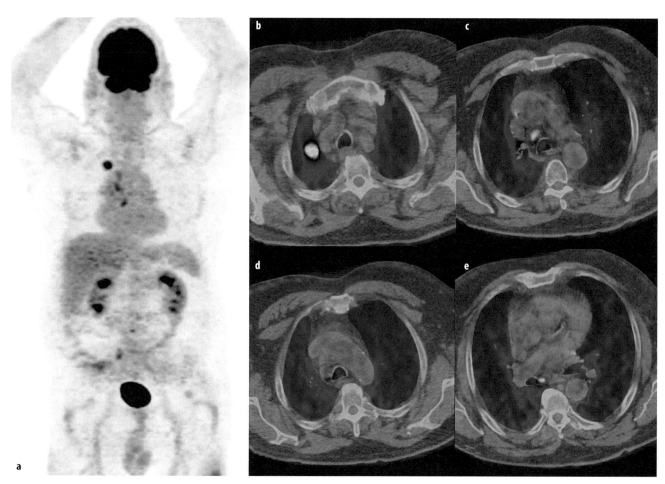

Fig. 1 a-e. FDG-PET/CT in a 76-year-old man. Images display an FDG-avid squamous cell carcinoma in the right upper lobe (**a, b**) as well as pretracheal (**c**), right paratracheal (**d**), and subcarinal (**e**) lymph node metastases. The classification pT1B pN2 cM0 was proven by histology. Notably, the left lateral border of the trachea differentiates left from right paratracheal lymph nodes. Thus, the pretracheal lymph node metastases (**c**) would not mean N2 but N3 disease if the lung tumor was in the left lung. Subcarinal lymph node metastases (**e**) are always considered N2 disease regardless of the location of the primary lung tumor

but N3 disease if the primary is located in the left lung (Fig. 1).

The M descriptor has been divided into M1a and M1b, for intrathoracic and distant spread, respectively. Patients with malignant pleural effusions have been up-staged from T4 to M1 (Table 1).

The labeling of stages also was revised between the 6th and 7th editions (Table 2). For example, T2bN0 has moved from stage IB to stage IIA, and T2aN1 from stage IIB to stage IIA. Patients with tumors >7 cm move from IB to IIB if there is no lymph node metastasis, and from IIB to IIIA if they have N1 lymph nodes. Patients without N3 lymph nodes but with an additional nodule in the same lobe have been moved from stage IIIB to stage IIIA.

The new TNM staging system for lung cancer directly impacts treatment algorithms. Treatment approaches for NSCLC are being constantly adapted and may be shifted from standardized to personalized strategies. Formerly, stages I to IIIA were considered "operable," while stages IIIB and VI were considered "not to be operable". This

is no longer in line with current treatment guidelines. For instance, stage IIIA with N2 lymph node metastasis may be considered inoperable if lymph node metastases are bulky or in multiple lymph node levels that lie in the ipsilateral mediastinum. A curative operation may be considered if down-staging of N3 disease with neoadjuvant chemotherapy is successful. In stage IV disease, curative treatment approaches may be considered today even if oligometastatic disease is found with involvement of the adrenal glands or the brain. Last but not least, standardized treatment strategies are to be defined in adenocarcinomas with EGFR mutations or ALK rearrangements.

This brief summary demonstrates the complexity of tumor staging in lung cancer and thus shows the need for a multidisciplinary approach.

T Staging

CT and FDG-PET/CT are important imaging modalities in the evaluation of the primary tumor (T staging). CT is known to have a low accuracy in the evaluation of invasion of the pleura, the chest wall, and/or the mediastinum, and the correct differentiation between tumor and peritumoral atelectasis is often difficult [6, 7]. FDG-PET/CT may improve accuracy in the detection of tumor invasion into the chest wall [8-10]. This is important particularly in patients with a poor cardio-pulmonary reserve, since the preoperative determination of chest wall infiltration is desirable in order to avoid extended en bloc resection.

To evaluate infiltration of the mediastinum (T4), contrast-enhanced CT may be employed but it has a relatively low sensitivity, specificity, and accuracy (68%, 72%, and 70%, respectively) [7]. According to our experience, PET/CT is not accurate in clearly identifying direct invasion of the mediastinal vasculature and airways even if the CT component of FDG-PET/CT is performed with contrast medium.

FDG-PET/CT is helpful for the differentiation between tumor and peritumoral atelectasis. This allows for a more precise determination of the T stage and thereby impacts surgical planning – as sleeve lobectomy is preferred over pneumonectomy – and radiotherapy planning – as the accurate information of tumor extent provided by FDG-PET/CT contributes to a change in the radiation field in 30–40% of patients [11].

N Staging

Accurate lymph node staging in patients with NSCLC is particularly important for patient management. Surgical resection is the treatment of choice for early stages (stage I or a subset of stage II T1-2, N1). Patients with ipsilateral mediastinal lymph nodes metastases (N2 disease) are still considered to have potentially resectable disease if lymph node metastases are not bulky, multilevel, or technically unresectable. Induction chemotherapy is usually recommended with or without combined radiation therapy. Surgery is generally not indicated if contralateral mediastinal scalene or supraclavicular lymph node metastases are present (N3).

Both the sensitivity and specificity of CT in the determination of lymph node metastases from NSCLC are between 60% and 70% [6, 12]. Thus, CT scanning will erroneously suggest the presence of mediastinal lymph node metastases but miss lymph node metastases in as many as 30–40% of cases. Several studies have demonstrated that FDG-PET/CT is significantly more accurate than CT in the determination of lymph node metastases [13-15]. State-of-the-art PET scanners have a fairly high spatial resolution (4-6 mm), and even small lesions with an increased FDG uptake may be detected. A meta-analysis of FDG-PET/CT and CT in the mediastinal staging of NSCLC demonstrated an accuracy of 86% for FDG-PET/CT and of 73% for CT. Sensitivity, specificity, positive and negative predictive values were 73%, 91%, 71%, and 90% for FDG-PET/CT and 74%, 73%, 52%, and 88% for CT, respectively [16]. Thus,

FDG-positive lymph nodes, suspicious for metastases, should generally be confirmed by biopsy, if relevant for patient management.

M Staging

Distant metastatic disease is already present in 18–36% of patients with newly diagnosed NSCLC [17]. The ability to detect distant metastases with a high sensitivity, specificity, and accuracy (94%, 97%, and 96%, respectively) [18] is the main advantage of FDG-PET/CT and renders PET/CT superior to other imaging modalities. The high sensitivity of FDG-PET/CT to detect distant metastases changes patient management in a considerable number of patients, mostly by the up-staging of disease. Thus, FDG-PET/CT becomes a cost effective imaging modality despite its high operational cost due to a significant reduction of morbidity though undesired surgeries [19-21].

The American National Comprehensive Cancer Network guidelines advocate FDG-PET/CT for all patients with newly diagnosed NSCLC provided that there is no evidence of distant metastases. An additional magnetic resonance imaging (MRI) study of the brain is recommended in patients with stage II-IV disease to complete accurate whole-body tumor staging. This is mandatory because the ability to detect brain metastases is low in FDG-PET/CT (see below).

False Negative and False Positive FDG-PET/CT Results

False-negative results in FDG-PET/CT may occur in small lesions since the spatial resolution is limited; PET is usually not able to detect metastases <4–6 mm. Carcinoid tumors and adenocarcinomas with lepidic growth (formally called BAC) [22, 23] may be false-negative on FDG-PET/CT, as these tumors often metabolize only small amounts of FDG. Finally, false-negative findings may occur in organs with a high metabolic turn-over, such as the kidneys or the brain.

False-positive results may occur in states of inflammation and other neoplasms [24] (Fig. 2). For example, sarcoidosis often presents with FDG-positive lymphadenopathy that may be interpreted as lymph node metastasis or rarely that will imitate distant metastasis [25]. If there is doubt, the findings must be confirmed histologically if considered relevant for patient management.

Therapy Monitoring

Quantitative assessment of therapy-induced changes has shown that tumoral FDG uptake predicts both response and outcome [26]. Moreover, cancer therapy may be adjusted according to the chemosensitivity of the primary tumor as assessed on follow-up FDG-PET/CT (Fig. 3).

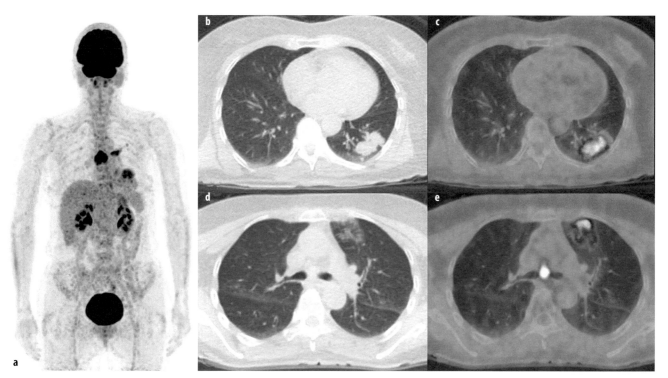

Fig. 2 a-e. FDG-PET/CT in a 69-year-old woman with an FDG-avid adenocarcinoma of the left lower lobe (**a-c**). FDG-PET/CT shows not only N2 disease (**a, e**) but also an FDG-avid pneumonia in the right upper lobe (**d, e**), which may be misinterpreted as metastasis, resulting in upstaging to T4 disease (i.e., nodule in another lobe on the same side) and thus in total pneumonectomy. Final tumor classification after resection of the left lower lobe and mediastinal lymphadenectomy was pT1B pN2 cM0

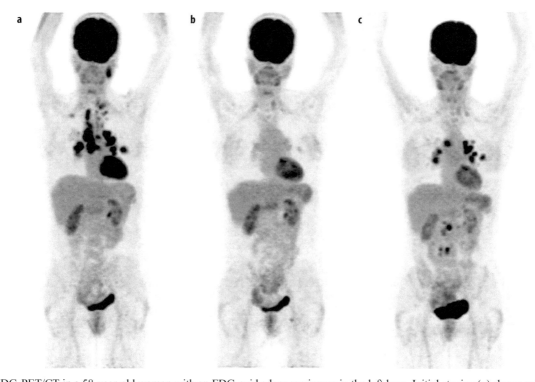

Fig. 3 a-c. FDG-PET/CT in a 58-year-old woman with an FDG-avid adenocarcinoma in the left lung. Initial staging (**a**) shows extensive lymph node metastases (N3); TNM stage was cT1 pN3 cM0. First follow-up (**b**) 2 months after the scan in (**a**) shows the complete metabolic response of both the lung cancer and all lymph nodes metastases after first line chemotherapy with cisplatin and alimta. Second PET/CT follow-up (**c**) 5 months after the scan in (**b**) and while the asymptomtic patient was on maintenance therapy with alimta. The recurrence of hilar and mediastinal lymph nodes metastases and new abdominal lymph nodes metastases are seen. Chemotherapy with taxotere was started

Hence, FDG-PET/CT has the potential to reduce side effects and costs when therapy is ineffective [27].

Recurrent Lung Cancer

Patients with NSCLC who have been treated with curative intent are usually followed up with CT every 6–12 months. FDG-PET/CT is used to evaluate equivocal CT findings, due to its very high accuracy in distinguishing recurrent disease from benign treatment effects. If tumor recurrence is suspected or confirmed, a FDG-PET/CT for restaging is indicated to differentiate local from distant recurrence, and thus to plan local or systemic treatment [28, 29] (Fig. 3). Moreover, initial data suggests that FDG-PET/CT is useful in the detection of recurrences in asymptomatic NSCLC patients after potentially curative operations [28-30].

References

1. Charloux A, Quoix E, Wolkove N et al (1997) The increasing incidence of lung adenocarcinoma: reality or artefact? A review of the epidemiology of lung adenocarcinoma. Int J Epidemiol 26:14-23.
2. Travis WD, Brambilla E, Noguchi M et al (2011) International association for the study of lung cancer/american thoracic society/european respiratory society international multidisciplinary classification of lung adenocarcinoma. J Thorac Oncol 6:244-285.
3. Janne PA, Meyerson M (2012) ROS1 rearrangements in lung cancer: a new genomic subset of lung adenocarcinoma. J Clin Oncol 30:878-879.
4. Sobin L, Gospodarowisz M, Wittekind C (eds) (2010) TNM classification of malignant tumours, 7th Ed. Blackwell Publishing, Oxford, UK.
5. Mountain CF, Dresler CM (1997) Regional lymph node classification for lung cancer staging. Chest 111:1718-1723.
6. Webb WR, Gatsonis C, Zerhouni EA et al (1991) CT and MR imaging in staging non-small cell bronchogenic carcinoma: report of the Radiologic Diagnostic Oncology Group. Radiology 178:705-713.
7. Rendina EA, Bognolo DA, Mineo TC et al (1987) Computed tomography for the evaluation of intrathoracic invasion by lung cancer. J Thorac Cardiovasc Surg 94:57-63.
8. Antoch G, Stattaus J, Nemat AT et al (2003) Non-small cell lung cancer: dual-modality PET/CT in preoperative staging. Radiology 229:526-533.
9. Lardinois D, Weder W, Hany TF et al (2003) Staging of non-small-cell lung cancer with integrated positron-emission tomography and computed tomography. N Engl J Med 348:2500-2507.
10. Shim SS, Lee KS, Kim BT et al (2005) Non-small cell lung cancer: prospective comparison of integrated FDG PET/CT and CT alone for preoperative staging. Radiology 236:1011-1019.
11. Nestle U, Walter K, Schmidt S et al (1999) 18F-deoxyglucose positron emission tomography (FDG-PET) for the planning of radiotherapy in lung cancer: high impact in patients with atelectasis. Int J Radiat Oncol Biol Phys 44:593-597.
12. McLoud TC, Bourgouin PM, Greenberg RW et al (1999) Bronchogenic carcinoma: analysis of staging in the mediastinum with CT by correlative lymph node mapping and sampling. Radiology 182:319-323.
13. Steinert HC, Hauser M, Allemann F et al (1997) Non-small cell lung cancer: nodal staging with FDG PET versus CT with correlative lymph node mapping and sampling. Radiology 202:441-446.
14. Vansteenkiste JF, Stroobants SG, De Leyn PR et al (1998) Lymph node staging in non-small-cell lung cancer with FDG-PET scan: a prospective study on 690 lymph node stations from 68 patients. J Clin Oncol 16:2142-2149.
15. Pieterman RM, van Putten JW, Meuzelaar JJ et al (2000) Preoperative staging of non-small-cell lung cancer with positron-emission tomography. N Engl J Med 343:254-261.
16. Chao F, Zhang H (2012) PET/CT in the staging of the non-small-cell lung cancer. J Biomed Biotechnol 2012:783739.
17. Quint LE (2007) Staging non-small cell lung cancer. Cancer Imaging 7:148-159.
18. Hellwig D, Ukena D, Paulsen F et al (2001) [Meta-analysis of the efficacy of positron emission tomography with F-18-fluorodeoxyglucose in lung tumors. Basis for discussion of the German Consensus Conference on PET in Oncology 2000]. Pneumologie 55:367-377.
19. van Tinteren H, Hoekstra OS, Smit EF et al (2002) Effectiveness of positron emission tomography in the preoperative assessment of patients with suspected non-small-cell lung cancer: the PLUS multicentre randomised trial. Lancet 359:1388-1393.
20. Kelly RF, Tran T, Holmstrom A et al (2004) Accuracy and cost-effectiveness of [18F]-2-fluoro-deoxy-D-glucose-positron emission tomography scan in potentially resectable non-small cell lung cancer. Chest 125:1413-1423.
21. Fischer B, Lassen U, Mortensen J et al (2009) Preoperative staging of lung cancer with combined PET-CT. N Engl J Med 361:32-39.
22. Higashi K, Ueda Y, Seki H et al (1998) Fluorine-18-FDG PET imaging is negative in bronchioloalveolar lung carcinoma. J Nucl Med 39:1016-1020.
23. Erasmus JJ, McAdams HP, Patz EF, Jr. et al (1998) Evaluation of primary pulmonary carcinoid tumors using FDG PET. AJR Am J Roentgenol 170:1369-1373.
24. Lardinois D, Weder W, Roudas M et al (2005) Etiology of solitary extrapulmonary positron emission tomography and computed tomography findings in patients with lung cancer. J Clin Oncol 23:6846-6853.
25. Soussan M, Augier A, Brillet PY et al (2014) Functional imaging in extrapulmonary sarcoidosis: FDG-PET/CT and MR features. Clin Nucl Med 39:e146-159.
26. Tiseo M, Ippolito M, Scarlattei M et al (2014) Predictive and prognostic value of early response assessment using 18FDG-PET in advanced non-small cell lung cancer patients treated with erlotinib. Cancer Chemother Pharmacol 73:299-307.
27. Skoura E, Datseris IE, Platis I et al (2012) Role of positron emission tomography in the early prediction of response to chemotherapy in patients with non-small-cell lung cancer. Clin Lung Cancer 13:181-187.
28. Jimenez-Bonilla JF, Quirce R, Martinez-Rodriguez I et al (2013) Diagnosis of recurrence and assessment of post-recurrence survival in patients with extracranial non-small cell lung cancer evaluated by 18F-FDG PET/CT. Lung Cancer 81:71-76.
29. Kanzaki R, Higashiyama M, Maeda J et al (2010) Clinical value of F18-fluorodeoxyglucose positron emission tomography-computed tomography in patients with non-small cell lung cancer after potentially curative surgery: experience with 241 patients. Interact Cardiovasc Thorac Surg 10:1009-1014.
30. Toba H, Sakiyama S, Otsuka H et al (2012) 18F-fluorodeoxyglucose positron emission tomography/computed tomography is useful in postoperative follow-up of asymptomatic non-small-cell lung cancer patients. Interact Cardiovasc Thorac Surg 15:859-864.

How To Approach Incidental Findings on Computed Tomography Images of the Lungs Obtained in Hybrid Imaging

Jeffrey P. Kanne

Department of Radiology, University of Wisconsin School of Medicine and Public Health, Madison, WI, USA

Cross-sectional imaging has become an important component in nuclear medicine, as it can be used for more precise anatomic localization as well as attenuation correction. Positron emission tomography (PET) performed in conjunction with computed tomography (CT) is commonly used in staging and restaging malignancies and occasionally used for other imaging purposes such as evaluating larger lung nodules and for myocardial imaging. Single photon emission computed tomography (SPECT) is also performed in conjunction with CT to improve anatomic localization. Very recently, hybrid imaging with PET and magnetic resonance imaging (MRI) has become available and may prove to have many applications beyond oncologic imaging.

Interpreting hybrid imaging studies requires not only an understanding of nuclear imaging but also knowledge of cross-sectional anatomy. Furthermore, the individual interpreting hybrid imaging studies must be aware of the range of incidental findings encountered on hybrid imaging studies. Some incidental findings may have important clinical significance whereas others may require no further attention.

This chapter focuses primarily on the incidental thoracic findings encountered in the chest on PET/CT.

Lungs

Although CT performed for attenuation correction with PET or SPECT is typically not optimized to evaluate the lungs, many incidental findings are still encountered on nuclear medicine hybrid studies. Optimal imaging of the lungs is performed with thin-section (<1.5 mm) volumetric helical CT of the chest during full inspiration. Coronal and sagittal reformations are often generated and reviewed. This technique provides high spatial resolution and a detailed anatomic evaluation of the lungs. Typically, attenuation correction CT is performed with thick (~5 mm) contiguous (non-helical) sections acquired during quiet breathing. This results in decreased spatial resolution and artifact from respiratory motion.

Lung Nodules

A lung nodule is defined as a rounded or ovoid soft-tissue opacity in the lung, surrounded by air, and measuring no more than 30 mm in maximum diameter. Nodules can have mineral (calcium), soft tissue, fat, or mixed attenuation. Subsolid nodules, or those containing ground-glass opacity, are extremely difficult to detect or fully characterize on CT performed as part of nuclear imaging studies and are best evaluated with dedicated thin-section chest CT.

Calcified Nodules

Calcified nodules (Fig. 1) are usually the result of remote granulomatous infection, particularly histoplasmosis (in North America) and tuberculosis (the rest of the world). Larger nodules may be only partially calcified. To be considered benign, a partially calcified nodule should fall into one of the following four patterns: diffusely calcified, centrally calcified, lamellated (concentric rings) calcification, or dystrophic ("popcorn") calcification. Eccentric or stippled patterns of calcification are considered indeterminate. In patients with a history of matrix-forming sarcoma (osteosarcoma or chondrosarcoma) or adenocarcinoma (especially mucinous), metastases can present on CT as calcified nodules. Comparison to previous imaging and correlation with metabolic imaging are usually sufficient to determine the nature of these nodules.

Soft-Tissue Attenuation Nodules

Most soft-tissue attenuation nodules on CT are indeterminate. In the absence of a known malignancy, the vast majority of tiny (<5 mm) solid nodules are benign. The rate of malignancy increases with size. Guidelines exist for the management of incidental small solid nodules. However, they are not applicable to patients with known malignancy. In most cases, if not recently performed, a dedicated non-contrast chest CT is warranted to fully characterize incidental nodules on hybrid imaging.

Pattern	Schematic	Behavior
Diffuse		Benign[a]
Central	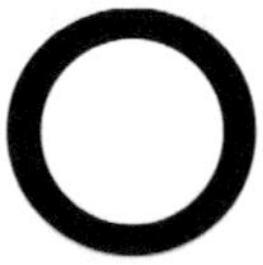	Benign
Lamellated	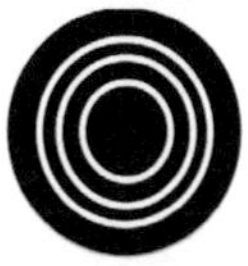	Benign
Dystrophic ("popcorn")	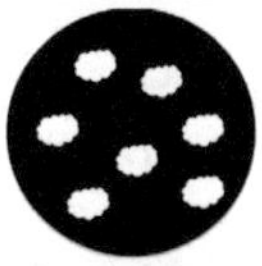	Benign
Eccentric	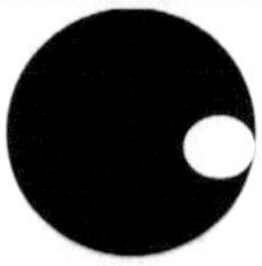	Indeterminate
Stippled	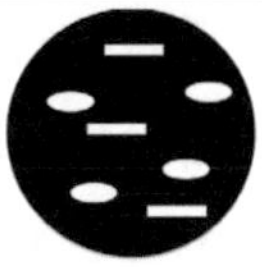	Indeterminate

[a] Except in the setting of matrix-forming sarcoma or metastatic adenocarcinoma.

Fig. 1. Patterns of lung nodule calcification

Fat-Attenuation Nodules

Nodules with macroscopic fat apparent on chest CT often represent pulmonary hamartomas (mesenchymomas). These nodules can be purely fat, primarily soft tissue, or contain coarse "popcorn" calcification. Hamartomas typically show no increased metabolic activity on nuclear imaging, although they can grow slowly over several years.

Diffuse Micronodules

The differential diagnosis of diffuse micronodules (<10 mm diameter) depends on their distribution in the lungs. The spatial resolution of CT technique used in hybrid imaging is typically not sufficient enough to fully characterize the morphology and distribution of diffuse micronodules. However, occasionally, small branching (Y- or V-shaped) opacities (tree-in-bud) may be apparent on hybrid imaging studies. Tree-in-bud opacities are a CT finding of bronchiolitis and nearly always reflect infection. Occasionally, tree-in-bud opacities reflect bronchiolitis from aspiration and may be encountered in patients

undergoing hybrid imaging for esophageal carcinoma or head and neck malignancies. Clues to the diagnosis include a gravitationally dependent distribution as well as ancillary findings such as a large hiatus hernia or fluid in the esophagus.

Emphysema

Emphysema (Fig. 2) is the process of airspace expansion and alveolar destruction with minimal fibrosis. Most emphysema is the result of cigarette smoking. Emphysema is frequently encountered in patients undergoing hybrid imaging for lung cancer staging. Emphysema is classified based on its histopathologic morphology, but strong correlation with CT appearances allows for use of the same classification scheme.

Centrilobular Emphysema

Centrilobular emphysema occurs in the central portion of the pulmonary lobule, around the lobular bronchiole and lobular pulmonary artery. It is almost always the result of cigarette smoking and has a predilection for the upper lobes and superior segments of the lower lobes. On CT, centrilobular emphysema appears as round foci of low attenuation. A punctate opacity may be visible within the emphysematous lesion, representing the lobular artery.

Pattern	Schematic	Distribution
Centrilobular	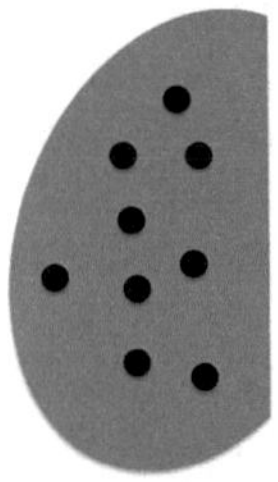	Upper lobe predominant, patchy
Panlobular		Lower lobe, diffuse
Paraseptal	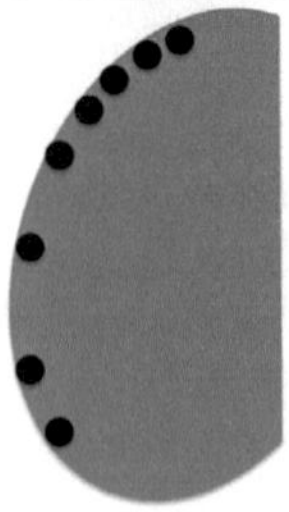	Upper and mid lungs, subpleural

Fig. 2. Patterns of emphysema

Panlobular Emphysema

Panlobular emphysema reflects emphysematous destruction of an entire pulmonary lobule and often affects most if not all of an entire segment or lobe. Panlobular emphysema is most commonly associated with alpha-1 antitrypsin deficiency and predominates in the lower lobes. CT shows large foci of low attenuation, hyperinflation, and attenuated pulmonary vasculature.

Paraseptal Emphysema

Paraseptal emphysema occurs in the periphery of the pulmonary lobule and usually develops along pleural spaces. It may occur in isolation but more often in conjunction with centrilobular emphysema. Large (<10 mm) paraseptal emphysematous lesions are termed bullae and can become quite large.

Linear Opacities

Fine linear (or reticular) opacities (Fig. 3) may be identified on CT performed as part of hybrid imaging studies. These opacities can be described as interlobular (or septal) or irregular (intralobular).

Interlobular Septal Thickening

Interlobular septal thickening occurs when fluid, cells, or fibrosis fill and expand the normal septum that surrounds the pulmonary lobule. It is usually apparent on CT performed in conjunction with PET. Septal thickening most commonly reflects lung edema and may be seen in patients with congestive heart failure or other causes of lung edema. The primary differential diagnosis is lymphangitic carcinomatosis, which occurs when tumor cells invade and obstruct the pulmonary lymphatics. Whereas septal thickening from lung edema is typically bilateral, symmetric, and gravitationally dependent, septal thickening from lymphangitic carcinomatosis is more often randomly distributed. In the setting of a centrally obstructing mass (usually lung carcinoma), septal thickening may be observed in the affected lobe(s) as a result of central lymphatic and venous obstruction.

Intralobular Lines

Intralobular lines occur within a pulmonary lobule and are nearly always the result of pulmonary fibrosis. These irregular lines may be more difficult to detect on attenuation correction CT but can be seen when fibrosis is more extensive. Most pulmonary fibrosis occurs in the lung bases. Other findings associated with pulmonary fibrosis include traction bronchiectasis and honeycomb cysts. Pulmonary fibrosis may be encountered in patients with a history of cigarette smoking and in those with collagen vascular diseases. If clinically appropriate, full characterization can be performed with dedicated noncontrast thin-section chest CT.

Cysts

Lung cysts (Table 1) are low attenuation foci in the lungs surrounded by a thin, smooth wall. Single or a small number of cysts can be found in healthy patients and require no further evaluation. However, some lung diseases can primarily manifest by the development of extensive lung cysts.

Pulmonary Langerhans Cell Histiocytosis

Pulmonary Langerhans cell histiocytosis (PLCH) occurs almost exclusively in adult smokers and is characterized by the formation of nodules and cysts that predominate in the upper lungs. With progressive disease, the number and size of cysts increase as the profusion of nodules diminishes. Larger cysts may have bizarre shapes. PLCH may be encountered in hybrid imaging in patients being staged for lung cancer and should not be mistaken for metastases.

Lymphoid Interstitial Pneumonia

Lymphoid interstitial pneumonia (LIP) is part of the spectrum of pulmonary lymphoproliferative disorders and is characterized by infiltration and expansion of the pulmonary interstitium by a polyclonal mix of lymphoid cells. In adults, it is most commonly associated with Sjögren syndrome and thus may be encountered on hybrid imaging performed for staging of lymphoma. On CT, LIP is characterized by the presence of basal-predominant cysts, ranging up to approximately 30 mm in diameter. Frequently, a vessel can be observed coursing along the wall of the cyst. Other CT features of LIP include nodules (soft tissue or calcified, the latter often reflecting amyloid deposition), septal lines, and ground-glass opacity.

Pattern	Schematic	Causes
Interlobular	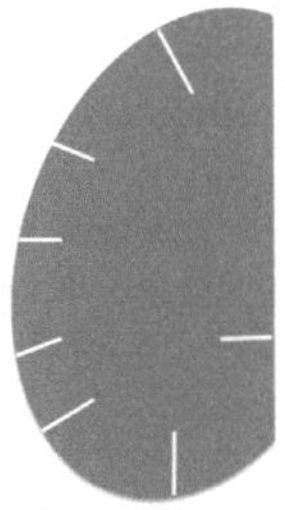	Edema Lymphangitic carcinomatosis Central venous and lymphatic obstruction
Intralobular	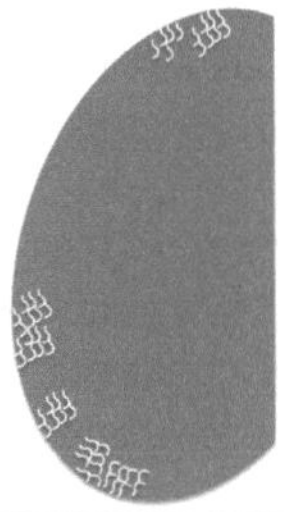	Fibrosis

Fig. 3. Fine linear (reticular) opacities

Table 1. Causes of lung cysts

Disease	Distribution	Other features and associationss
Pulmonary Langerhans cell histiocytosis	Upper lungs	Bizarre shapes Nodules Cigarette smoking (>97%)
Lymphoid interstitial pneumonia	Basal predominant	Perivascular Nodules (± calcification) Septal lines Ground-glass opacity Collagen-vascular disease (especially Sjögren syndrome)
Birt-Hogg-Dubé syndrome	Basal predominant	Bilenticular Renal neoplasms Skin lesions on face and upper trunk

Birt-Hogg-Dubé Syndrome

This autosomal dominant disease is characterized by the development of soft-tissue lesions on the face and upper trunk (primarily fibrofolliculomas), lung cysts, and renal neoplasms. Many patients report a personal or family history of spontaneous pneumothorax. The lung cysts in Birt-Hogg-Dubé syndrome have a characteristic bilenticular shape and a predilection for the lower lobes, along the pulmonary fissures, pulmonary veins, and septopleural junction. These cysts may be encountered in patients undergoing hybrid imaging for renal cell carcinoma, and the diagnosis should be suggested given the implications for nephron-sparing therapy and the screening of family members.

Lung Consolidation

Lung consolidation (Table 2) is defined as increased attenuation of the lung parenchyma such that the underlying architecture is obscured. CT typically cannot establish the cause of lung consolidation but common causes include infection, hemorrhage, neoplasm, edema, and noninfectious inflammation such as organizing or eosinophilic pneumonia. Typically, obtaining additional clinical information is sufficient to establish a cause for the consolidation.

Lung Carcinoma Presenting as Consolidation

Non-resolving, slowly progressive lung consolidation is an uncommon manifestation of lung carcinoma. Many of these neoplasms are mucinous adenocarcinomas and can grow slowly over several years. It is often the case that patients are initially diagnosed as having recurrent infection. Documenting slow progression across serial examinations usually suggests the diagnosis. Percutaneous or transbronchial biopsy usually confirms the diagnosis. Clues to the diagnosis on CT include lucencies within areas of consolidation (pseudocavitation), small solid and subsolid nodules adjacent to larger areas of consolidation, and distortion (stretching) of the involved bronchi.

Lymphoma Presenting as Lung Consolidation

Whether primary or secondary, lymphoma can present as single or multiple mass-like areas of consolidation on CT. Distinguishing lymphoma from other causes of consolidation can be extremely difficult without previous imaging or tissue confirmation.

Organizing Pneumonia

Organizing pneumonia (OP) is defined as the accumulation of newly synthesized collagen in the airspaces (alveoli and alveolar ducts) of the lung. OP is a normal healing mechanism of the lung and typically occurs in conjunction with other processes, such as infection or hemorrhage. It can also be an immunologic response to an extrinsic (drug, inhaled antigen) or intrinsic (autoimmune) stimulus. In the setting of oncologic imaging, OP most commonly results from drug reaction, as many antibiotics and chemotherapeutic agents can trigger an OP response in the lung. On

Table 2. Causes of lung consolidation

Cause	Other clues
Hemorrhage	Acute hypoxia and dyspnea Hemoptysis (~50%)
Infection	Fever Leukocytosis Purulent sputum
Edema	Other signs of heart or kidney failure Pleural effusion Cardiomegaly
Neoplasm (lung adenocarcinoma or lymphoma)	Slowly progressive Pseudocavitation (adenocarcinoma) Bronchial stretching (adenocarcinoma)
Organizing pneumonia (OP) and eosinophilic pneumonia	Peripheral and peribronchial distribution Reversed halo sign (OP) Drug reaction (antibiotics and chemotherapeutic agents)
Large opacities of pneumoconiosis	Background of small pneumoconiotic nodules Upper lung predominant Coalescence of small nodules Lateral margins typically smooth Volume loss in affected lobe(s)

CT, OP manifests as peripheral and peribronchial foci of consolidation. Air bronchograms are usually visible within the foci of consolidation. In approximately 20% of patients, the "reversed halo" or "atoll" sign is present, defined as a focus of peripheral consolidation with central ground-glass opacity. In a small number of patients undergoing chest wall radiation for breast carcinoma, OP can develop outside the small portion of irradiated lung, even affecting the contralateral lung. The CT appearance of OP in this setting is similar to that of other causes.

Eosinophilic Pneumonia

This inflammatory condition of the lung is associated with tissue (and sometimes peripheral) eosinophilia. The CT findings of eosinophilic pneumonia (EP) are very similar to those of OP and the two entities should be considered in the differential diagnosis of multifocal lung consolidation. However, the reversed halo sign is not a feature of EP. The most common cause of EP encountered in hybrid imaging is drug reaction.

Large Opacities of Pneumoconiosis

Silicosis and coal worker's pneumoconiosis (CWP) are associated with lung carcinoma and may be encountered on PET/CT studies of patients undergoing staging. Simple pneumoconiosis is characterized by the formation of small nodules (<10 mm) in the lungs in response to inhalation of silica or coal dusts. Simple silicosis and CWP are readily diagnosed by a combination of occupational exposure and findings on chest radiography and/or chest CT. Complicated pneumoconiosis (progressive massive fibrosis, PMF) is defined by the formation of large opacities (>10 mm in diameter) in the lungs, resulting from the coalescence of small pneumoconiotic nodules into mass-like areas of consolidation. These large opacities can be misinterpreted as lung carcinoma if the typical appearance and background of small nodules are overlooked. Large opacities usually have lateral margins that parallel the chest wall and are associated with significant volume loss (recognized by displacement of the pulmonary fissure(s) and hilar distortion). Large pneumoconiotic opacities are often bilateral, especially as PMF becomes more advanced.

Airways

Evaluation of the airways is usually the purview of volumetric thin-section CT. However, abnormalities of larger airways, especially the bronchi, can be encountered on hybrid imaging.

Bronchiectasis

Bronchiectasis is a chronic condition characterized by local, irreversible dilation of the bronchi, usually associated with inflammation. Bronchiectasis results from chron-ic bronchial obstruction, bronchial wall damage, or parenchymal fibrosis. With parenchymal fibrosis, the dilation of bronchi, termed traction bronchiectasis, occurs by the maturation and retraction of fibrous tissue formed adjacent to an airway. The CT findings of bronchial dilation include lack of tapering of bronchial lumena (the primary sign of bronchiectasis), internal diameter of bronchi greater than that of the adjacent pulmonary artery (signet ring sign), bronchi visible within 1 cm of the costal pleura or abutting the mediastinal pleura, and mucus-filled dilated bronchi. Bronchiectasis can be described as cylindrical, varicose, or cystic, depending on the morphology.

Pleura

Aside from the pulmonary fissures and an occasional thin pleural stripe along the chest wall, the normal pleura is not visible on CT, particularly on the thicker section images that are typically used with PET/CT. For many oncology patients, the presence of pleural effusion or soft tissue involvement will be part of the malignant process. However, some pleural findings may be benign.

Pleural Effusion

Pleural effusions are classified as transudative or exudative depending on their content. Malignant pleural effusions are almost always exudative and can even be bloody. By contrast, pleural effusions associated with heart failure are typically transudative. Malignant pleural effusion often shows ^{18}F-fluorodeoxyglucose (FDG) avidity on PET/CT, and occasionally tumor deposits are apparent in the pleural space. Small, layering pleural effusions that are not hypermetabolic, especially when bilateral, may reflect congestive heart failure or fluid overload from treatment-related renal toxicity.

Pleural Plaque

Pleural plaques appear as focal thickening of the pleura, usually the parietal surface, and are almost always the result of asbestos exposure. Pleural plaques are acellular and contain hyaline. They typically form along the hemidiaphragms, costal pleura anterolaterally and posteromedially, and occasionally along the mediastinal pleura. Pleural plaques have no malignant potential and are usually not associated with altered respiratory physiology.

Diffuse Pleural Thickening

There is no specific definition of diffuse pleural thickening as seen on CT. The causes of diffuse pleural thickening vary but commonly include instrumentation (e.g., pleural drainage, thoracic or cardiac surgery), healed empyema, pleural hemorrhage (hemothorax), and asbestos exposure.

Fibrothorax

Extensive pleural thickening can result in a restrictive physiology in the affected lung, a condition termed fibrothorax. Thickened pleura can also calcify as well, either in focal areas or diffusely. Densely calcified pleura is usually the result of previous hemithorax or empyema.

Rounded Atelectasis

Rounded atelectasis develops when there is progressive infolding of lung adjacent to thickened visceral pleura. Over time, the infolded lung becomes mass like. The characteristic feature of rounded atelectasis on cross-sectional imaging is a soft-tissue nodule or mass located immediately adjacent to thickened visceral pleura. Vessels and bronchi can be seen swirling into the focus of rounded atelectasis, giving the "comet tail" sign. Other signs of volume loss include displacement of the nearby fissure and decreased volume in the affected lobe.

Talc Pleurodesis

Pleurodesis is often used to palliate malignant pleural effusion by inducing fusion of the pleural layers and subsequently obliterating the pleural space. Pleurodesis can be performed through mechanical or chemical means, but for malignant effusions, instillation of talc slurry into the pleural space is the most commonly used method. Talc pleurodesis has a characteristic appearance on CT, manifesting as nodular high-attenuation pleural thickening, similar to faint calcification. Importantly, the pleura can remain hypermetabolic for many years following talc pleurodesis and should not be mistaken for malignant pleural disease.

Pleural Lipoma

Pleural lipomas are benign neoplasms containing fat and a thin capsule. Occasionally, they are large enough to be visible on chest radiographs, and most are easily detectable on cross-sectional imaging. On CT, pleural lipomas have fat attenuation and lie in contact with the chest wall. A thin capsule may be visible.

Mediastinum

Normal Thymus

The normal thymus is large at birth and gradually atrophies, usually replaced primarily with fat in early adulthood. However, normal thymic tissue may be apparent in middle-age adults as well. On CT, the normal thymus consists of two triangular or ellipsoid lobes, one typically larger than the other. A trapezoidal configuration can also occur, particularly in young women. Strands of fat coursing through normal thymic tissue are often apparent.

Thymic Hyperplasia

The thymus can increase in size and weight after an immunologic insult to the body. This may occur following a severe illness, chemotherapy, or other injury. Cross-sectional imaging will show enlargement of the thymus. This may be seen on PET/CT performed for restaging of malignancy.

Lymphoid Thymic Hyperplasia

Lymphoid thymic hyperplasia occurs when lymphoid follicles with germinal centers develop in the thymus. Lymphoid hyperplasia is often associated with autoimmune disease such as myasthenia gravis. Distinguishing true hyperplasia from lymphoid hyperplasia on CT is typically not possible.

Foregut Duplication Cysts

Foregut duplication cysts are congenital remnants of foregut tissue and are usually lined with either bronchial or esophageal mucosa. Over time they can enlarge, producing mass effect, resulting in symptoms such as pain. Usually the diagnosis is readily apparent on CT, but dedicated MRI can be used in cases in which there is diagnostic uncertainty. Symptomatic cysts are usually resected.

Bronchogenic Cysts

Bronchogenic cysts most commonly occur in the subcarinal space and less commonly in the paratracheal spaces and inferior pulmonary ligaments. On CT, bronchogenic cysts are typically spheroid and have homogeneous attenuation. Attenuation may exceed that of water secondary to accumulation of proteinaceous fluid. FDG activity is typically nil unless there is active inflammation.

Esophageal Duplication Cysts

Esophageal duplication cysts usually occur in the lower mediastinum adjacent to the esophagus. Esophageal duplication cysts can also be lined with pancreatic or gastric mucosa, and intracystic hemorrhage can occur.

Esophageal Diverticula

Esophageal diverticula are described as either pulsion or traction, depending on the underlying cause. Pulsion diverticula usually occur in the superior or inferior mediastinum whereas traction diverticula typically form in the central mediastinum, usually from adjacent inflammation such as tuberculous lymphadenitis.

Neurogenic Neoplasm

Neurogenic neoplasms are the most common posterior mediastinal masses. The vast majority of mediastinal neurogenic neoplasms are benign and include schwannoma and neurofibromas. Neurofibromas commonly course along the intercostal nerves and can lead to bone remodeling. Schwannomas may be seen extending into and widening the neural foramen, taking on a "dumbbell" appearance. These lesions are best characterized with dedicated MRI.

Heart, Pericardium, and Aorta

The heart is frequently overlooked on hybrid nuclear imaging for a variety of reasons. First, cardiac metabolic activity is quite variable and detecting malignant disease can be challenging. Second, because attenuation correction CT is performed during free breathing and at slower acquisitions, cardiac motion can be extensive. Nevertheless, several important findings may still be apparent on CT, especially if a higher quality CT is performed in conjunction with PET.

Coronary Arteries

Coronary artery disease remains the number one cause of death, both for men and for women, in the developed world. CT has been shown to be effective in detecting the presence of coronary calcification, a marker of coronary artery atherosclerosis. Extensive research has confirmed that quantifying coronary calcification on CT can be used to risk-stratify patients for subsequent major adverse cardiac events. While most CT performed for attenuation correction and anatomic localization may be insufficient to accurately quantify coronary calcium, the images typically show the presence of moderate or severe coronary calcium and its distribution. In patients with a known diagnosis of coronary artery disease, reporting the presence of coronary calcium is probably not necessary on hybrid nuclear imaging. However, it may be an unexpected finding in other, particularly younger patients, and should be commented on in the body of the report and in the conclusions.

Cardiac Valves

Calcification of the cardiac valve leaflets and annuli may be apparent on hybrid nuclear imaging. In most patients, the clinical significance is little or none, but leaflet calcification in particular can reflect valvular stenosis.

Mitral Annular Calcification

This is an extremely common incidental finding on CT of the chest, and its prevalence increases with age. Women are affected more than men. The characteristic appearance of mitral annular calcification (MAC) on CT is a crescent- or C-shape band of calcium outlining the lateral and inferior margins of the mitral valve annulus. More extensive MAC can involve the septal and anterior portions of the mitral annulus. In a minority of patients,

MAC can be exuberant, with milk of calcium deposition and a tumefactive appearance. MAC is typically an incidental finding and is only rarely associated with dysrhythmias. However, studies have correlated the presence of MAC with an increased risk of atherosclerotic disease of the coronary arteries.

Aortic Valve Leaflet Calcification

Aortic valve leaflet calcification usually indicates aortic valvular stenosis. While it is commonly present in patients older than 70 years of age, its presence in young individuals is an important finding that may suggest abnormal valve structure, particularly a bicuspid aortic valve, which leads to premature stenosis. Long-standing aortic stenosis can lead to both left ventricular hypertrophy and ascending aortic aneurysm.

Pericardium

The normal pericardium is visible as a thin ($\leqslant 4$ mm) structure surrounding the heart, separating mediastinal fat (superficial to pericardium) from epicardial fat (deep to pericardial fat). A small amount of liquid (usually <50 mL) distributes throughout the pericardium, most commonly seen on cross-sectional imaging along the right heart border, anterior pericardium, base of the heart, and in the superior pericardial recesses.

Pericardial Effusion

As with pleural effusions, pericardial effusions can be transudative or exudative. Pericardial effusions can be a sign of pericarditis or pericardial malignancy. Effusions associated with nodular pericardial thickening are usually malignant. High-attenuation pleural effusions usually reflect the presence of blood.

Pericardial Thickening

Pericardial thickness >4 mm is considered to be abnormal. Pericardial thickening is the sequela of pericarditis and can either cause no physiologic impact or result in constrictive pericarditis. CT findings of constrictive pericarditis include pericardial thickening with large atria and small ventricles, the latter reflecting the inability of the ventricles to relax during diastole. Pericardial calcification may present in addition to thickening and indicates remote pericarditis. Constrictive physiology may or may not be present in patients with pericardial calcification.

Pericardial Cyst

Pericardial cysts form from a pinched off portion of pericardium during embryogenesis. Approximately 90% occur in the right cardiophrenic space, with the remainder occurring anywhere adjacent to the pericardium. On CT they have homogeneous water attenuation ($\leqslant 10$ HU).

Pericardial cysts can change shape depending on the patient position during imaging and rarely result in symptoms. Treatment is rarely indicated.

Aorta

The aorta can be readily assessed on hybrid nuclear imaging studies involving CT or MRI. The thoracic aorta is divided into root (valve plane, sinuses of Valsalva), ascending aorta (sinotubular junction until the first arch vessel), arch, and descending (just distal to the last arch vessel until the diaphragmatic hiatus). The normal adult aorta measures up to 40 mm in transverse diameter, typically largest in the ascending segment and gradually tapering toward the diaphragm.

Atherosclerosis

Aortic atherosclerosis is apparent on hybrid imaging by the presence of mural calcification. Similar to coronary calcification, it should be reported on if it has not been previously documented or if the patient is younger, typically <55 years of age for men and <67 years of age for women.

Aortic Aneurysm

When the aortic diameter is between 40 and 50 mm, it is termed ectatic (dilated). A diameter >50 mm is considered to be an aneurysm. Aneurysms are classified as either fusiform or saccular. Fusiform aneurysms are characterized by diffuse dilation of the affected segment whereas saccular aneurysms are characterized by an eccentric outpouching. Fusiform aneurysms usually result from atherosclerosis and less commonly aortitis whereas saccular aneurysms, which are often pseudoaneurysms, can result from infection (mycotic aneurysm), trauma, or subsequent to the rupture of an ulcerative atherosclerotic plaque. FDG uptake may be apparent if an aortic aneurysm is associated with infection or inflammation (aortitis).

Chest Wall

The chest wall consists of the bones of the thorax, the supporting and surrounding musculature, subcutaneous fat, and the skin. Incidental findings, particularly those of the skeleton, are common and the majority of these findings require neither mentioning nor further workup.

Bones

The ribs, thoracic vertebrae, clavicles, sternum (including manubrium and xyphoid) constitute the bones of the chest wall. The bones of the shoulder girdle (scapula and proximal humerus) are typically included, as well.

Ribs

The normal thorax contains twelve paired ribs. Incidental findings may include healed fractures, hypoplastic ribs (usually one or both of the first ribs), or fused ribs. In patients who have had thoracotomy, portions of one or more ribs may have been resected. Cervical ribs, either single or bilateral, may be present, arising from the C7 vertebral body. These ribs can be fused to the first ribs, either through an osseous or fibrous bridge. In some patients, cervical ribs can cause thoracic outlet syndrome, in which there is neural (most common), venous, or arterial (least common) compression. Dense sclerotic lesions (bone islands or enostoses) are commonly found in the ribs and should not be mistaken for metastases.

Thoracic Vertebrae

Degenerative findings such as disc-space narrowing, osteophytes, and endplate sclerosis are commonly encountered on cross-sectional imaging of the chest. Endplate sclerosis can be mistaken for osteoblastic metastases; however, recognizing the associated findings of disc-space narrowing and osteophytes should help in distinguishing degenerative sclerosis from metastases. Sagittal reformations are especially useful for depicting lesions of the spine. Bone islands are commonly encountered on cross-sectional imaging of the thoracic spine. As in other bones, they present as dense sclerotic foci with irregular, often spiculated margins. Osteoblastic metastases are usually less dense, with smoother margins.

Other Bones

Bone islands may be seen in the sternum, clavicle, and scapula. Additionally, subchondral cysts may be apparent in the humeral head. In the latter, they appear as well-corticated lucencies located just below its articulating surface. Osteophytes may be present along the corresponding scapular glenoid. With severe osteoarthritis of the glenohumeral joint, intra-articular loose bodies ("joint mice") may be seen, and fluid may be seen accumulating in the bursae of the shoulder joints. Increased FDG activity may be apparent depending on the degree of inflammation.

Soft Tissues

Lipoma

Chest wall lipomas are commonly identified on cross-sectional CT. Most are small and are clinically silent. They are commonly seen within a chest wall muscle as an encapsulated, homogeneous fat-attenuation mass.

Sebaceous Cyst

Sebaceous cysts are occasionally seen on cross-sectional imaging of the chest. They may result from inflammation or infection of a sebaceous gland, resulting in obstructing of the normal drainage route. On CT, they have a defined capsule, central low attenuation, and occur immediately deep to the skin. They can become infected or inflamed and may have increased FDG uptake. Targeted ultrasound can be used if the diagnosis is uncertain.

Breast Tissue

CT does not perform well in evaluating breast tissue. Abnormalities encountered on CT are best evaluated with mammography with or without additional imaging with breast ultrasound or MRI. Patients with abnormal hybrid imaging findings in the breast, such as soft-tissue nodules or fluid collections, should be referred for dedicated breast imaging if it has not been recently performed.

Suggested Reading

Andreu J, Mauleon S, Pallisa E et al (2002) Miliary lung disease revisited. Current problems in diagnostic radiology 31:189-197.

Bogaert J, Francone M (2013) Pericardial disease: value of CT and MR imaging. Radiology 267:340-356.

Cox CW, Rose CS, Lynch DA (2014) State of the art: Imaging of occupational lung disease. Radiology 270:681-696.

Date H (2009) Diagnostic strategies for mediastinal tumors and cysts. Thoracic surgery clinics 19:29-35, vi.

Einstein AJ, Johnson LL, Bokhari S et al (2010) Agreement of visual estimation of coronary artery calcium from low-dose CT attenuation correction scans in hybrid PET/CT and SPECT/CT with standard Agatston score. Journal of the American College of Cardiology 56:1914-1921.

Elicker B, Pereira CA, Webb R, Leslie KO (2008) High-resolution computed tomography patterns of diffuse interstitial lung disease with clinical and pathological correlation. Jornal brasileiro de pneumologia: publicacao oficial da Sociedade Brasileira de Pneumologia e Tisilogia 34:715-744.

Holloway BJ, Rosewarne D, Jones RG (2011) Imaging of thoracic aortic disease. Br J Radiol 84 Spec No 3:S338-354.

Jeong YJ, Kim KI, Seo IJ et al (2007) Eosinophilic lung diseases: a clinical, radiologic, and pathologic overview. Radiographics 27:617-637; discussion 637-619.

MacMahon H, Austin JH, Gamsu G et al (2005) Guidelines for management of small pulmonary nodules detected on CT scans: a statement from the Fleischner Society. Radiology 237:395-400.

Naidich DP, Bankier AA, MacMahon H et al (2013) Recommendations for the management of subsolid pulmonary nodules detected at CT: a statement from the Fleischner Society. Radiology 266:304-317.

Roberton BJ, Hansell DM (2011) Organizing pneumonia: a kaleidoscope of concepts and morphologies. European Radiology 21:2244-2254.

Sayyouh M, Vummidi DR, Kazerooni EA (2013) Evaluation and management of pulmonary nodules: state-of-the-art and future perspectives. Expert Opin Med Diagn 7:629-644.

Seaman DM, Meyer CA, Gilman MD, McCormack FX (2011) Diffuse cystic lung disease at high-resolution CT. AJR Am J Roentgenol 196:1305-1311.

Shahrzad M, Le TS, Silva M (2014) Anterior mediastinal masses. AJR Am J Roentgenol 203:W128-138.

Integrated Cardiac Imaging

Philipp A. Kaufmann, Tobias A. Fuchs

Nuclear Medicine, University Hospital Zurich, Switzerland

Introduction

Noninvasive cardiac imaging has evolved substantially over the past few years. New reconstruction algorithms and a new generation of y-cameras with cadmium-zinc telluride (CZT) semiconductor detectors have shortened scan time and improved image quality in myocardial perfusion imaging (MPI) by single photon emission computed tomography (SPECT). In addition, technical refinements in coronary computed tomography angiography (CCTA) have led to a substantial dose reduction while image quality has improved. However, invasive coronary angiography has remained the anatomic standard of reference even though it is associated with a nonnegligible perioperative morbidity and mortality that suggests confining its use to patients who will benefit from a subsequent revascularization procedure. The poor agreement between the severity of coronary artery stenosis (morphological assessment) and the hemodynamical relevance of the stenosis (functional assessment) has been shown; thus, the coronary anatomy rarely allows estimation of the pathophysiologic relevance of a coronary lesion.

The potential of cardiac hybrid imaging, which offers a comprehensive evaluation of coronary artery disease (CAD) by combining both morphological and functional information after fusion of SPECT with CCTA, is well established, as documented in the emerging guidelines for cardiac hybrid imaging presented by several societies [1, 2]. Hybrid imaging with SPECT-CT can provide entirely noninvasively, unique information that helps to improve diagnostic assessment and risk stratification in addition to impacting decision-making with regard to revascularization in patients with CAD [3].

Functional Versus Morphological Assessment of CAD

Despite its considerable morbidity (1.5%) [4] and mortality (0.3%) rates [5], invasive coronary angiography has remained the most widely used method for visualizing the coronary arteries and is the standard of reference for diagnosing coronary stenosis. However, its accuracy is severely hampered by a large intra- and interobserver variability (up to 50%) in defining the anatomic relevance of the stenosis [6]. Furthermore, the poor agreement between the severity of coronary artery stenosis (morphological assessment) and the hemodynamic relevance of the stenosis (functional assessment) has been shown [7]. Thus, invasive coronary angiography not only is affected by limitations regarding anatomical evaluation but the anatomic findings of angiographically documented coronary artery stenosis are known to be poor predictors of a lesion's physiologic relevance [6]. The low yield of invasive coronary angiography (approximately 38%) [8] has stimulated the search for strategies of noninvasive coronary angiography, of which CCTA has emerged as the most promising and well established in large series of patients such as the COronary CT angiography evaluatioN For clinical outcomes InteRnational Multicentre (CONFRIM) registry [9]. However, in intermediate lesions, many factors influence the relationship between anatomic findings and hemodynamic consequence in ways that cannot be fully elucidated by anatomic evaluation alone, not even with the use of quantitative coronary angiography [10]. Accordingly, the actual guidelines on myocardial revascularization recommend the documentation of ischemia using functional testing in patients with suspected stable CAD before elective invasive procedures [11]. The large gap between these evidence-based guidelines and the above-mentioned reality in daily clinical routine emphasizes the need to increase both awareness of the importance and availability of noninvasive testing by SPECT for CAD. Fusion of SPECT-MPI and CCTA for cardiac hybrid imaging is a unique technique combining both functional and morphological assessment of CAD.

Morphological Assessment: CCTA

CCTA is an important non-invasive tool for the evaluation of CAD. Technical refinements in CCTA have led to the rapid implementation of CCTA in daily clinical routine and its high accuracy compared to invasive coronary angiography has been demonstrated [12]. With the increasing acceptance of CCTA, the associated radiation exposure has been the focus of growing attention. However, the introduction of prospective ECG-triggering, including high-pitch spiral acquisition, has led to a substantial dose reduction [13, 14]. Recently, iterative reconstruction algorithms for CCTA have demonstrated significant noise reduction, allowing tube current and tube voltage reduction without degradation of image quality such that in some settings CCTA can be performed using a radiation exposure similar to a chest X-ray [15].

Functional Assessment: MPI with SPECT

MPI with SPECT represents the most widely available, robust, and by far best established noninvasive method for the evaluation of ischemic heart disease [16]. A perfect agreement of MPI SPECT and coronary angiography, however, is inherently precluded because the main role of SPECT is not to correctly predict or exclude epicardial coronary lesions but rather to evaluate the physiological relevance of a given lesion. In fact, only 40% of coronary lesions with a luminal narrowing of 50–70% induce ischemia, as documented in the FAME sub study by Tonino et al. [17]. Despite this wisdom, SPECT MPI has often been compared with findings of coronary angiography, as this is the generally accepted standard of reference for coronary lesions. One of the largest reports, the British Royal Brompton and UCL study of Thallium and Technetium (ROBUST), assessed 2,560 patients who were randomized to one of the commonly used tracers (thallium, sestamibi, or tetrofosmin) during stress, mainly adenosine-induced. This study documented a sensitivity of 91% and a specificity of 87% without differences among the tracers [18].

Several attempts to improve MPI by using iterative reconstruction algorithms, early-imaging protocols, or different tracers have provided valuable benefits. However, the novel CZT detector systems have the potential to represent the much awaited milestone in the technical improvement of MPI. The CZT technique has enabled a substantial miniaturization of the detectors, a development exploited by new cameras in that a stationary positioning of numerous CZT detectors can be chosen, with pinhole geometry around the heart. As a result, the scan on the CZT camera covers the entire heart, allowing very fast acquisition times, comparable to those of cardiac PET imaging. The first clinical studies reported very encouraging results [19], a high accuracy for the detection of angiographically documented CAD [20], and the feasibility of fast acquisition protocols [21].

Integrated Cardiac Imaging

The feasibility of cardiac hybrid imaging with the use of PET and CT for noninvasive simultaneous visualization of individual myocardial-wall territories with impaired myocardial perfusion by the subtending coronary artery was initially described by Namdar and colleagues [22]. The added diagnostic clinical value beyond that of either technique alone or that of side-by-side analysis has been demonstrated [23, 24]. In low-risk populations, hybrid imaging may increase the confidence to rule out CAD; for example, in the stepwise evaluation of CAD, when equivocal results were obtained with the first study and a second modality is needed to finally rule out disease. Many of these patients would end up having invasive coronary angiography, whereas hybrid imaging increases diagnostic confidence by avoiding equivocal findings, which helps to reduce the number of patients unnecessarily exposed to the risk associated with invasive coronary procedures. It was recently shown that cardiac hybrid imaging (by SPECT and CCTA) in CAD evaluation has a profound impact on patient management and may contribute to optimal downstream resource utilization [25]. At the other end of the spectrum, i.e., in older patients, who often suffer from multivessel disease with more jeopardized myocardium, hybrid imaging provides important comprehensive information to allow timely and appropriate treatment. In these settings, the value of hybrid imaging lies far beyond the simple addition of a further diagnostic test, as it allows the accurate spatial association of perfusion defects with their subtending coronary stenosis (Fig. 1).

The CT part of hybrid imaging has an excellent ability to rule out anatomic CAD, but an abnormal CCTA (or an abnormal conventional angiography) is a poor predictor of ischemia. Therefore, MPI testing is recommended to identify patients who might benefit from a revascularization procedure, i.e., those with an ischemic

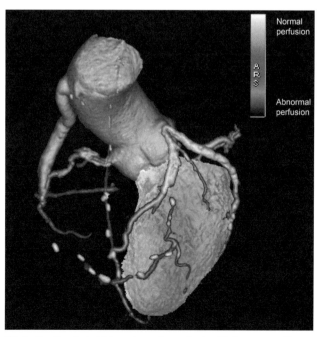

Fig. 1. Cardiac hybrid imaging of a patient with bypass grafts revealed a perfusion defect in the territory of the diagonal branch

burden >10% [26, 27]. The technologic refinements implemented in the latest generation of CT scanners have reduced the number of non-evaluable coronary segments, and further improvements may be expected. However, the two pieces of information obtained with perfusion imaging versus morphology are difficult to compare and will likely remain complementary. By contrast, the receiver operator characteristic analysis for detecting perfusion defects (by SPECT) has been shown to result in a similar area under the curve for the reference standard (conventional angiography) as for CCTA, documenting the comparable performance and limitations of both anatomic and morphologic techniques [28].

Results from a multicenter study emphasize the value of a combined functional and anatomical approach even without image fusion, i.e., without creating a hybrid image, showing that this combination allows improved risk stratification [29]. The added value of hybrid imaging seems most pronounced for functionally relevant lesions in distal segments and diagonal branches and in vessels with extensive coronary lesions of heavy calcification on CCTA. The prognostic value of cardiac hybrid imaging has been confirmed, and matched defects on hybrid imaging have been shown to be a strong predictor of major adverse cardiovascular events [30]. Cardiac hybrid imaging in CAD evaluation may have the potential to optimize the downstream resource utilization [25].

References

1. Flotats A, Knuuti J, Gutberlet M et al (2011) Hybrid cardiac imaging: SPECT/CT and PET/CT. A joint position statement by the European Association of Nuclear Medicine (EANM), the European Society of Cardiac Radiology (ESCR) and the European Council of Nuclear Cardiology (ECNC). Eur J Nucl Med Mol Imaging 38:201-212.
2. Dorbala S, Di Carli MF, Delbeke D et al (2013) SNMMI/ASNC/SCCT guideline for cardiac SPECT/CT and PET/CT 1.0. J Nucl Med 54:1485-1507.
3. Hodler J, Schulthess GK, Zollikofer CL (2011) Diseases of the Heart, Chest & Breast. Diagnostic Imaging and Interventional Techniques. Springer, pp 199-202.
4. Achenbach S, Daniel WG (2001) Noninvasive coronary angiography—an acceptable alternative? N Engl J Med 345:1909-1910.
5. Shaw LJ, Shaw RE, Merz CN et al (2008) Impact of ethnicity and gender differences on angiographic coronary artery disease prevalence and in-hospital mortality in the American College of Cardiology-National Cardiovascular Data Registry. Circulation 117:1787-1801.
6. White CW, Wright CB, Doty DB et al (1984) Does visual interpretation of the coronary arteriogram predict the physiologic importance of a coronary stenosis? N Engl J Med 310:819-824.
7. Uren NG, Melin JA, De Bruyne B et al (1994) Relation between myocardial blood flow and the severity of coronary-artery stenosis. N Engl J Med 330:1782-1788.
8. Patel MR, Peterson ED, Dai D et al (2010) Low diagnostic yield of elective coronary angiography. N Engl J Med 362:886-895.
9. Cheng VY, Berman DS, Rozanski A et al (2011) Performance of the traditional age, sex, and angina typicality-based approach for estimating pretest probability of angiographically significant coronary artery disease in patients undergoing coronary computed tomographic angiography: results from the multinational coronary CT angiography evaluation for clinical outcomes: an international multicenter registry (CONFIRM). Circulation 124:2423-2432, 2421-2428.
10. Bartunek J, Sys SU, Heyndrickx GR et al (1995) Quantitative coronary angiography in predicting functional significance of stenoses in an unselected patient cohort. J Am Coll Cardiol 26:328-334.
11. Windecker S, Kolh P, Alfonso F et al (2014) 2014 ESC/EACTS Guidelines on myocardial revascularization: The Task Force on Myocardial Revascularization of the European Society of Cardiology (ESC) and the European Association for Cardio-Thoracic Surgery (EACTS) Developed with the special contribution of the European Association of Percutaneous Cardiovascular Interventions (EAPCI). EuroIntervention [Epub ahead of print].
12. Budoff MJ, Dowe D, Jollis JG et al (2008) Diagnostic performance of 64-multidetector row coronary computed tomographic angiography for evaluation of coronary artery stenosis in individuals without known coronary artery disease: results from the prospective multicenter ACCURACY (Assessment by Coronary Computed Tomographic Angiography of Individuals Undergoing Invasive Coronary Angiography) trial. J Am Coll Cardiol 52:1724-1732.
13. Buechel RR, Husmann L, Herzog BA et al (2011) Low-dose computed tomography coronary angiography with prospective electrocardiogram triggering: feasibility in a large population. J Am Coll Cardiol 57:332-336.
14. Achenbach S, Marwan M, Ropers D et al (2010) Coronary computed tomography angiography with a consistent dose below 1 mSv using prospectively electrocardiogram-triggered high-pitch spiral acquisition. Eur Heart J 31:340-346.
15. Fuchs TA, Stehli J, Bull S et al (2014) Coronary computed tomography angiography with model-based iterative reconstruction using a radiation exposure similar to chest X-ray examination. Eur Heart J 35:1131-1136.
16. Underwood SR, Anagnostopoulos C, Cerqueira M et al (2004) Myocardial perfusion scintigraphy: the evidence. Eur J Nucl Med Mol Imaging 31:261-291.
17. Tonino PA, Fearon WF, De Bruyne B et al (2010) Angiographic versus functional severity of coronary artery stenoses in the FAME study fractional flow reserve versus angiography in multivessel evaluation. J Am Coll Cardiol 55:2816-2821.
18. Kapur A, Latus KA, Davies G et al (2002) A comparison of three radionuclide myocardial perfusion tracers in clinical practice: the ROBUST study. Eur J Nucl Med Mol Imaging 29:1608-1616.
19. Buechel RR, Pazhenkottil AP, Herzog BA et al (2010) Real-time breath-hold triggering of myocardial perfusion imaging with a novel cadmium-zinc-telluride detector gamma camera. Eur J Nucl Med Mol Imaging 37:1903-1908.
20. Fiechter M, Ghadri JR, Kuest SM et al (2011) Nuclear myocardial perfusion imaging with a novel cadmium-zinc-telluride detector SPECT/CT device: first validation versus invasive coronary angiography. Eur J Nucl Med Mol Imaging 38:2025-2030.
21. Herzog BA, Buechel RR, Katz R et al (2010) Nuclear myocardial perfusion imaging with a cadmium-zinc-telluride detector technique: optimized protocol for scan time reduction. J Nucl Med 51:46-51.
22. Namdar M, Hany TF, Koepfli P et al (2005) Integrated PET/CT for the assessment of coronary artery disease: a feasibility study. J Nucl Med 46:930-935.
23. Gaemperli O, Kaufmann PA. (2008), Hybrid cardiac imaging: more than the sum of its parts? J Nucl Cardiol 15:123-126.
24. Gaemperli O, Schepis T, Valenta I et al (2007) Cardiac image fusion from stand-alone SPECT and CT: clinical experience. J Nucl Med 48:696-703.
25. Fiechter M, Ghadri JR, Wolfrum M et al (2012) Downstream resource utilization following hybrid cardiac imaging with an

integrated cadmium-zinc-telluride/64-slice CT device. Eur J Nucl Med Mol Imaging 39:430-436.

26. Hachamovitch R, Hayes SW, Friedman JD et al (2003) Comparison of the short-term survival benefit associated with revascularization compared with medical therapy in patients with no prior coronary artery disease undergoing stress myocardial perfusion single photon emission computed tomography. Circulation 107:2900-2907.

27. Shaw LJ, Berman DS, Maron DJ et al (2008) Optimal medical therapy with or without percutaneous coronary intervention to reduce ischemic burden: results from the Clinical Outcomes Utilizing Revascularization and Aggressive Drug Evaluation (COURAGE) trial nuclear substudy. Circulation 117:1283-1291.

28. Gaemperli O, Schepis T, Valenta I et al (2008) Functionally relevant coronary artery disease: comparison of 64-section CT angiography with myocardial perfusion SPECT. Radiology 248:414-423.

29. van Werkhoven JM, Schuijf JD, Gaemperli O et al (2009) Prognostic value of multislice computed tomography and gated single-photon emission computed tomography in patients with suspected coronary artery disease. J Am Coll Cardiol 53:623-632.

30. Pazhenkottil AP, Nkoulou RN, Ghadri JR et al (2011) Prognostic value of cardiac hybrid imaging integrating single-photon emission computed tomography with coronary computed tomography angiography. Eur Heart J 32:1465-1471.

FDG PET/CT in the Imaging of Mediastinal Masses

Pek-Lan Khong

Department of Diagnostic Radiology, The University of Hong Kong, Queen Mary Hospital, Hong Kong, China

Anterior mediastinal tumors that may be encountered on ^{18}F-fluorodeoxyglucose-positron emission tomography/ computed tomography (FDG-PET/CT) scans include malignant lymphoma, benign and malignant germ cell tumors, thymoma, and thymic carcinoma. Of these, lymphomas that involve the mediastinum are the most common.

Lymphomas that involve the anterior mediastinum may be Hodgkin lymphoma (HL) (Figs. 1, 2) or non-

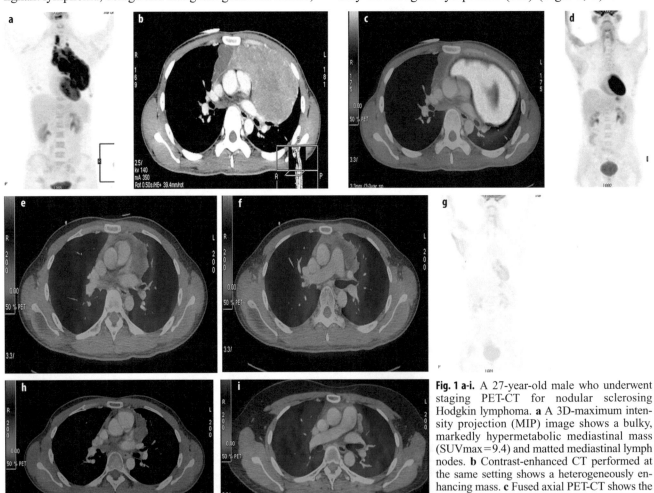

Fig. 1 a-i. A 27-year-old male who underwent staging PET-CT for nodular sclerosing Hodgkin lymphoma. **a** A 3D-maximum intensity projection (MIP) image shows a bulky, markedly hypermetabolic mediastinal mass (SUVmax=9.4) and matted mediastinal lymph nodes. **b** Contrast-enhanced CT performed at the same setting shows a heterogeneously enhancing mass. **c** Fused axial PET-CT shows the hypermetabolic mass with central area of reduced uptake. **d-f** End-chemotherapy PET-CT scans of the MIP image (**d**), and fused PET-CT of two axial sections (**e, f**) show a residual anterior mediastinal mass with minimal residual uptake (Deauville 5-point score=3). The patient underwent radiation therapy (RT) of the mediastinal mass. A post-RT treatment scan 3 months after the end of RT was performed. MIP image (**g**) and fused axial PET-CT image (**h**) show a reduction in the size of the mass and a complete metabolic response (CMR). Routine surveillance PET-CT scan was obtained 5 years later. Fused axial PET-CT image (**i**) shows a persistent residual mediastinal mass that has further reduced in size and CMR

Diseases of the Chest and Heart 2015-2018,
DOI: 10.1007/978-88-470-5752-4_27 © Springer-Verlag Italia 2015

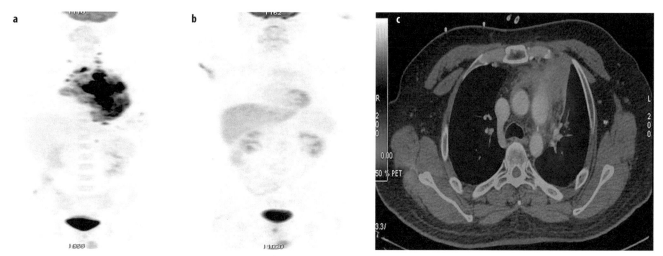

Fig. 2 a-c. A 31-year-old male with nodular sclerosing Hodgkin lymphoma. **a** Staging PET-CT was performed. MIP image (**b**) shows a hypermetabolic mediastinal mass with lower cervical, mediastinal, and diaphragmatic lymphadenopathy (SUVmax=11.7). He was treated with ABVD (adriamycin, bleomycin, vinblastine and darcarbacine) × 8 and radiotherapy. Subsequent recurrent disease in the left lower chest wall was treated with DHAP (dexamethasone, cytarabine, cisplatin) and autologous bone marrow transplantation (BMT). PET-CT was performed post-BMT. MIP image (**b**) and fused axial PET-CT image (**c**) show a residual mediastinal mass with minimal residual uptake (Deauville 5-point score=2). Punch biopsy showed fibrofatty tissue only, with no malignancy

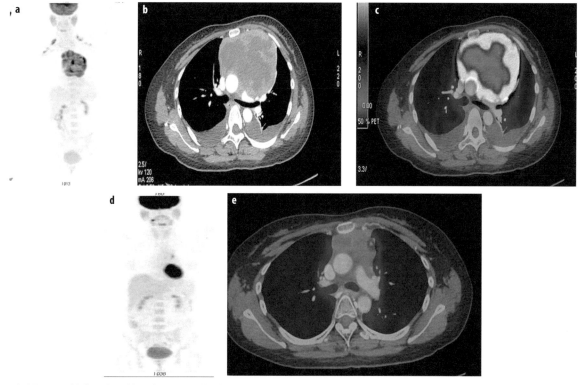

Fig. 3 a-e. A 37-year-old female with primary mediastinal B-cell lymphoma. Staging PET/CT was performed. MIP image (**a**), contrast-enhanced CT (**b**) and fused axial PET-CT image (**c**) show a heterogeneously contrast-enhancing mass in the anterior and middle mediastinum that extends from the thoracic inlet to the lower end of the sternum. The lesion shows central necrosis and peripheral contrast enhancement (SUVmax=10.6). The end-chemotherapy PET scan shows a complete metabolic response with residual mass. The mediastinal mass was treated with radiotherapy (RT). PET-CT was performed 3 months after end of RT. MIP image (**d**) and fused axial PET-CT image (**e**) show suspicious focal uptake in the mass. Follow-up PET-CT 3 months later shows resolution of the focal uptake suggesting false positive findings in the previous scan (**d, e**)

Hodgkin lymphoma subtypes, with the latter including diffuse large B-cell lymphoma (DLBCL), primary mediastinal B-cell lymphoma (PMBCL) (Fig. 3), gray-zone lymphoma (B-cell lymphoma, unclassifiable, with features intermediate between DLBCL and classical HL), and T-cell lymphoblastic lymphoma [1] (Fig. 4).

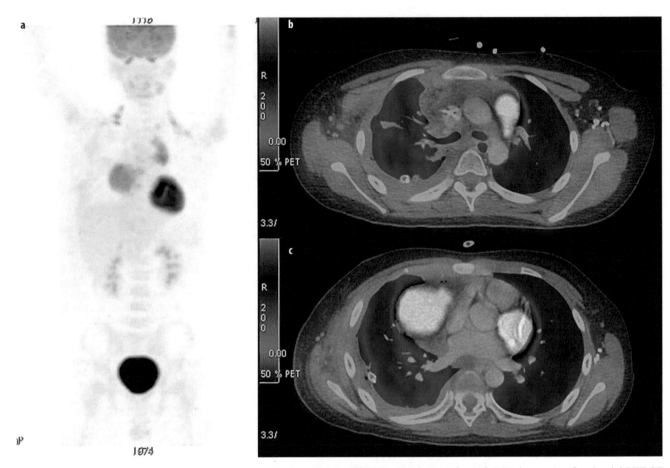

Fig. 4 a-c. A 10-year-old male with T-lymphoblastic lymphoma. Staging PET/CT scan was performed. MIP image (**a**), fused axial PET-CT image of 2 sections (**b, c**) show a hypermetabolic anterior mediastinal mass (SUVmax=6.4). The patient responded poorly to chemotherapy and died from progressive disease 2 years later

In about 5% of these cases, the anterior mediastinum is the only site of disease and may manifest as isolated thymic involvement, as isolated nodal involvement, or as a combination of both [2]. HL accounts for the majority of mediastinal lymphomas. Lymphoblastic lymphomas mainly occur in children and adolescents, while DLBCL is usually seen in young to middle-aged adults. Diagnosis is made based on the pathological examination, with mandatory immunohistochemical staining, and a typical clinical presentation. PMBCL belongs to the group of aggressive DLBCLs but was distinguished as a separate entity in the WHO 2008 classification due to its specific clinical and pathological features, namely, gene expression profile studies showing common features with classical HL and thus having an impact on the choice of therapy [1]. Since all the above-mentioned lymphomas that involve the mediastinum fall into the subtypes are FDG-avid [3], FDG-PET/CT is the imaging modality of choice for staging and treatment response assessment.

For disease staging, compared to conventional CT, FDG-PET/CT may lead to a change in disease stage, more often upstaging [4, 5]. This is particularly important before consideration of radiotherapy (RT), because the PET/CT findings may have an impact on RT planning and design of the RT field. A single nodal mass/mediastinal mass should be measured on the CT scan across the longest measurement. In HL, tumor bulk ≥10 cm is defined as bulky disease and has prognostic and therapeutic implications. Moreover, contrast-enhanced CT, if not already performed, should ideally be done as part of a "one-stop" approach during a single imaging session combined with PET/CT [6]. Baseline findings should be used to determine whether contrast-enhanced CT or lower dose and non-enhanced PET/CT will suffice for additional imaging examinations. A bone marrow biopsy is no longer indicated for routine staging of HL or most DLBCLs [7].

For response assessment, conventional morphologic imaging using CT or magnetic resonance imaging was shown to lack specificity in the characterization of residual masses that often remain after treatment. However, FDG-PET allows better discrimination between viable tissue and fibrotic residual masses, by showing the altered metabolism of the former (Figs. 1–3). Thus, FDG-PET/CT was incorporated into the 2007 International

Working Group guidelines for response assessment of these malignant lymphomas [8]. In the previous guidelines, visual interpretation of positive or negative PET/CT scans was based on comparison with the mediastinal blood pool for end-of-treatment response assessment [8]. For HL, end-of-treatment scans were shown to carry a high negative predictive value (80–100%), although the positive predictive value is more variable (25–100%). In the recent updated recommendation, a 5-point scale (5-PS) based on visual assessment is used to assess response to PET/CT [7]. The 5-PS score assesses uptake at the site of initial disease as follows: 1, no uptake; 2, uptake ≤mediastinum, 3, uptake >mediastinum but ≤liver; 4, uptake moderately higher than liver; 5, uptake markedly higher than liver (2-to 3-fold higher than a large region of normal liver) and/or new lesions. In the recommendation, a score of 1 or 2 represents a complete metabolic response (CMR); a score 3 of represents a probable CMR in patients receiving standard treatment (Fig. 1); and a score of 4 or 5 with reduced uptake from baseline is considered a partial metabolic response, but if the assessment is at the end of treatment it represents residual metabolic disease. An increase in FDG uptake to a score of 5, or a score of 5 with no decrease in uptake, and new FDG-avid foci consistent with lymphoma represent treatment failure and/or progression.

For interim assessment, patients should undergo scanning as long after the previous chemotherapy administration as possible, since non-specific FDG uptake may occur with treatment-related inflammation. A minimum of 3 weeks but preferably 6–8 weeks after the completion of the last chemotherapy cycle, 2 weeks after granulocyte colony-stimulating factor treatment, or 3 months after RT is recommended (Fig. 3).

Early treatment assessment is potentially of importance for response-adapted treatment, both to optimize treatment and to avoid unnecessary toxicity. For HL, it has been found that early metabolic changes are highly predictive of final treatment response and progression-free survival [9]. Currently, based on interim PET findings after two courses of ABVD (adriamycin, bleomycin, vinblastine, and darcarbacine) chemotherapy, early treatment intensification with BEACOPPesc (bleomycin, etoposide, adriamycin, cyclophosphamide, vincristine, procarbazine, and prednisone escalated regimen) should be instituted in patients with a positive PET scan. Multiple clinical trials are on-going to determine the value of early PET in response-adapted therapy for the identification of patients with poor treatment response who may benefit from escalation to more aggressive therapy, and for patients with good treatment response who can be cured with less than standard therapy, including omission of RT to the mediastinum.

In children, FDG accumulation in the thymus is a common, normal finding and thymic rebound hyperplasia can be observed after chemotherapy (Fig. 5), which may be a potential pitfall in the interpretation of FDG-PET/CT in pediatric patients. Thymic rebound may reflect a hematological rebound phenomenon, characterized by lymph follicles with large nuclear centers and plasma cell infiltration. Although thymic rebound usually appears within 6–12 months after cessation of chemotherapy, it can develop over a period as short as 1 week. The time course of FDG uptake in the thymus is such that it is usually not apparent at cessation of therapy, with uptake reaching a peak within 12 months after treatment (10 months in a few reported series), with a slow decline thereafter [10, 11]. Moreover, there is often a concurrent increase in bone marrow uptake due to increased bone marrow

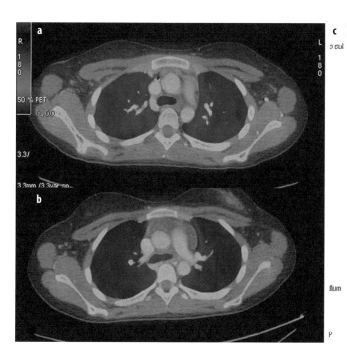

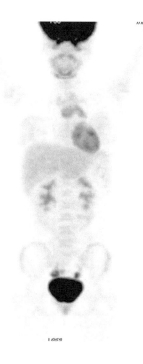

Fig. 5 a-c. A 10-year-old boy with rebound thymic hyperplasia after chemotherapy. **a** Mid-treatment PET-CT scan, **b** fused axial PET-CT image, **c** MIP image. **a, b** show that the thymus gland is enlarged, with a convex border, and low-grade diffuse uptake, increased compared to the mid-treatment PET-CT scan (**a**)

stimulation from cytokine therapy [11]. Generally, it is of diffuse low metabolic activity compared to malignant mediastinal soft tissue. Although there is considerable overlap in SUV values, thymic rebound is of homogenous soft-tissue density, with a typical shape and convex margins [12] (Fig. 5). It is important to also be aware of normal-variant, whereby thymic tissue extends superiorly and thus appears as a superior mediastinal nodule, in which case it may be confused with superior mediastinal adenopathy (Fig. 6).

Other potential pitfalls are inflammatory or infective lesions in the form of mediastinal lymphadenopathy, which occur more frequently after chemotherapy, and brown fat activity in the anterior mediastinum.

The differential diagnosis of mediastinal lymphoma includes thymic epithelial tumors, i.e., thymoma, thymic carcinoma, and thymic carcinoid, and benign and malignant germ-cell tumors. Differentiation of these tumors based solely on imaging can be challenging. Findings of associated thoracic nodal disease are rare in thymomas and instead usually suggest lymphoma. Thymomas are soft-tissue-density tumors although they may have areas of cysts, hemorrhage, necrosis, and calcification (Fig. 7). They are classified as high-risk (WHO type B2 and B3) or low-risk (WHO type A, AB, B1) and non-invasive or invasive depending on whether the capsule of the gland has been transgressed. Thymomas typically spread along pleural and pericardial surfaces, and may spread into regional lymph nodes, but hematogenous metastasis

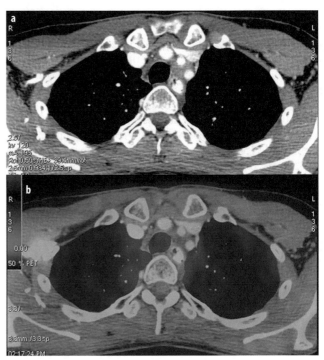

Fig. 6 a, b. A 17-year-old female with Hodgkin lymphoma who completed treatment 2 years earlier. Surveillance PET/CT shows superior extension of the thymus between the left brachiocephalic vein and the left common carotid artery in the superior mediastinum (**a**), with low-grade FDG uptake (**b**). No interval change was noted in the subsequent follow-up scans. The findings are in keeping with rebound thymic hyperplasia with extension into the superior mediastinum

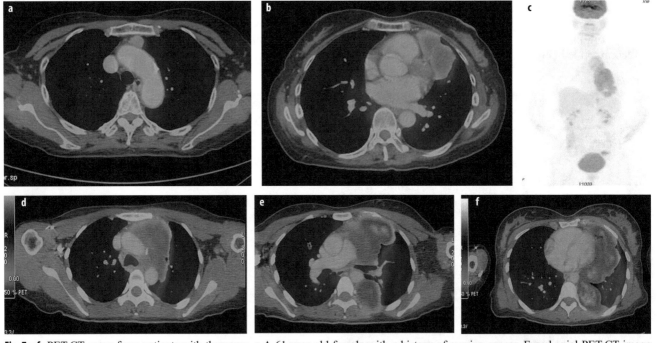

Fig. 7 a-f. PET-CT scans from patients with thymoma. **a** A 61-year-old female with a history of ovarian cancer. Fused axial PET-CT image shows an anterior mediastinal nodule with low grade uptake (SUVmax=1.6) which was detected as an incidental finding. Biopsy showed a type AB thymoma with microscopic foci of capsular invasion. **b** A 51-year-old female with an incidental finding of an anterior mediastinal mass (SUVmax=2.0). Biopsy showed a type AB thymoma. **c-f** A 45-year-old female with invasive thymoma type B2. MIP image (**c**) and fused axial PET-CT images at 3 sections of the mediastinum (**d-f**) show a moderately hypermetabolic anterior mediastinal mass with mediastinal invasion (**d**) and extension to the left posterior pleura and hemidiaphragm (**e, f**) (SUVmax=5.2)

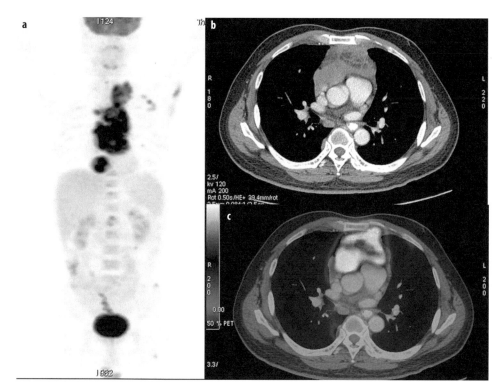

Fig. 8 a-c. PET-CT scan of a 46-year-old male with metastatic thymic carcinoma who presented with hoarseness and dyspnea. MIP image (**a**), contrast-enhanced CT image (**b**) and fused axial PET-CT image (**c**) show the invasive tumor has a necrotic center (SUVmax =12.7). Additional nodules were detected in the lower anterior mediastinum; skeletal metastases were also present (**a**)

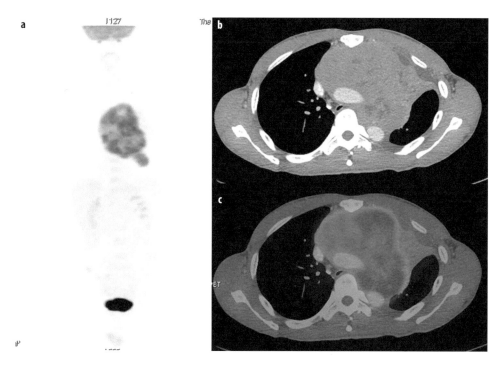

Fig. 9 a-c. A 48-year-old male with a mediastinal germ cell tumor (seminoma). Staging PET/CT was performed. MIP image (**a**), contrast-enhanced CT image (**b**) and fused axial PET-CT image (**c**) show an invasive mediastinal mass with a necrotic component (SUVmax=7.7)

is very rare. Thymic carcinomas are aggressive in appearance, can be associated with vessel invasion and/or the invasion of mediastinal fat, and may present with nodal and distant metastases [13] (Fig. 8). FDG uptake is significantly higher in thymic carcinoma than in thymoma and can be used to differentiate between high-grade and low-grade thymomas [14, 15]. This can aid in selecting patients with low-risk tumors, who are eligible for up front surgery, and those with high-risk tumors, who will need to have an open biopsy for histological diagnosis before surgery and for neoadjuvant therapy, if appropriate. Cystic changes may be found in thymomas, thymic carcinoma, and germ-cell tumors (Fig. 9) and rarely in lymphoma before treatment. Calcifications are sometimes seen in lymphoma post-therapy and in teratomas, which may also contain fat. Clinical history, e.g., B-cell symptoms in malignant lymphoma, the association of myasthenia gravis in thymic epithelial tumors, and biochemical tests are helpful, e.g., elevated serum α-fetoprotein levels in patients with malignant germ-cell tumors.

References

1. Dabrowska-Iwanicka A, Walewski JA (2014) Primary mediastinal large B-cell lymphoma. Curr Hematol Malig Rep 9:273-283.
2. Priola AM, Galetto G, Priola SM (2014) Diagnostic and functional imaging of thymic and mediastinal involvement in lymphoproliferative disorders. Clin Imaging 38:771-784.
3. Weiler-Sagie M, Bushelev O, Epelbaum R et al (2010) F-18-FDG avidity in lymphoma readdressed: a study of 766 patients. J Nucl Med 51:25-30.
4. Schaefer NG, Hany TF, Taverna C et al (2004) Non-Hodgkin lymphoma and Hodgkin disease: coregistered FDG PET and CT at staging and restaging—do we need contrast-enhanced CT? Radiology 232:823-829.
5. Isasi CR, Lu P, Blaufox MD (2005) A metaanalysis of 18F-2-deoxy-2-fluoro-D-glucose positron emission tomography in the staging and restaging of patients with lymphoma. Cancer 104:1066-1074.
6. Barrington SF, Mikhaeel NG, Kostakoglu L et al (2014) Role of imaging in the staging and response assessment of lymphoma: consensus of the International conference on Malignant lymphomas imaging working group. J Clin Oncol 32:3048-3058.
7. Cheson BD, Fisher RL, Barrington SF et al (2014) Recommendations for initial evaluation, staging and response assessment of Hodgkin and Non-Hodgkin lymphoma: The Lugano Classification. J Clin Oncol 32:3059-3067.
8. Cheson BD, Pfistner B, Juweid ME et al (2007) Revised response criteria for malignant lymphoma. J Clin Oncol 25:579-586.
9. Biggi A, Gallamini A, Chauvie S et al (2013) International validation study for interim PET in ABVD-treated advanced-stage Hodgkin lymphoma: interpretation criteria and concordance rate among reviewers. J Nucl Med 54: 683-690.
10. Goethals I, Hoste P, Vriendt CD et al (2010) Time-dependent changes in ^{18}F-FDG activity in the thymus and bone marrow following combination chemotherapy in paediatric patients with lymphoma. Eur J Nucl Med Mol Imaging 37:462-467.
11. Gawande RS, Khurana A, Messing S et al (2012) Differentiation of normal thymus from anterior mediastinal lymphoma and lymphoma recurrence at pediatric PET/CT. Radiology 262:613-622.
12. Quint LE (2007) Imaging of anterior mediastinal masses. Cancer Imaging 7:S56-S62.
13. Lococo F, Cesario A, Okami J et al (2013) Role of combined ^{18}F-FDG-PET/CT for predicting the WHO malignancy grade of thymic epithelial tumors: a multicenter analysis. Lung Cancer 82:245-251.
14. Luzzi L, Campione A, Gorla A (2009) Role of fluorine-flurodeoxyglucose positron emission tomography/computed tomography in preoperative assessment of anterior mediastinal masses. Eur J Cardiothorac Surg 36:475-479.
15. Treglia G, Sadeghi R, Giovanella L et al (2014) Is ^{18}F-FDG PET useful in predicting the WHO grade of malignancy in thymic epithelial tumors? A meta-analysis. Lung Cancer 86: 5-13.

Integrated Cardiovascular PET/MR: Lessons Learned

Christoph Rischpler, Stephan G. Nekolla, Markus Schwaiger

Nuklearmedizinische Klinik und Poliklinik, Klinikum rechts der Isar, Technische Universität München, Munich, Germany

Introduction

Before the wide distribution of positron emission tomography/computed tomography (PET/CT) systems, nuclear cardiology was mainly restricted to single-photon emission computed tomography (SPECT) scanners. With the broader availability of PET/CT systems which was mainly caused by their tremendous success in oncology, a variety of imaging strategies, using different PET tracers such as ^{18}F-fluorodeoxyglucose (FDG) for viability imaging or ^{13}N-ammonia for perfusion imaging, became feasible. Furthermore, PET/CT systems with multislice CT components increased the interest in hybrid imaging strategies, since combined metabolic imaging with assessment of the coronary anatomy finally became feasible [1]. Another advantage of the CT component is the fast and simple determination of the attenuation correction map, which is an important prerequisite for (quantitative) myocardial perfusion imaging. A disadvantage of hybrid imaging systems, however, is the increased complexity of the workflow, which may result in a higher susceptibility to errors. Given the markedly higher complexity of magnetic resonance imaging MRI compared to CT, this might particularly hold true for integrated PET/MRI systems. Nonetheless, with the advantages of MRI, such as higher soft-tissue spatial resolution, the lack of ionizing radiation, and the better tolerated contrast agents, it was generally expected that the positive aspects would outweigh the constraints. In this review we provide an overview of the technical and workflow peculiarities and describe initial experiences with common imaging strategies, especially in patients with particular cardiac diseases, using integrated simultaneous PET/MRI systems.

Commercially Available PET/MRI Systems

Currently, three different architectures of PET/MRI systems are commercially available. In the first, the PET and MRI components are arranged in direct proximity and connected via a common rail system (Philips Ingenuity

TF PET/MR) [2]. In the second approach, which comprises a truly integrated system, simultaneous PET and MRI scans are feasible (Siemens Biograph mMR) [3]. As part of a major instrumentation initiative of the German Research Foundation, the latter was installed in our institution by the end of 2010. Photodetectors that are insensitive to the magnetic field had to be designed for this architecture and the feasibility of avalanche photodiodes (APDs) for this purpose, even at high field strengths, were proven [4]. Eventually APD-lutetium oxyorthosilicate crystal PET detectors were used for the construction of the Siemens Biograph mMR.

The newest system on the market is the SIGNA PET/MRI, constructed by General Electric Healthcare. This scanner also operates in a fully integrated fashion but instead uses silicon photomultiplier detectors. An advantage of this system is the capability of time-of-flight PET imaging [5].

Approaches to and Issues with Attenuation Correction Using MRI

Generation of a μ-Map

One of the major hurdles using this novel scanner technology was the requirement to assess a μ-map for 511-keV photons. The generation of an appropriate μ-map is of great importance as it is essential for quantitative PET imaging (such as the absolute quantification of myocardial blood flow) [6]. Inaccuracies in the μ-map may result in significant errors in the resulting PET images [7, 8]. In stand-alone PET systems which are no longer available commercially, the μ-map was generated by a rotating rod source, while in state-of-the-art PET/CT systems the μ-map is derived from X-rays emitted by the CT tube. A disadvantage of the latter approach is an additional radiation dose of about 0.8 mSv to the patient per stress/rest scan [9].

There is no direct connection between MRI or MRI-based parameters and tissue density. Therefore, novel

Diseases of the Chest and Heart 2015-2018,
DOI: 10.1007/978-88-470-5752-4_28 © Springer-Verlag Italia 2015

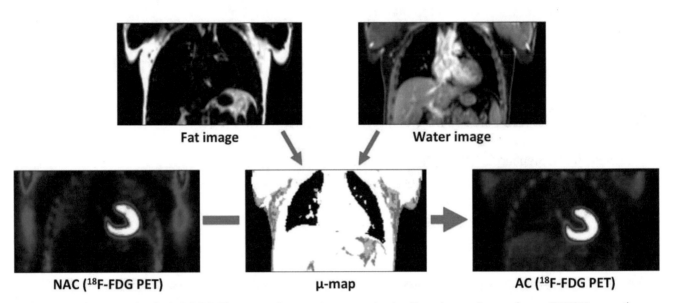

Fig. 1. Attenuation correction in PET/MRI. The attenuation map is generated using fat and water images from a DIXON magnetic resonance sequence. The μ-map only differentiates between air, lung, fat, and soft tissue. Using this μ-map NAC (non-attenuation-corrected) PET images are then corrected according to the respective tissue-specific attenuation coefficients

ways to generate a μ-map had to be found [6], resulting in the development of different approaches.
1. The segmentation-based approach using individual attenuation coefficients for specific tissue classes; this approach was already described in 1981 [10]. It was adopted by our group, who proposed using it for the generation of a μ-map for whole-body PET/MRI [11]. By making use of water- and fat-weighted images from a Dixon magnetic resonance sequence, each voxel can be assigned to one of the following tissue classes: air, lung, fat, or soft tissue [12] (Fig. 1). Cortical bone is ignored because it is virtually impossible to segment this tissue class from these data. Data acquisition usually requires about 18 s per bed position during one breath-hold. The obvious major disadvantage of this approach is the limited number of tissue classes with fixed attenuation coefficients. This is particularly relevant in cardiac imaging, as there is significant inter-patient variability in lung structure and location. The neglecting of bone may result in differences in tumor uptake between PET/CT and PET/MRI that can be as high as 23% [11, 13, 14]. Other disadvantages of this approach are that contrast agents may cause inaccuracies due to reduced T1 values, and metal implants do not contribute to the attenuation map [15]. This segmentation-based approach is used in currently commercially available PET/MRI scanners, such as the Biograph mMR [11] or the Ingenuity TF [13]. Our group demonstrated a good correlation between PET/MRI and PET/CT data in oncologic studies [16].
2. The second route to μ-map generation is the template- (or atlas-) based approach. Here, the model-based known μ-map is adjusted to the patient's real anatomy.

The first application of this approach was in imaging of the head, where a rigid model is sufficient [17, 18]. For whole-body imaging, however, an elastic model is necessary, which remains a problem regarding the translation into clinical use. The combined use of a template- and segmentation-based approach has been described [19].
3. It is also possible to generate μ-maps using PET emission data [20, 21]. The underlying principle of this approach is that any voxel exhibiting at least some tracer uptake has to be part of the body and must thus add to the attenuation. An undesirable property of many tracers, namely, their unspecific uptake in non-targeted tissues, is thus a prerequisite for this technique. This approach is particularly useful in combination with the segmentation-based approach, to address motion and truncation problems when body parts are outside the field of view (FOV) [7, 22]. Actually, this combined approach is used in the Siemens Biograph mMR, where the FOV of the magnetic resonance device is only 45 cm [22, 23]. The extension of the field of view is the most obvious solution to this problem [24].

Another source of photon scatter and attenuation in PET/MRI are artificial components outside the body but within the FOV, such as coils, patient monitoring devices, positioning aids, earphones, cables, and the patient bed itself. For the MRI system these objects are "invisible" and thus do not contribute to the μ-map. Only the patient bed and the fixed coils are implanted in the precalculated attenuation models [25]. Consequently, vendors have redesigned their hardware, although the effects are still detectable. Whether there is a relevant impact on diagnostic scans is not yet known [26].

Cardiac Devices

Cardiac devices, such as pacemakers, implantable cardioverter defibrillators (ICDs), or cardiac resynchronization therapy (CRT), cause artifacts on CT that result in an overestimation of the attenuation. The effect on the quantification of tracer uptake seems to be negligible in PET/CT [27]. Analogously, non-magnetic metals cause a signal void in MRI that exceeds the actual size of the object, possibly resulting in an underestimation of the attenuation. More importantly, these devices may interact with the radiofrequency, which may result in their malfunction or heating. Therefore, many subjects cannot be examined using MRI (and thus by PET/MRI); this is a growing problem because the number of patients with diseases qualifying for the implantation of such cardiac devices is increasing [28, 29]. Phase analysis using nuclear medicine studies (such as PET or SPECT) has been proposed to better identify patients who might respond to CRT implantation [30, 31]; however, larger clinical trials are still warranted.

Workflows for Cardiac PET/MRI

As mentioned above, attenuation correction is a crucial aspect of imaging and so is the exact alignment of the μ-map and the acquired PET data. One major advantage of MRI over CT is that the attenuation correction scan may be repeated as often as necessary without any radiation. Unfortunately, the subsequent necessary choice of the ideal μ-map is a time-consuming, inconvenient matter. According to our experience, however, in the vast majority of cases there is satisfactory alignment between PET data and the μ-map.

Another important consideration regarding PET/MRI is that most data are acquired in "parallel" and not truly "simultaneously". PET acquires a volume with frame lengths ranging from a few seconds up to 20–30 min (or more) depending on the chosen protocol (tracer, half-life, injected activity, endurance of the patient, etc.). Consequently, the acquired PET data comprise motion that took place during the scan (e.g., heart beat, ventilation and "true" patient motion) whereas in MR data are usually acquired sequentially (even in 3D acquisitions), with acquisition times ranging from about 50 ms for dynamic scans to several breath-holds for high-resolution images. A major problem with sequential imaging is that the data are acquired over several breath-holds; since the reproducibility of breath-holding is limited, this results in partially overlapping (or partially lacking) data. However, the imaging of moving objects with MRI would result in enormous, unacceptable artifacts. With cardiac PET/MRI, this raises the issue, that ungated (cardiac cycle and ventilation) PET images are compared to or fused with, for example, end-diastolic magnetic resonance images that are acquired during breath-hold. Another inconvenient and time-consuming matter is that the PET

volume data have to be coregistered with the MRI data in various (partially overlapping) slices of various positions (e.g., short axes; two-, three-, and four-chamber view). However, researchers are aware of this problem and techniques such as motion-triggered acquisition [32] and software corrections [33] are being developed that allow free-breathing during imaging.

Still, parallel PET/MRI is much more favorable than sequential PET/MRI. The sequential approach (either on separate scanners or on scanners connected via a common rail system) is not only inconvenient for the patient and personnel; it is also logistically demanding. Parallel PET/MRI, on the other hand, can not only improve patient compliance and comfort, it can also increase patient throughput and thus cost-efficiency. Two potential work flows are depicted in Fig. 2.

An application that might benefit from the truly simultaneous acquisition of PET and MRI data is myocardial perfusion imaging (MPI). The initial benefit would be the capability to cross-validate one modality with the other (which is of research interest). Taking into consideration PET, with its vast variety of specific tracers and its good volume-coverage, and MRI, with its high in-plane resolution, a synergistic effect would, for example, be the separate investigation of epicardial and endocardial perfusion. However, some hurdles still need to be overcome: (1) MRI usually only acquires a few slices of the heart, (2) Gd-chelate based contrast medium, used in most applications, has properties that are unfavorable for truly quantitative perfusion assessment, such as a low extraction fraction and a non-specific (only partially perfusion-dependent) uptake by the myocardium. The major advantage is, however, that PET and MRI data can be acquired under truly identical conditions, even though the injection speed of the imaging agent (PET: $\approx$30 s, MRI: $\approx$5 s) as well as the acquisition time (MRI: $\approx$1 min, PET: $\approx$10 min) differ significantly.

Cardiovascular Applications Using Hybrid PET/MRI

Myocardial Perfusion Imaging

The diagnosis of flow-limiting coronary artery disease (CAD) and the investigation of the hemodynamic significance of known CAD are the most regularly conducted studies in nuclear cardiology, due to its high sensitivity and specificity [34] and its high value in patient management [35-37]. PET MPI helps in clinical decision-making as the extent of ischemic tissue determined by this imaging modality allows patients to be assigned to optimal therapy, either revascularization or medical therapy [38]. Furthermore, there is increasing evidence that PET MPI offers advantages over SPECT MPI due to the absolute quantification of myocardial blood flow (MBF), attenuation correction, and superior image quality, especially in obese patients [39]. So far, several PET perfusion tracers have been established: N-13 ammonia, O-15

STRESS/REST PERFUSION

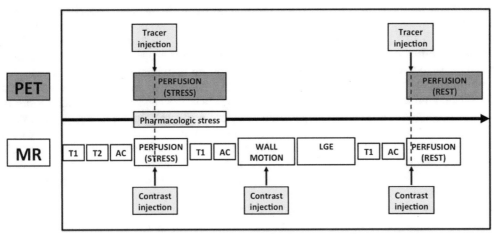

Inside scanner (≈50-60 minutes)

VIABILITY (including PET perfusion)

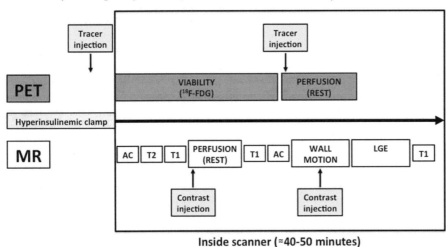

Inside scanner (≈40-50 minutes)

Fig. 2. Two potential workflows (stress/rest perfusion, viability including perfusion) for simultaneous PET/MRI

water, rubidium-82 (Rb-82), and F-18 flurpiridaz. The relatively short half-lives of N-13 ammonia (≈10 min), O-15 water (122 s) and Rb-82 (76 s) allow rapid PET MPI with only short lag times between the stress and the at-rest studies. The disadvantages of these tracers are, however, the high positron energies, resulting in decreased image quality (Rb-82), the need of an on-site cyclotron (N-13 ammonia, O-15 water) or of a generator, which is only cost-effective when a certain patient-throughput can be guaranteed (Rb-82), or the fact that stress imaging is only feasible when the patient is administered the pharmacological agent and the tracer while inside the scanner (N-13 ammonia, O-15 water, Rb-82). F-18 flurpiridaz offers some advantages, e.g. a low positron energy, a half-life that is long enough to enable tracer distribution even to hospitals and clinics in rural areas, the option of ergometer exercise with tracer injection outside the scanner, and possibly a simplified MBF estimation approach [40, 41]. Despite the above-

mentioned advantages of PET MPI and its use in many centers, MRI has also been evaluated recently for the purpose of MPI. The underlying principle that first-pass MRI with gadolinium-based contrast agents (e.g., Gd-DTPA) can be used to detect CAD was shown about 20 years ago [42]; since then, a multitude of studies have investigated its value in flow-limiting CAD [43, 44]. While these studies consisted almost exclusively of visual analysis, the absolute quantification of MBF is known to be of great value in patients suffering from extensive CAD and balanced ischemia [45, 46]. The feasibility of quantifying MBF using MRI has been investigated. One study evaluated a rather simple approach, namely, the upslope ratio as an index of coronary flow reserve [47]. However, in a subsequent study, this approach was definitively shown to result in an underestimation of the flow reserve when compared to N-13 ammonia PET MPI [48]. Subsequently, a more complex model, using the central volume principle, was investigated for absolute MBF

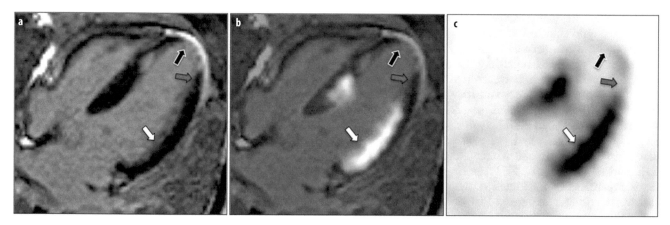

Fig. 3 a-c. FDG PET/MRI "viability" imaging shortly after acute myocardial infarction (MI). Example from a patient who was imaged a few days after acute MI by FDG PET/MRI (hyperinsulinemic/euglycemic clamp). Four-chamber views of late gadolinium enhancement (LGE) MRI (**a**), FDG PET (**c**), and fusion of LGE MRI and FDG PET (**b**) are depicted. Early after acute MI, different patterns of FDG uptake and LGE transmurality can be observed: (1) normal FDG uptake and no LGE (*white arrows*), (2) reduced/absent FDG uptake and transmural LGE (*black arrows*), and (3) reduced FDG uptake and non-transmural LGE (*red arrows*)

quantification [49]. This approach was recently studied in 41 patients who underwent PET and MRI MPI separately [50]. Good agreement for the coronary flow reserve between these two modalities was obtained; the correlation was weak for absolute MBF values, though. It should be noted, however, that a rare quantification method for N-13 ammonia was applied [51] and that differences in absolute MBF may also be due to the fact that Gd-chelates do not enter the cells and thus show a distribution only in the interstitial space (also in increased interstitial spaces such as scarred myocardium) [52].

There are patients in whom even extremely well-tolerated MRI contrast agents cannot be used and alternative approaches, without the use of any contrast medium, are being developed. For example, arterial spin labeling (ASL), which originates from techniques to determine cerebral blood flow, has been investigated in a preclinical study, where it demonstrated a good correlation with the results of O-15 water PET [53]. In patients, ASL was able to measure the increase in blood flow induced by adenosine [54]. The obvious advantages of ASL are the possibility of repetitive and continuous measurements of MBF without need for any contrast agents

In summary, cardiac MPI using simultaneous PET/MRI might be valuable to detect subendocardial ischemia by MRI and to quantify absolute MBF using PET.

Myocardial Viability Imaging

Another potential application of PET/MR in cardiology is myocardial viability imaging. Hypoperfused myocardium exhibits a shift of its metabolism from fatty acids towards glucose, a state called "hibernation" [55]. Several studies have shown that myocardium in this state is prone to recover after revascularization [56]. Usually, FDG PET is the method of choice for non-invasive viability imaging [55]. Recently, cardiac MRI using the late gadolinium enhancement (LGE) technique has emerged as a possible

alternative. Notably, however, unlike FDG PET, this approach images non-viable, scarred myocardium, information used to draw conclusions regarding the potential of non-scarred myocardium to recover. The enrichment of Gd-chelates in increased extracellular space (such as scarred myocardium) results in a reduced wash-out of the contrast agent compared to remote myocardium which may be visualized in cardiac MRI using inversion recovery sequences, in which the signal of the remote myocardium is nulled [57]. Despite the fundamental difference in these approaches (imaging viable vs. non-viable tissue) there is good agreement between the two modalities [58]. One essential property of MRI is its high in-plane resolution (1–3 mm), which enables the differentiation between transmural (>50%) and non-transmural (<50%) scarred myocardium [59]. Another interesting finding is that in patients with suspected CAD but without known myocardial infarction, even small areas of scarred myocardium carry prognostic significance [60]. A similar observation was described in a study comparing areas of non-transmural LGE with SPECT MPI [61]. Since small areas of infarction may be overlooked by PET because of partial volume effects, this fact is relevant in hybrid PET/MRI, as an improved tissue classification can be expected. Our group made similar observations in patients shortly after myocardial infarction, in whom severely reduced FDG uptake was accompanied by non-transmural LGE signal only (Fig. 3). Accordingly, hybrid PET/MRI might ultimately result in an improved prediction of wall motion recovery after revascularization, when information such as wall motion and thickening, FDG uptake, perfusion, and LGE transmurality are integrated.

As mentioned above, the assessment of global and regional wall motion is a relevant surrogate marker for myocardial vitality and therapy response after revascularization. Several studies have shown that left ventricular parameters, such as ejection fraction, end-systolic volume, and end-diastolic volume carry prognostic significance. MRI is the gold standard for the assessment of these parameters and it has been extensively validated [62]. The disadvantages of MRI regarding the assessment of left ventricular function are, however, that data are acquired in multiple slices in short- and long axis orientations (usually in 20–30 phases) and thus do not provide fully volumetric data. Gated PET, however, is fully volumetric and acquired at typically 8–12 phases; it has been validated in patients with and without cardiac diseases [63, 64]. Furthermore, gated PET can be performed in patients regardless of implanted cardiac devices. Another fact worth noting is that gated PET data are analyzed using highly automated software, which results in high intra- and interobserver reproducibility, whereas MRI usually requires at least some manual interaction for segmentation of the myocardium.

Atherosclerotic Plaque Imaging

While coronary artery and plaque imaging are still the domain of CT angiography, there is increasing interest in the use of MRI in this setting. Besides the fact that MR angiography can be performed without any radiation whereas the radiation dose of CT angiography, depending on the protocol and scanner, is $\approx$1–20 mSv [65, 66]. Moreover, MRI can provide additional valuable information, such as characterization of the vessel wall or the plaque itself [67, 68]. An interesting finding by our group was the observation of Gd-contrast enhancement in the vessel wall following myocardial infarction that correlated with the degree of stenosis; the enhancement resolved in a 3-month follow-up scan, possibly representing reduced inflammatory activity [69]. Also, several PET tracers have been used to image atherosclerotic plaques, especially FDG. It is assumed that an increased FDG uptake is related to an intense macrophage infiltration, representing a high vulnerability [70, 71]. Another tracer that has recently been investigated in 80 patients with myocardial infarction or stable angina is F-18 fluoride (F-18 NaF) [72]. In 93% of the patients with myocardial infarction, F-18 NaF uptake was highest in the culprit lesion whereas FDG uptake was obscured by the myocardial uptake. Furthermore, 45% of the patients with stable angina had plaques with focal F-18 NaF uptake that were associated with high-risk features on intravascular ultrasound. However, whether this tracer can be useful to improve patient management remains to be determined in future studies. Potentially valuable tracers targeting integrins, such as $\alpha_V\beta_3$, have also been investigated in preclinical models and are currently being translated into clinical applications [73-75]. Because tracer uptake in atherosclerotic plaques and the vessel wall is usually rather low, cardiac and respiratory motion is an issue, which might ultimately be addressed using MRI. Hybrid PET/MRI might help to make molecular PET imaging of the coronary arteries and culprit lesions feasible, through the use of novel tracers.

Conclusion

For a long time, the integration of PET and MRI seemed practically impossible. Accordingly, following the recent introduction of hybrid PET/MRI systems, expectations were high. Yet, almost 4 years after the introduction of the first clinically available hybrid PET/MRI scanner, studies with a cardiovascular focus are scarce. The main advantages of this novel technique are the reduction of the radiation dose to the patient, increased patient comfort and throughput compared to sequential imaging, and the capability to simultaneously investigate biological processes under the same physiological conditions. The major downside is a complex workflow requiring additional personnel and training, which results in extra costs. In summary, PET/MRI systems represent a superb research tool, and first studies demonstrating their additional value in clinical routine are being conducted.

References

1. Kajander S, Ukkonen H, Sipila H et al (2009) Low radiation dose imaging of myocardial perfusion and coronary angiography with a hybrid PET/CT scanner. Clinical physiology and functional imaging 29:81-88.
2. Zaidi H, Ojha N, Morich M et al (2011) Design and performance evaluation of a whole-body Ingenuity TF PET-MRI system. Physics in medicine and biology 56:3091-3106.
3. Delso G, Furst S, Jakoby B et al (2011) Performance measurements of the Siemens mMR integrated whole-body PET/MR scanner. J Nucl Med 52:1914-1922.
4. Pichler BJ, Judenhofer MS, Catana C et al (2006) Performance test of an LSO-APD detector in a 7-T MRI scanner for simultaneous PET/MRI. J Nucl Med 47:639-647.
5. Levin C, Deller T, Peterson W (2014) Initial results of simultaneous whole-body ToF PET/MR. J Nucl Med 55 (Suppl 1):660.
6. Hofmann M, Pichler B, Scholkopf B, Beyer T (2009) Towards quantitative PET/MRI: a review of MR-based attenuation correction techniques. Eur J Nucl Med Mol Imaging 36 (Suppl 1):S93-104.
7. Martinez-Moller A, Souvatzoglou M, Navab N et al (2007) Artifacts from misaligned CT in cardiac perfusion PET/CT studies: frequency, effects, and potential solutions. J Nucl Med 48:188-193.
8. Gould KL, Pan T, Loghin C et al (2007) Frequent diagnostic errors in cardiac PET/CT due to misregistration of CT attenuation and emission PET images: a definitive analysis of causes, consequences, and corrections. J Nucl Med 48:1112-1121.
9. Koepfli P, Hany TF, Wyss CA et al (2004) CT attenuation correction for myocardial perfusion quantification using a PET/CT hybrid scanner. J Nucl Med 45:537-542.
10. Huang SC, Carson RE, Phelps ME (1981) A boundary method for attenuation correction in positron computed tomography. J Nucl Med 22:627-637.
11. Martinez-Moller A, Souvatzoglou M, Delso G et al (2009) Tissue classification as a potential approach for attenuation correction in whole-body PET/MRI: evaluation with PET/CT data. J Nucl Med 50:520-526.

12. Coombs BD, Szumowski J, Coshow W (1997) Two-point Dixon technique for water-fat signal decomposition with B0 inhomogeneity correction. Magn Reson Med 38:884-889.

13. Schulz V, Torres-Espallardo I, Renisch S et al (2011) Automatic, three-segment, MR-based attenuation correction for whole-body PET/MR data. Eur J Nucl Med Mol Imaging 38:138-152.

14. Samarin A, Burger C, Wollenweber SD et al (2012) PET/MR imaging of bone lesions—implications for PET quantification from imperfect attenuation correction. Eur J Nucl Med Mol Imaging 39:1154-1160.

15. Fürst S, Souvatzoglu M, Rischpler C (2012) Effects of MR contrast agents on attenuation map generation and cardiac PET quantification in PET/MR. J Nucl Med 53 (Suppl 1):139.

16. Drzezga A, Souvatzoglou M, Eiber M et al (2012) First clinical experience with integrated whole-body PET/MR: comparison to PET/CT in patients with oncologic diagnoses. J J Nucl Med 53:845-855.

17. Hofmann M, Steinke F, Scheel V et al (2008) MRI-based attenuation correction for PET/MRI: a novel approach combining pattern recognition and atlas registration. J Nucl Med 49:1875-1883.

18. Schreibmann E, Nye JA, Schuster DM et al (2010) MR-based attenuation correction for hybrid PET-MR brain imaging systems using deformable image registration. Medical physics 37:2101-2109.

19. Hofmann M, Bezrukov I, Mantlik F et al (2011) MRI-based attenuation correction for whole-body PET/MRI: quantitative evaluation of segmentation- and atlas-based methods. J Nucl Med 52:1392-1399.

20. Nuyts J, Dupont P, Stroobants S et al (1999) Simultaneous maximum a posteriori reconstruction of attenuation and activity distributions from emission sinograms. IEEE Trans Med Imaging 18(393-403.

21. Censor Y, Gustafson D, Lent A, Tuy H (1979) A new approach to the emission computerized tomography problem: Simultaneous calculation of attenuation and activity coefficients. IEEE Trans Nucl Sci 26:2275-2279.

22. Nuyts J, Michel C, Fenchel M et al (2010) Completion of a truncated attenuation image from the attenuated PET emission data. IEEE Nucl Sci Symp Conf Record (NSS/MIC) 2123-2127.

23. Delso G, Martinez-Moller A, Bundschuh RA et al (2010) The effect of limited MR field of view in MR/PET attenuation correction. Medical physics 37:2804-2812.

24. Blumhagen JO, Ladebeck R, Fenchel M, Scheffler K (2012) MR-based field-of-view extension in MR/PET: B(0) homogenization using gradient enhancement (HUGE). Magn Reson Med 70:1047-1057.

25. Delso G, Martinez-Moller A, Bundschuh RA et al (2010) Evaluation of the attenuation properties of MR equipment for its use in a whole-body PET/MR scanner. Physics in medicine and biology 55:4361-4374.

26. MacDonald LR, Kohlmyer S, Liu C et al (2011) Effects of MR surface coils on PET quantification. Medical physics 38:2948-2956.

27. DiFilippo FP, Brunken RC (2005) Do implanted pacemaker leads and ICD leads cause metal-related artifact in cardiac PET/CT? J Nucl Med 46:436-443.

28. Marinskis G, Bongiorni MG, Dagres N et al (2012) Performing magnetic resonance imaging in patients with implantable pacemakers and defibrillators: results of a European Heart Rhythm Association survey. Europace 14:1807-1809.

29. Cohen JD, Costa HS, Russo RJ (2012) Determining the risks of magnetic resonance imaging at 1.5 tesla for patients with pacemakers and implantable cardioverter defibrillators. Am J Cardiol 110:1631-1636.

30. Henneman MM, van der Wall EE, Ypenburg C et al (2007) Nuclear imaging in cardiac resynchronization therapy. J Nucl Med 48:2001-2010.

31. Uebleis C, Ulbrich M, Tegtmeyer R et al (2011) Electrocardiogram-gated 18F-FDG PET/CT hybrid imaging in patients with unsatisfactory response to cardiac resynchronization therapy: initial clinical results. J Nucl Med 52:67-71.

32. Adluru G, Chen L, Kim SE et al (2011) Three-dimensional late gadolinium enhancement imaging of the left atrium with a hybrid radial acquisition and compressed sensing. J Magn Reson Imaging 34:1465-1471.

33. Xue H, Zuehlsdorff S, Kellman P et al (2009) Unsupervised inline analysis of cardiac perfusion MRI. Medical image computing and computer-assisted intervention: MICCAI International Conference on Medical Image Computing and Computer-Assisted Intervention 12:741-749.

34. Klocke FJ, Baird MG, Lorell BH et al (2003) ACC/AHA/ASNC guidelines for the clinical use of cardiac radionuclide imaging–executive summary: a report of the American College of Cardiology/American Heart Association Task Force on Practice Guidelines (ACC/AHA/ASNC Committee to Revise the 1995 Guidelines for the Clinical Use of Cardiac Radionuclide Imaging). J Am Coll Cardiol 42:1318-1333.

35. Schwaiger M, Melin J (1999) Cardiological applications of nuclear medicine. Lancet 354:661-666.

36. Yoshinaga K, Chow BJ, Williams K et al (2006) What is the prognostic value of myocardial perfusion imaging using rubidium-82 positron emission tomography? J Am Coll Cardiol 48:1029-1039.

37. Merhige ME, Breen WJ, Shelton V et al (2007) Impact of myocardial perfusion imaging with PET and (82)Rb on downstream invasive procedure utilization, costs, and outcomes in coronary disease management. J Nucl Med 48:1069-1076.

38. Hachamovitch R, Hayes SW, Friedman JD et al (2003) Comparison of the short-term survival benefit associated with revascularization compared with medical therapy in patients with no prior coronary artery disease undergoing stress myocardial perfusion single photon emission computed tomography. Circulation 107:2900-2907.

39. Flotats A, Bravo PE, Fukushima K et al (2012) (82)Rb PET myocardial perfusion imaging is superior to (99m)Tc-labelled agent SPECT in patients with known or suspected coronary artery disease. Eur J Nucl Med Mol Imaging 39:1233-1239.

40. Rischpler C, Park MJ, Fung GS et al (2012) Advances in PET myocardial perfusion imaging: F-18 labeled tracers. Annals of nuclear medicine 26:1-6.

41. Sherif HM, Nekolla SG, Saraste A et al (2011) Simplified quantification of myocardial flow reserve with flurpiridaz F 18: validation with microspheres in a pig model. J Nucl Med 52:617-624.

42. Manning WJ, Atkinson DJ, Grossman W et al (1991) First-pass nuclear magnetic resonance imaging studies using gadolinium-DTPA in patients with coronary artery disease. J Am Coll Cardiol 18:959-965.

43. de Jong MC, Genders TS, van Geuns RJ et al (2012) Diagnostic performance of stress myocardial perfusion imaging for coronary artery disease: a systematic review and meta-analysis. Eur Radiol 22:1881-1895.

44. Nandalur KR, Dwamena BA, Choudhri AF et al (2007) Diagnostic performance of stress cardiac magnetic resonance imaging in the detection of coronary artery disease: a meta-analysis. J Am Coll Cardiol 50:1343-1353.

45. Kajander SA, Joutsiniemi E, Saraste M et al (2011) Clinical value of absolute quantification of myocardial perfusion with (15)O-water in coronary artery disease. Circ Cardiovasc Imaging 4:678-684.

46. Parkash R, deKemp RA, Ruddy TD et al (2004) Potential utility of rubidium 82 PET quantification in patients with 3-vessel coronary artery disease. J Nucl Cardiol 11:440-449.

47. Schwitter J, Nanz D, Kneifel S et al (2001) Assessment of myocardial perfusion in coronary artery disease by magnetic resonance: a comparison with positron emission tomography and coronary angiography. Circulation 103:2230-2235.

48. Ibrahim T, Nekolla SG, Schreiber K et al (2002) Assessment of coronary flow reserve: comparison between contrast-enhanced magnetic resonance imaging and positron emission tomography. J Am Coll Cardiol 39:864-870.

49. Jerosch-Herold M (2010) Quantification of myocardial perfusion by cardiovascular magnetic resonance. J Cardiovasc Magn Res 12:57.

50. Morton G, Chiribiri A, Ishida M et al (2012) Quantification of absolute myocardial perfusion in patients with coronary artery disease: comparison between cardiovascular magnetic resonance and positron emission tomography. J Am Coll Cardiol 60:1546-1555.

51. Choi Y, Huang SC, Hawkins RA et al (1993) A simplified method for quantification of myocardial blood flow using nitrogen-13-ammonia and dynamic PET. J Nucl Med 34:488-497.

52. Zierler K (2000) Indicator dilution methods for measuring blood flow, volume, and other properties of biological systems: a brief history and memoir. Annals of biomedical engineering 28:836-848.

53. McCommis KS, Zhang H, Herrero P et al (2008) Feasibility study of myocardial perfusion and oxygenation by noncontrast MRI: comparison with PET study in a canine model. Magn Reson Imaging 26:11-19.

54. Zun Z, Varadarajan P, Pai RG et al (2011) Arterial spin labeled CMR detects clinically relevant increase in myocardial blood flow with vasodilation. JACC Cardiovasc Imaging 4:1253-1261.

55. Ghosh N, Rimoldi OE, Beanlands RS, Camici PG (2010) Assessment of myocardial ischaemia and viability: role of positron emission tomography. Eur Heart J 31:2984-2995.

56. Di Carli MF (2008) Predicting improved function after myocardial revascularization. Current opinion in cardiology 13:415-424.

57. Klein C, Schmal TR, Nekolla SG et al (2007) Mechanism of late gadolinium enhancement in patients with acute myocardial infarction. J Cardiovasc Magn Res 9:653-658.

58. Klein C, Nekolla SG, Bengel FM et al (2002) Assessment of myocardial viability with contrast-enhanced magnetic resonance imaging: comparison with positron emission tomography. Circulation 105:162-167.

59. Kim RJ, Wu E, Rafael A et al (2000) The use of contrast-enhanced magnetic resonance imaging to identify reversible myocardial dysfunction. N Engl J Med 343:1445-1453.

60. Kwong RY, Chan AK, Brown KA et al (2006) Impact of unrecognized myocardial scar detected by cardiac magnetic resonance imaging on event-free survival in patients presenting with signs or symptoms of coronary artery disease. Circulation 113:2733-2743.

61. Wagner A, Mahrholdt H, Holly TA et al (2003) Contrast-enhanced MRI and routine single photon emission computed tomography (SPECT) perfusion imaging for detection of subendocardial myocardial infarcts: an imaging study. Lancet 361:374-379.

62. Bellenger NG, Davies LC, Francis JM (2000) Reduction in sample size for studies of remodeling in heart failure by the use of cardiovascular magnetic resonance. J Cardiovasc Magn Res 2:271-278.

63. Rajappan K, Livieratos L, Camici PG, Pennell DJ (2002) Measurement of ventricular volumes and function: A comparison of gated PET and cardiovascular magnetic resonance. J Nucl Med 43:806-810.

64. Boyd HL, Gunn RN, Marinho NVS et al (1996) Non-invasive measurement of left ventricular volumes and function by gated positron emission tomography. Eur J Nucl Med 23:1594-1602.

65. Fink C, Krissak R, Henzler T et al (2011) Radiation dose at coronary CT angiography: second-generation dual-source CT versus single-source 64-MDCT and first-generation dual-source CT. AJR Am J Roentgenol 196:W550-557.

66. Hausleiter J, Meyer T, Hermann F et al (2009) Estimated radiation dose associated with cardiac CT angiography. JAMA 301:500-507.

67. Fayad ZA, Fuster V, Fallon JT et al (2000) Noninvasive in vivo human coronary artery lumen and wall imaging using black-blood magnetic resonance imaging. Circulation 102:506-510.

68. Kim WY, Stuber M, Bornert P (2002) Three-dimensional black-blood cardiac magnetic resonance coronary vessel wall imaging detects positive arterial remodeling in patients with nonsignificant coronary artery disease. Circulation 106:296-299.

69. Ibrahim T, Makowski MR, Jankauskas A et al (2009) Serial contrast-enhanced cardiac magnetic resonance imaging demonstrates regression of hyperenhancement within the coronary artery wall in patients after acute myocardial infarction. JACC Cardiovasc Imaging 2:580-588.

70. Rudd JH, Warburton EA, Fryer TD et al (2002) Imaging atherosclerotic plaque inflammation with [18F]-fluorodeoxyglucose positron emission tomography. Circulation 105:2708-2711.

71. Davies JR, Rudd JH, Weissberg PL, Narula J (2006) Radionuclide imaging for the detection of inflammation in vulnerable plaques. J Am Coll Cardiol 47:C57-68.

72. Joshi NV, Vesey AT, Williams MC et al (2014) 18F-fluoride positron emission tomography for identification of ruptured and high-risk coronary atherosclerotic plaques: a prospective clinical trial. Lancet 383:705-713.

73. Saraste A, Laitinen I, Weidl E et al (2012) Diet intervention reduces uptake of alphavbeta3 integrin-targeted PET tracer 18F-galacto-RGD in mouse atherosclerotic plaques. J Nucl Cardiol 19:775-784.

74. Laitinen I, Notni J, Pohle K et al (2013) Comparison of cyclic RGD peptides for alphavbeta3 integrin detection in a rat model of myocardial infarction. EJNMMI research 3:38.

75. Beer AJ, Pelisek J, Heider P et al (2014) PET/CT imaging of integrin alphavbeta3 expression in human carotid atherosclerosis. JACC Cardiovasc Imaging 7:178-187.

PEDIATRIC RADIOLOGY SATELLITE COURSE
"KANGAROO"

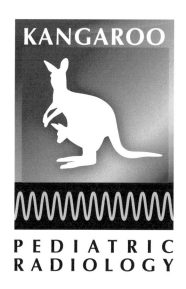

Pediatric Chest Tumors Including Lymphoma

Alexander Oshmyansky, Thierry A.G.M. Huisman

Division of Pediatric Radiology and Pediatric Neuroradiology, Russell H. Morgan Department of Radiology and Radiological Science, Baltimore, MD, USA

Introduction

Pediatric chest neoplasms are heterogeneous in etiology and presentation and their diagnosis is often challenging. Radiography, ultrasonography, computed tomography (CT), and magnetic resonance imaging (MRI) are all of utility in the diagnosis of pediatric chest neoplasms. In this chapter we review the imaging appearance of various common and rare pediatric chest neoplasms.

In the following, chest neoplasms are categorized as chest wall malignancies, mediastinal masses, metastatic disease, and primary lung parenchymal neoplasms. We emphasize the imaging features of neoplasms, which can be used to obtain an accurate diagnosis of visualized masses prior to pathologic evaluation.

We also discuss the distinguishing characteristics that differentiate neoplastic processes from congenital malformation or other non-neoplastic mass lesions that occur in the chest. Differentiation between these categories is often challenging, but a consideration of clinical information may facilitate this process.

We begin with a discussion of the various methods of imaging pediatric chest neoplasms.

Imaging of Chest Neoplasms

Radiography

Radiography is a common initial method for imaging the pediatric chest and for evaluating pediatric chest neoplasms. It is widely available in a variety of settings and inexpensive. However, it is limited in its inherent contrast resolution between different soft-tissue structures and for precise anatomic localization of the extent of a pathologic process. Nonetheless, radiography remains useful in both the initial evaluation and follow-up of pediatric chest neoplasms [1].

Ultrasound

Ultrasound can often be of great utility in evaluating neoplasms that arise from or abut the chest wall. It is relatively inexpensive, widely available, and does not require the use of ionizing radiation. It allows for the assessment of tissue characteristics and vascularity in many superficial chest lesions. However, evaluating the mediastinal structures through a trans-thoracic approach, especially structures in the middle and posterior mediastinum, is often difficult because of difficulties in finding acoustic windows between ribs and issues with depth of penetration [2]. Ultrasound is also often problematic for intrapulmonary lesions. Lung parenchymal processes can be difficult to evaluation due to acoustic reflections from the air-containing lungs. Also, any process that does not abut/reach the chest wall is usually difficult to evaluate.

Computed Tomography

The mainstay of imaging lesions originating from or within the lung parenchyma is chest CT. CT offers a high spatial resolution, excellent contrast to noise ratio, and a high speed of acquisition such that imaging can usually be done within a single, short, patient breath hold. It permits a higher level of anatomic resolution and tissue characterization than radiography and, unlike MRI, is not impeded by respiratory motion. However, CT necessitates the use of ionizing radiation, and radiation dose issues often arise in pediatric patients who require serial follow-up evaluations. New, low dose CT dose techniques have reduced the radiation dose required for diagnostic imaging, but concerns remain regarding repeated radiation exposure in diagnostic imaging [1].

Magnetic Resonance Imaging

MRI allows high levels of contrast and anatomic resolution in the pediatric chest without the use of ionizing radiation. By applying various magnetic resonance pulse

Diseases of the Chest and Heart 2015-2018,
DOI: 10.1007/978-88-470-5752-4_29 © Springer-Verlag Italia 2015

sequences and imaging techniques, a broad spectrum of tissue characteristics can be visualized. In particular, hypercellularity in malignant neoplastic structures often manifests as restricted diffusion on diffusion-weighted imaging (DWI). Thus, DWI can be useful in the initial evaluation and staging of pediatric malignancies. However, even though DWI sequences are typically relatively rapid, issues with motion artifacts during respiration and susceptibility artifact from air in the lungs remain [3].

Another matter of concern is that MRI in the pediatric population often requires the use of general anesthesia in order to prevent patient motion during longer imaging sequences. In these instances, MRI thus brings with it the inherent risks of general anesthesia. This is countered, however, by the lack of ionizing radiation in MRI, an advantage over CT.

Neoplasms of the Pediatric Mediastinum

Anterior Mediastinum

Hodgkin's and Non-Hodgkin's Lymphoma

Hodgkin's lymphoma is the most common mediastinal mass in the pediatric population. Malignant lymphoma overall accounts for 23% of all mediastinal masses in children [4, 5]. Presentation with an anterior mediastinal mass occurs with lymphomatous infiltration of the thymus and lymph nodes (Fig. 1). Hodgkin's disease is typically nodal and spreads in direct continuity, whereas non-Hodgkin's lymphoma tends to be extranodal and to spread hematogenously. A mediastinal mass occurs in <50% of patients with non-Hodgkin's lymphoma [4-6]. In both processes, invasion of the pericardium can result in pericardial effusion. Pleural effusion, on the other hand, can result from venous or lymphatic compromise and does not necessarily indicate direct tumor extension [4].

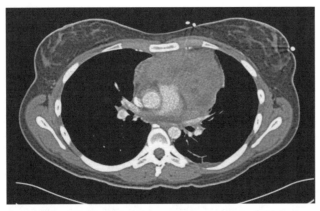

Fig. 1. An 18-year-old-female presenting with Hodgkin's lymphoma as a mediastinal mass. The mass is irregular in shape, having lost the normal morphology of the thymus, and is heterogeneous in appearance

On radiography, lymphoma frequently presents as a large anterior mediastinal mass. CT is critical in the initial diagnosis, to evaluate for potential tracheobronchial compromise. Life threatening airway obstruction is seen in up to 10% of patients with mediastinal lymphoma. Endotracheal anesthesia is reported to be safe in patients with lymphoma in the anterior mediastinum when the expected cross-sectional area of the trachea is reduced by no more than 50% [7].

The role of MRI in the initial diagnosis of lymphoma is generally considered to be limited. However, some reports indicate that whole body DWI may be useful in the staging of lymphoma. MRI may also be of value in determining the amount of fibrous stroma in a lymphomatous mass, which can indicate the expected residual mass after treatment [6].

Germ-Cell Tumors

Germ cell tumors are less common masses of the anterior mediastinum, accounting for 6–18% of all mediastinal masses [6]. The majority are benign teratomas (80% of all mediastinal germ cell tumors) [4, 5]. Malignant germ cell tumors in the pediatric population include both seminomatous and non-seminomatous lesions. Seminomatous lesions typically lack serologic markers and usually do not contain internal calcifications. For this reason, seminomas typically require histologic diagnosis. Non-seminomatous germ cell tumors can usually be identified through a combination of imaging appearance, serum markers such as β-human chorionic gonadotropin and α-fetoprotein, and clinical symptoms such as precocious puberty [8].

Thymic Neoplasms

Primary thymic neoplasms are typically benign in the pediatric population, with thymolipomas as the most common lesions. Thymolipomas usually present as fat- and soft-tissue-containing lesions of the anterior mediastinum. They typically do not have internal calcifications [9, 10].

Most of the other mass-type lesions arising from the thymus are non neoplastic. Of these, perhaps the most important to consider is benign thymic hyperplasia. In infants, the mean thickness of the thymus is 1.50 cm, with a standard deviation of 0.46 cm. In children over the age of 10 years, the mean thickness of the thymus is 1.05 cm, with a standard deviation of 0.36. An abnormal process should be considered when thymic thickness on cross-sectional imaging is over two standard deviations above normal (upper limits of normal thymic thickness are 2.42 cm from ages 0–10 and 1.77 cm respectively) [4, 11].

The thymus normally atrophies as a result of cytotoxic injury, but may undergo secondary, benign hyperplasia thereafter. This period is referred to as "thymic rebound." The smooth contours of the hypertrophied thymus and a homogeneous soft-tissue density distinguish thymic rebound from tumor recurrence [6] (Fig. 2).

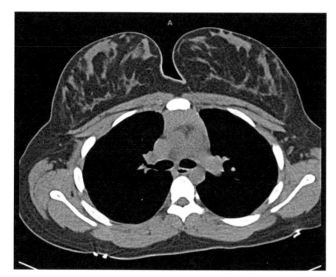

Fig. 2. A 16-year-old female with thymic rebound after undergoing chemotherapy for a sarcoma of the lower extremity. The margins of the thymus are preserved and the thymus is homogenous in appearance

Thymic cysts are another potential non-neoplastic lesion that involve the anterior mediastinum. These are fluid density, smooth, well-demarcated lesions found within otherwise normal thymic tissue [6, 12].

Middle Mediastinal Neoplasms

The most common primary pediatric middle mediastinal neoplasms are lymphomatous or leukemic [4, 5]. Otherwise, primary middle mediastinal neoplasms are unusual in the pediatric population. Other neoplasms of the middle mediastinum include cardiac tumors, which are rare, and metastatic disease, which is more common. The majority of middle mediastinal masses in the pediatric population are either infectious, inflammatory, or congenital (such as bronchopulmonary foregut cysts; discussed below) in origin.

Cardiac Tumors

Cardiac tumors are rare in the pediatric population. The most common pediatric tumor is a cardiac rhabdomyoma which is usually seen in association with tuberous sclerosis. In one series, 91% of cardiac rhabdomyomas were found in association with tuberous sclerosis. In general, any intracavitary mass found in infants should be considered a rhabomyoma until proven otherwise [13, 14].

Other tumors include cardiac fibroma, which is thought to be a hamartomatous lesion, and cardiac myxoma. The latter are typically found in association with myxoma syndrome, a familial disorder [13, 14].

Foregut Cysts

The most frequently encountered developmental anomaly of the pediatric middle mediastinum is the foregut cyst,

which may be bronchogenic, enteric, or neurenteric. As a group, foregut cysts comprise 11% of mediastinal masses in children [4, 5]. It can be difficult to precisely determine the structure of origin associated with a foregut cyst, but it is often the structure that the cyst is most closely associated with anatomically. The CT appearance of foregut cysts is typically diagnostic. Most foregut cysts are well-defined, well-circumscribed, homogeneous, fluid-density structures, although internal proteinacious debris can confer them with a hyperdense CT appearance [4, 5].

Lymphadenopathy

Lymphadenopathy, either in association with lymphoma or with an infectious or inflammatory process, is often encountered in the middle mediastinum. Identifiable mediastinal lymph nodes in infants are typically abnormal. In adolescents, lymph nodes >1 cm in their short axis are typically considered abnormal [4, 15].

Posterior Mediastinal Neoplasms

Neurogenic Tumors

Neurogenic tumors make up approximately 90% of posterior mediastinal masses in the pediatric population [6]. Tumors of ganglion-cell origin include neuroblastoma, ganglioneuroblastoma, and ganglioneuroma. Neuroblastoma is most common amongst infants and young children with a median patient age at presentation of 2 years (Figs. 3, 4). Ganglioneuroma, typically a benign lesion, occurs in older children with a median age at presentation of 10 years. For ganglioneuroblastoma, the median age at presentation is 5.5 years [6, 16].

All three tumors of ganglion cell origin typically appear as a vertically elongated mass with tapered superior and inferior margins. Internal calcifications are seen in 30% of ganglion cell origin tumors and adjacent bony changes are common [17].

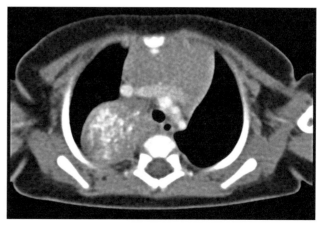

Fig. 3. A 3-month-old male with a partially calcified posterior mediastinal mass found to be a neuroblastoma. Normal thymic tissue is seen anteriorly

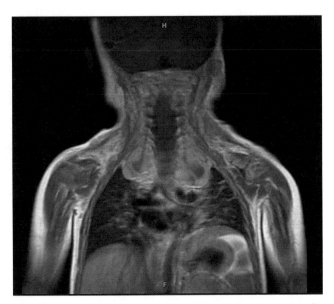

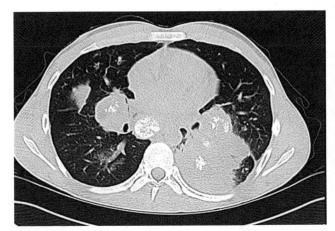

Fig. 5. Multiple osteosarcoma metastatic lesions seen on axial CT scan through the chest without contrast

Fig. 4. Bilateral apical masses in a 2-year-old male with neurofibromatosis type I. Post-contrast coronal MRI shows prominent peripheral enhancement in both lesions.

Peripheral nerve sheath tumors, schwannomas, and neurofibromas, are generally indistinguishable by imaging criteria alone. Schwannomas are encapsulated tumors that lack nerve fibers. Neurofibromas are non-encapsulated and contain nerve fibers. Both masses are generally well-demarcated and spherical/lobulated in appearance. Both are associated with a "target-sign" appearance on T2 weighted MRI sequences, consisting of peripheral T2 bright sequences and internal T2 dark signal. Schwannomas and neurofibromas are usually associated with the diagnosis of neurofibromatosis [4, 6, 18].

Approximately 5% of peripheral nerve sheath tumors undergo malignant degeneration, characterized by large size, central necrosis, and restricted diffusion on DWI sequences [6].

Primary Pulmonary Neoplasms

Pleuropulmonary Blastoma

Pleuropulmonary blastoma (PPB) is a rare entity that has recently been separated from the adult pulmonary blastoma. It is considered to be a dysontogenetic tumor, such as Wilms' tumor of the kidney, neuroblastoma, or hepatoblastoma [19]. The imaging appearance of PPB has been described primarily in a series of case reports. PPB is typically quite large on presentation, probably because of the late diagnosis. These tumors can be a solid lesion, mixed solid and cystic, or predominantly cystic. Most are heterogeneous in appearance and pleural-based. For reasons that are unclear, PBB most frequently occurs in the right hemithorax, with 70% of reported cases being right-sided [19].

Carcinoid Tumor

The vast majority (80–85%) of primary malignant lung tumors in children are carcinoid tumors, with approximately 85%, of them occurring within the tracheobronchial tree [20, 21]. These are endoluminal lesions that are often associated with internal calcifications, and therefore with post-obstructive atelectasis or pneumonia. Presenting symptoms typically include cough, hemoptysis, or recurrent pneumonia. Carcinoid tumors are often spherical, lobulated, or elongated along the axis of the associated bronchi. Their typically prominent internal contrast enhancement is helpful in distinguishing these tumors from mucus plugs [20, 22].

Metastatic Pulmonary Neoplasms

The most common pediatric pulmonary neoplasm is metastatic disease (Fig. 5). Metastatic disease can involve the pulmonary structures through hematogenous spread, lymphatic spread, or direct extension. Renal malignancies in particular, such as Wilms' tumor, can invade the chest by direct extension in the renal veins and inferior vena cava [15].

Distinguishing infectious or inflammatory pulmonary nodules from metastatic disease in the pediatric chest is often a challenging proposition. Inflammatory and neoplastic pulmonary nodules are often indistinguishable on both CT and MRI. Reports in the literature suggest that in a patient with a known primary malignancy a nodule with a sharp contour is more likely to represent a metastatic lesion than is a nodule with a less well-defined, hazy border. However, this distinction is somewhat controversial [23]. Other potentially distinguishing characteristics, such as anatomic location and distribution, have not been demonstrated to be useful in the differentiating benign from malignant nodules.

Chest Wall Neoplasms

Benign Soft-Tissue Lesions

Lipomas are benign masses consisting of adipose tissue that commonly occurs in the chest wall. Lipoblastoma is a tumor of fetal embryonic fat; despite its rapid growth it is typically benign. After resection, a lipoblastoma can recur years later as a mature lipoma. The two lesions are typically differentiated histologically and are usually easily identified on CT or MRI by the presence of macroscopic fat within the lesion [24, 25].

Other benign neoplastic lesions include neurofibromas, discussed above, and fibromas. Fibromas associated with Gardner's syndrome are nodular subcutaneous lesions that contain hyaline or collagen. They are soft-tissue-density structures on CT and slightly T1 and T2 bright on MRI. However, histologic diagnosis is normally required [24, 26].

Mesenchymal hamartomas are benign lesions resulting from the overgrowth of normal skeletal elements of the rib (Fig. 6). They are well defined, extra-pleural, and often cystic. Hemorrhagic and cystic findings with associated fluid-fluid levels and partial calcification are said to be diagnostic [24, 27].

Vascular malformations of the chest wall are a heterogeneous group of congenital lesions that include venous sascular malformations, hemangiomas, arteriovenous malformations/fistula, and lymphatic malformations (Fig. 7). A complete discussion of vascular malformations is beyond the scope of this review. However, vascular malformations can typically be diagnosed based on their avidly bright signal on T2 weighted MRI sequences as well as their prominent vascular flow. Phleboliths can often be seen with venous malformations. In most cases, the dynamic contrast enhancement features of vascular malformations readily allow their differentiation [28].

Malignant Soft-Tissue Lesions

Rhabdomyosarcoma is the most common pediatric sarcoma, although it is generally uncommon in the chest wall (Fig. 8). Rhabdomyosarcoma accounts for 2–4% of pediatric malignancies. On imaging, it presents as an enhancing, aggressive mass with imaging characteristics similar to that of skeletal muscle [24, 28].

Neuroblastoma can also occur in the chest wall in addition to the posterior mediastinum and has similar imaging characteristics.

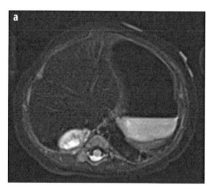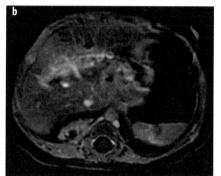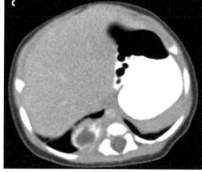

Fig. 6 a-c. A 16-year-old male with a chest wall hamartoma of the right lower chest. **a** Axial T2 fat-saturated image shows a heterogeneous, partially cystic mass, initially mistaken for a neuroblastoma; **b** axial post-contrast MRI; **c** axial post-contrast CT through the lesion

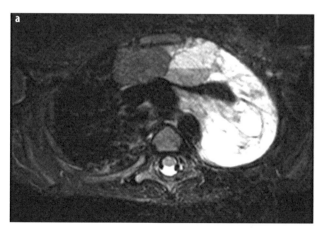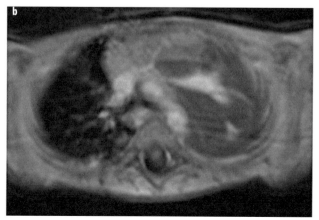

Fig. 7 a, b. A large lymphangioma extending from the mediastinum into the left chest on axial T2 fat-saturated sequence (**a**) and axial post-contrast MRI sequence (**b**)

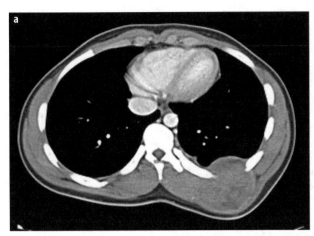
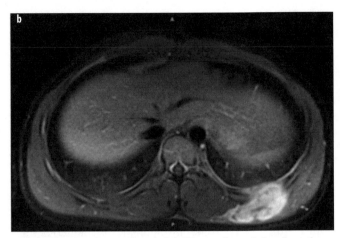

Fig. 8 a, b. A 16-year-old male with an alveolar rhabdomyosarcoma of the left posterior chest wall. **a** Axial CT scan through the chest shows a soft-tissue mass arising from the soft tissues of the right back. **b** Axial post-contrast MRI of the lesion shows avid contrast enhancement

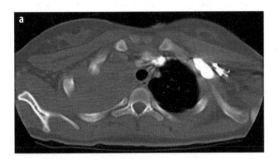
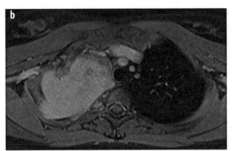
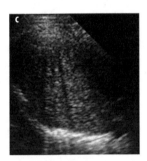

Fig. 9 a-c. A 15-year old female with a mass arising from right first rib, found to be Ewing's sarcoma. Axial CT (**a**), axial post-contrast MRI (**b**), and focused ultrasound (**c**) examinations

Small Round Blue Cell Tumors

Small round blue cell tumors, including Ewing's sarcoma and primitive neuroectodermal tumors (PNETs), can occur in the chest wall in both osseous and extraosseous locations (Fig. 9). These are collectively referred to as Askin tumors of the chest wall [24]. One-third of extraosseous Ewing's tumors and half of PNETs present in the chest wall. Both lesions are typically heterogeneous, enhancing lesions on CT and MRI [28]. However, the imaging appearance of either lesion is non-specific and histologic correlation is required for a definitive diagnosis. Cross-sectional imaging is useful for demarcating the extent of disease [29].

Osseous Neoplasms

Osseous malignancies such as osteosarcoma can occur in the chest wall and the spine, just as they do in other portions of the body. In particular, in the pediatric population, leukemia should be considered when multiple osseous lesions are seen. Osseous lymphoma is also a consideration when an osseous lesion is seen in children. However, it should be noted that primary osseous lymphoma is relatively uncommon in children [29].

Langerhans cell histiocytosis is a multisystem disease characterized by the proliferation of bone-marrow-derived Langerhans cells and eosinophils. Imaging features include lytic, expansive bone lesions that are typically T2 bright and T1 dark [30].

Conclusions

Pediatric chest neoplasms are a heterogeneous group of diseases. They can arise from any structure within the pediatric chest. Differentiation between malignant and benign processes such as congenital abnormalities is of essential importance. Overall, primary pediatric pulmonary malignancies are uncommon. However, mediastinal masses and chest wall masses are not and should prompt a thorough investigation.

References

1. Kuhn JP, Slovis TL, Haller JO et al (2004) Caffey's pediatric diagnostic imaging, 10th ed. Mosby, Philadelphia, PA.
2. Haller JO, Schneider M, Kassner EG et al (1980) Sonographic evaluation of the chest in infants and children. AJR Am J Roentgenol 134:1019-1027.

3. Siegel MJ, Acharyya S, Hoffer FA et al (2013) Whole-body MR imaging for staging of malignant tumors in pediatric patients: results of the American College of Radiology Imaging Network 6660 Trial. Radiology 266:599-609.

4. Merten DF (1992) Diagnostic imaging of mediastinal masses in children. AJR Am J Roentgenol 158:825-32.

5. King RM, Telander RL, Smithson WA et al (1982) Primary mediastinal tumors in children. J Pediatr Surg 17:512-520.

6. Franco A, Mody NS, and Meza MP (2005) Imaging evaluation of pediatric mediastinal masses. Radiol Clin North Am 43:325-353.

7. Shamberger RC, Holzman RS, Griscom NT et al (1991) CT quantitation of tracheal cross-sectional area as a guide to the surgical and anesthetic management of children with anterior mediastinal masses. J Pediatr Surg 26:138-142.

8. Shin MS, Ho KJ (1983) Computed tomography of primary mediastinal seminomas. J Comput Assist Tomogr 7:990-994.

9. Juanpere S, Canete N, Ortuno P et al (2013) A diagnostic approach to the mediastinal masses. Insights Imaging 4:29-52.

10. Gaerte SC, Meyer CA, Winer-Muram HT et al (2002) Fat-containing lesions of the chest. Radiographics 22 Spec No:S61-78.

11. St Amour TE, Siegel MJ, Glazer HS et al (1987) CT appearances of the normal and abnormal thymus in childhood. J Comput Assist Tomogr 11:645-650.

12. Mishra SK, Melinkeri SR, Dabadghao S (2001) Benign thymic hyperplasia after chemotherapy for acute myeloid leukemia. Eur J Haematol 67:252-254.

13. Becker AE (2000) Primary heart tumors in the pediatric age group: a review of salient pathologic features relevant for clinicians. Pediatr Cardiol 21:317-323.

14. Mader MT, Poulton TB, White RD (1997) Malignant tumors of the heart and great vessels: MR imaging appearance. Radiographics 17:145-153.

15. Lee JKT (2006) Computed body tomography with MRI correlation, 4th Ed. Lippincott Williams & Wilkins, Philadelphia, PA.

16. Lonergan GJ, Schwab CM, Suarez ES et al (2002) Neuroblastoma, ganglioneuroblastoma, and ganglioneuroma: radiologic-pathologic correlation. Radiographics 22:911-934.

17. Sofka CM, Semelka RC, Kelekis NL et al (1999) Magnetic resonance imaging of neuroblastoma using current techniques. Magn Reson Imaging 17:193-198.

18. Daldrup HE, Link TM, Wortler K et al (1998) MR imaging of thoracic tumors in pediatric patients. AJR Am J Roentgenol 170:1639-1644.

19. Senac MO, Jr., Wood BP, Isaacs H et al (1991) Pulmonary blastoma: a rare childhood malignancy. Radiology 179:743-746.

20. McCarville MB (2010) Malignant pulmonary and mediastinal tumors in children: differential diagnoses. Cancer Imaging 10 Spec no A:S35-41.

21. Neville HL, Hogan AR, Zhuge Y et al (2009) Incidence and outcomes of malignant pediatric lung neoplasms. J Surg Res 156:224-230.

22. Chong S, Lee KS, Chung MJ et al (2006) Neuroendocrine tumors of the lung: clinical, pathologic, and imaging findings. Radiographics 26:41-57.

23. McCarville MB, Lederman HM, Santana VM et al (2006) Distinguishing benign from malignant pulmonary nodules with helical chest CT in children with malignant solid tumors. Radiology 239:514-520.

24. Watt AJ (2002) Chest wall lesions. Paediatr Respir Rev 3:328-338.

25. Whyte AM and Powell N (1990) Mediastinal lipoblastoma of infancy. Clin Radiol 42:205-206.

26. Jabra AA, Taylor GA (1993) MRI evaluation of superficial soft tissue lesions in children. Pediatr Radiol 23:425-428.

27. Groom KR, Murphey MD, Howard LM et al (2002) Mesenchymal hamartoma of the chest wall: radiologic manifestations with emphasis on cross-sectional imaging and histopathologic comparison. Radiology 222:205-211.

28. David EA, Marshall MB (2011) Review of chest wall tumors: a diagnostic, therapeutic, and reconstructive challenge. Semin Plast Surg 25:16-24.

29. Faro SH, Mahboubi S, Ortega W (1993) CT diagnosis of rib anomalies, tumors, and infection in children. Clin Imaging 17:1-7.

30. Hashmi MA, Haque N, Chatterjee A et al (2012) Langerhans cell histiocytosis of long bones: MR imaging and complete follow up study. J Cancer Res Ther 8:286-288.

Pediatric Cardiovascular Diseases

Edward Y. Lee

Department of Radiology, Boston Children's Hospital and Harvard Medical School, Boston, MA, USA

Introduction

Cardiovascular diseases are important causes of morbidity and mortality in the pediatric population. Affected infants and children usually present with various clinical manifestations and imaging evaluation is often essential for early and accurate diagnosis. However, due to the inherent complexity of cardiovascular disease particularly in pediatric patients, imaging assessment continues to be a challenge for many radiologists. Therefore, the overarching goal of this chapter is to review the current imaging algorithm and techniques as well as the characteristic imaging appearance of some of the more commonly encountered congenital cardiovascular diseases in the pediatric population. Clear knowledge of underlying etiologies and their characteristic imaging appearances of pediatric cardiovascular diseases can help radiologists avoid potential pitfalls and render a more timely and accurate diagnosis.

Imaging Algorithm and Imaging Techniques

Three main radiological imaging modalities currently used in the evaluation of infants and children with congenital cardiovascular diseases are chest radiograph, computed tomography (CT), and magnetic resonance imaging (MRI) [1]. Echocardiography, which is helpful for real-time assessment of the intracardiac structures, with excellent temporal and spatial resolution, is typically within the domain of cardiologists rather than radiologists. Therefore, the following sections focus on radiographs, CT, and MRI.

Chest Radiographs

Chest radiograph is currently the initial imaging modality of choice for the infant or child with clinically suspected cardiovascular diseases. Standard chest posteroanterior and lateral views are useful for the optimal evaluation of cardiovascular diseases in children. For neonates and infants, in whom the lateral chest radiograph cannot be easily obtained, an anteroposterior view chest radiograph may suffice. Although the radiographic findings of cardiovascular diseases, particularly in cases of complex congenital heart diseases, may be varied and non-specific, some congenital cardiovascular conditions, such as transposition of the great arteries (TGA), Ebstein's anomaly, tetralogy of Fallot (TOF), and scimitar syndrome, have a classic radiographic appearance, as described later in this chapter [2].

Computed Tomography

In recent years, technical advances and the wide availability of CT angiography (CTA) have had a substantial impact on imaging evaluation of cardiovascular diseases in the pediatric population. In fact, CTA has largely replaced conventional diagnostic catheter-based angiography in this setting. Although CT is associated with potentially harmful ionizing radiation and nephrotoxic iodinated contrast media, careful attention to the proper selection of technical factors and optimal use of currently available dose reduction techniques can enable successful pediatric CTA with low radiation doses in the range of 1–3 mSv or less [3]. Common clinical indications of pediatric CTA include imaging evaluation of congenital mediastinal vascular anomalies (i.e., vascular rings and sling) and anomalous pulmonary veins [4]. In addition, CT can be used as an ancillary study to echocardiography or MRI in pediatric patients with limited acoustic window or indwelling MRI-incompatible metals. Specific CT technical factors depend on the type of CT scanners; however, in general, thin collimation (<1 mm), the lowest possible kilovoltage, weight- or age-based low-dose milliamperage, and pitch <1.5 can be used to evaluate most congenital (extra-cardiac and non-coronary) cardiovascular diseases [3, 4]. For the evaluation of intracardiac structures or anomalies of the coronary arteries, electrocardiographic gating is usually needed. Once an axial CT dataset is obtained, 2D and 3D reformatted CT images, which increase both diagnostic accuracy and the confidence level of detecting cardiovascular anomalies, can be generated.

Diseases of the Chest and Heart 2015-2018,
DOI: 10.1007/978-88-470-5752-4_30 © Springer-Verlag Italia 2015

Magnetic Resonance Imaging

Both anatomic and functional information on cardiovascular diseases can be obtained with MRI. It is a particularly useful imaging technique due to the lack of ionizing radiation exposure, unlike CT. Static spin echo "black blood" sequences (T1/T2) or cine gradient echo "bright blood" sequences (2D steady state free precession) are useful for evaluating cardiovascular morphology [1, 5]. Extracardiac thoracic vasculature can be assessed with spin echo black blood techniques. If there is a need for a dynamic assessment of the thoracic vessels, cine gradient echo imaging can be acquired throughout the cardiac cycle [1, 5]. Contrast-enhanced 3D magnetic resonance angiography (MRA), which can provide superb morphological evaluation of the thoracic vasculature with time resolved techniques, is useful in pediatric patients with underlying cardiovascular diseases [1, 5]. In fact, compared to CTA, MRA has the advantage of superior tissue characterization and direct multiplanar imaging. Furthermore, newer 3T MRA scanners can deliver improved signal-to-noise ratio, which can be traded for higher resolution and for decreased overall scanning times when a parallel imaging technique is employed. Once the MRA dataset is obtained, maximum intensity projection and 3D magnetic resonance images can enhance the visualization of cardiovascular anomalies and abnormalities.

Spectrum of Imaging Findings

This review focuses on congenital cardiovascular diseases that are considered to be of widespread clinical relevance and of current importance in pediatric cardiovascular imaging. These diseases include coarctation of the aorta, cardiac septal defects, TGA, Ebstein's anomaly, TOF, vascular rings and sling, and partial anomalous pulmonary venous return.

Coarctation of the Aorta

Coarctation of the aorta is the most common congenital anomaly of the thoracic aorta, occurring in 0.04% of newborns [5–7]. It is characterized by the presence of congenital narrowing of the aorta near the region where the ductus or ligamentum (after regression) arteriosus inserts (Fig. 1). Coarctation of the aorta is seen in approximately 7% of patients with congenital heart disease and has a strong male predominance (male-to-female ratio of 4:1) [5–7]. Although it has been historically categorized into two types: infantile (i.e., preductal) and adult (i.e., postductal) [5–7], this categorization is currently not favored because all aortic coarctations are juxtaductal in location, with various degrees and extension of aortic narrowing. Affected neonates typically present with congestive heart failure whereas affected older children usually come to medical attention during the evaluation of arterial hypertension in the upper extremities and normal-to-decreased blood pressure in the lower extremities [5–7].

In neonates with coarctation of the aorta, increased pulmonary vascularity with cardiomegaly is often seen on chest radiographs. In older children with delayed diagnosis of aortic coarctation, the "figure of 3" sign, which reflects pre-stenotic dilatation of the aortic arch and left subclavian artery, indentation at the coarctation site, and post-stenotic dilatation of the descending aorta, may be present [5-7]. Other typical concomitant findings are collateral

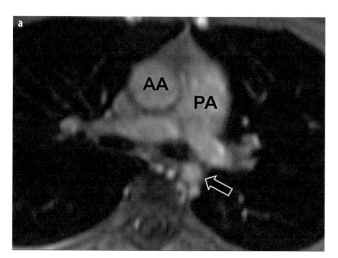
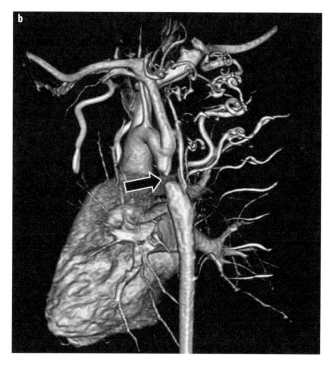

Fig. 1 a, b. Coarctation of the aorta in an 11-year-old male who presented with upper extremity hypertension. **a** Axial MRI shows a normal sized ascending aorta (*AA*) and a markedly small descending aorta (*arrow*) in the region of the aortic coarctation. *PA*, pulmonary artery. **b** 3D volume rendered image demonstrates marked focal narrowing (*arrow*) of the descending aorta, consistent with aortic coarctation. Enlarged collateral vessels, including those of the internal mammary artery and intercostal arteries, are also seen

vessel formations, including those of the internal mammary, intercostal, and superior epigastric arteries (Fig. 1b). In particular, enlarged intercostal arteries can result in the development of rib-notching under the posterolateral aspects of the fourth to eighth ribs [5–7]. Additionally, the bicuspid valve can be seen in 25–50% of patients with aortic coarctation [5–7]. In the evaluation of coarctation of the aorta using cross-sectional imaging studies such as multidetector CT, multiplanar (2D) and 3D images performed better than axial CT images alone [8].

Three currently used management options for aortic coarctation include surgical resection of the narrowed segment followed by primary end-to-end anastomosis, balloon angioplasty, and placement of a vascular stent. Imaging evaluation also plays an important role in the evaluation of residual or recurrent aortic coarctation as well as complications such as aortic dissection or pseudoaneurysm formation [5–7].

Cardiac Septal Defect

Cardiac septal defect refers to a hole or discontinuation in either the atrial or the ventricular septum, or both. Affected pediatric patients with small septal defects come to attention because of murmur on physical examination. By contrast, affected pediatric patients with moderate to large septal defects typically present early in life (1–3 months) with congestive heart failure due to pulmonary arterial overcirculation, which results from left-to-right shunt via the septal defect.

Ventricular Septal Defect

Ventricular septal defect (VSD) is the second most common congenital cardiac malformation, accounting for approximately 20% of all congenital cardiac anomalies [1–3]. On physical examination, systolic murmur is present because blood flow across the VSD is primarily during systole. Based on the location of the defect, VSD is classified into four different types: (1) subpulmonary type, caused by a deficiency of the conal septum; (2) membranous type, in which the defect is located posterior to the septal leaflet of the tricuspid valve; (3) atrioventricular canal, which is caused by a deficiency of the endocardial cushion component of the interventricular septum; and (4) muscular, which is the most common type of VSD and can occur in any portion of the muscular septum.

Although chest radiographs may be normal in affected pediatric patients with small VSDs, increased pulmonary vascularity due to an underlying left-to-right shunt (i.e., shunt vascularity), an enlarged main pulmonary artery, biventricular enlargement, and left atrial enlargement are present on chest radiographs in pediatric patients with moderate to large VSDs (Fig. 2). Shunt vascularity refers to an increase in the number and caliber of pulmonary vessels resulting from the increased arterial flow. CT and MRI can directly show the discontinuation of the ventricular septum in affected patients.

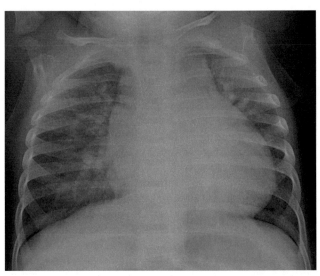

Fig. 2. Ventricular septal defect in a 13-month-old male. Chest radiograph shows increased pulmonary vascularity and cardiomegaly

While small VSDs (also called restrictive VSDs) often close spontaneously or can be managed with a percutaneous septal occlusion device, hemodynamically significant moderate to large VSD are usually treated surgically with a patch graft. Infectious endocarditis is a potential complication of untreated VSD.

Atrial Septal Defect

Atrial septal defect (ASD) is the most common shunt lesion detected in adults, accounting for approximately 10% of congenital heart anomalies [1–3].

On physical examination, diastolic murmur is present because blood flow across the VSD is primarily during diastole. Based on the location of the defect, there are three subtypes of ASD: (1) ostium primum, in which the defect is located in the anteroinferior portion of the septum; (2) ostium secundum, in which it is located in the midportion of the atrial septum; and (3) sinus venous defect, in which the defect is located at the superior portion of the interatrial septum, near the superior vena cava (SVC).

Although chest radiographs can be normal in affected pediatric patients with small ASDs, increased pulmonary vascularity due to underlying left-to-right shunt, an enlarged main pulmonary artery, right heart enlargement, and a normal size left atrium and aorta are typically seen in patients with moderate to large ASDs (Fig. 3a). CT and MRI can directly show the exact location and extent of an ASD as well as associated anomalies, such as anomalous drainage of the right superior pulmonary vein, which is highly associated with ASD of the sinus venous defect type (Fig. 3b).

Small ASDs often close on their own during infancy or early childhood or they can be managed with a septal occlusion device [9]. Surgical repair is typically necessary for managing large or multiple ASDs.

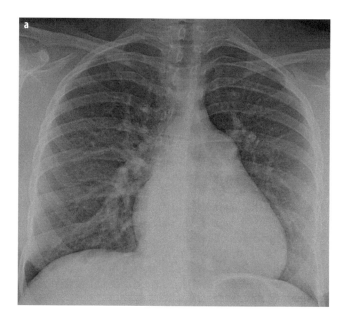

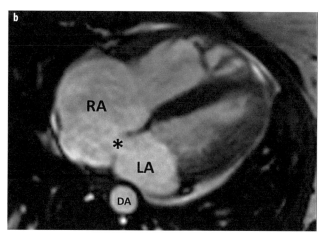

Fig. 3 a, b. Atrial septal defect in a 14-year-old female. **a** Chest radiograph shows increased pulmonary vascularity, a dilated main pulmonary artery, and cardiomegaly. **b** Axial MRI demonstrates an atrial septal defect (*asterisk*) along with enlargement of the right atrium (*RA*). *LA*, left atrium; *DA*, descending aorta

Transposition of the Great Arteries

TGA refers to a congenital malformation of the great arteries in which they are reversed in their origins from the heart (Fig. 4). There are two different types of TGA: D-transposition of the great arteries (D-TGA) and L-transposition of the great arteries (L-TGA) [1–3]. In D-TGA, the aorta arises from the morphologic systemic right ventricle and the pulmonary artery arises from the morphologic systemic right ventricle, resulting in ventricular arterial discordance. The pulmonary and systemic circulations exist in parallel, requiring bidirectional shunting between the two sides of the heart via an ASD, VSD, patent ductus arteriosus (PDA), or patent foramen ovale for survival. By contrast, congenitally corrected TGA, or L-TGA, is characterized by both ventriculoarterial and atrioventricular discordance. The pulmonary and systemic circulations are

in series rather than in parallel as in D-TGA. Systemic venous return flows to the right atrium, enters the morphologic left ventricle, and is eventually delivered to the pulmonary circulation via the main pulmonary artery. Pulmonary venous return subsequently flows to the left atrium, enters the morphologic right ventricle, and is delivered to the systemic circulation via the aorta. While patients with D-TGA usually present with cyanosis during the first day of life, those with L-TGA are typically asymptomatic.

On chest radiographs, increased pulmonary vascularity and mild to moderate cardiomegaly are usually seen in patients with D-TGA [1–3]. Additionally, the superior mediastinum is narrowed because of the abnormal position of the great vessels and a concave main pulmonary artery. The constellation of these findings results in the radiographic appearance of the cardiomediastinal silhouette, referred to as the "egg-on-a-string sign" [2]. CTA or MRA is useful for the assessment of postoperative complications including narrowing of the anastomosis of the aorta or pulmonary artery in addition to branch pulmonary artery stenosis and coronary artery narrowing.

Corrective surgery via a Jatene "arterial switch" procedure is required for managing patients with D-TGA in the first few days of life [1–3] (Fig. 5). By contrast, patients with congenitally corrected L-TGA may require pacemaker placement for progressive right ventricular dysfunction and conduction abnormalities in later life.

Ebstein's Anomaly

Ebstein's anomaly is the most common cause of marked cardiomegaly in the newborn period. It is characterized by the displacement of the septal and posterior leaflets of the tricuspid valve towards the apex of the right ventricle of the heart [10]. This results in "atrialization" of a portion of the morphologic right ventricle and subsequent

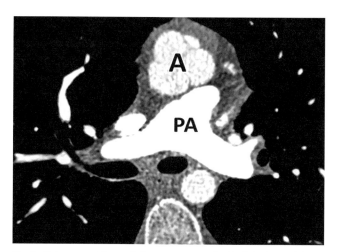

Fig. 4. D-transposition of the great vessels (D-TGA). Axial CT shows the aorta (*A*) located anterior to the pulmonary artery (*PA*)

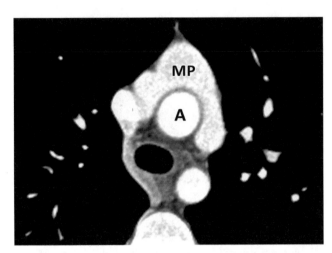

Fig. 5. Jatene procedure. Axial CT after an "arterial switch procedure" for TGA shows characteristic draping of the main pulmonary artery (*MP*) around the aorta (*A*)

enlargement of the right atrium and a reduction in the size of the anatomic right ventricle [10]. This condition may be an isolated finding or associated with other congenital heart defects, such as a patent foramen ovale or an atrial septal defect, allow the passage of a right-to-left shunt. Although patients with mild Ebstein's anomaly may be asymptomatic, in those with severer forms of the disease cyanosis and systolic murmur are often present [10].

On radiographs, decreased pulmonary vascularity, a concave pulmonary artery segment, and marked cardiomegaly due to underlying right atrial enlargement are characteristically seen [2, 10] (Fig. 6a). In affected patients with concomitant PDA, the pulmonary vascularity may be increased. CT and MRI can better demonstrate a small right ventricle and atrialized right ventricle (Fig. 6b), and MRI is better than echocardiography

in visualizing the morphology of the anterior leaflet of the tricuspid valve and right ventricular free wall.

Tricuspid annulopasty and plication of the atrialized portion of the right ventricle are the current management procedures of choice for symptomatic pediatric patients with severe Ebstein's anomaly.

Tetralogy of Fallot

Four anomalies of the cardiac structures comprise TOF: VSD, infundibular pulmonary stenosis, an overriding aorta, and right ventricular hypertrophy. It is the most common congenital heart defect resulting in cyanosis. A right aortic arch with a mirror-image branching, peripheral pulmonary arterial stenosis, and an anomalous anterior descending coronary artery that courses over the right ventricular outflow tract are also often associated with TOF. Affected pediatric patients typically present with cyanosis in the first 6 months of life.

The radiographic findings of TOF vary according to the severity of the obstruction of the pulmonary outflow tract. The classic appearance of TOF is a "boot-shaped" heart due to an underlying right-sided aortic arch, a small or concave main pulmonary artery, and right ventricular hypertrophy [2] (Fig. 7). Pulmonary vascularity can be either normal or diminished. The heart size is usually normal. However, increased pulmonary vascularity and cardiomegaly similar to that in patients with VSD can be seen in affected patients with very mild pulmonary stenosis, which is sometimes referred to as a pink tetralogy. MRI can be useful for evaluating the morphology and function of the cardiac chambers, calculating blood flow and velocities through the vessels to determine the presence of regurgitation, stenoses, and relative flow, and mapping collateral vessels in affected patients with pulmonary atresia [1, 2].

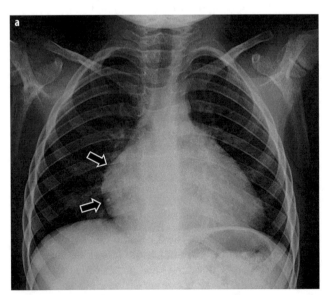

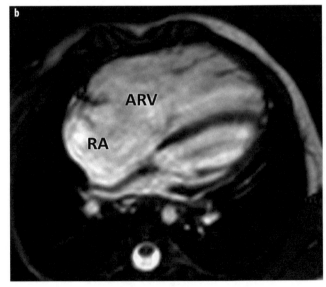

Fig. 6 a, b. Ebstein's anomaly in a 4-year-old female. **a** Chest radiograph shows decreased pulmonary vascularity and cardiomegaly with a prominent right heart (*arrows*). **b** Axial MRI demonstrates a large atrialized superior right ventricle (*ARV*). *RA*, right atrium

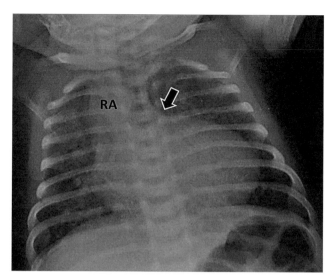

Fig. 7. Tetralogy of Fallot in a 3-day-old male. Chest radiograph shows uplifting of the cardiac apex and decreased underlying pulmonary vascularity. Concavity (*arrow*) is also seen in the region where the main pulmonary artery should be. Also note that the trachea is displaced toward the left side by the right aortic arch (*RA*)

After initial palliative surgery using a Blalock-Taussig anastomosis via the subclavian artery to the pulmonary artery, definitive surgical repair focuses on relieving the right ventricular outflow obstruction and closing the septal defect. During surgery, it is important to carefully assess the coronary arteries because an anomalous anterior descending coronary artery that courses over the right ventricular outflow tract can be present in pediatric patients with TOF and mistakenly incised at surgery.

Vascular Rings and Sling

Vascular rings and sling are congenital anomalies of the aortic arch and pulmonary artery. They account for 1–3%

of all congenital heart disease [4–6, 8, 11, 12]. Although relatively rare, they are important causes of respiratory and swallowing symptoms due to compression of the trachea and/or esophagus in infants and young children. Chest radiograph and esophagram may be used for the initial evaluation. More detailed preoperative assessment of vascular anomalies and associated large-airway malformation can be achieved with CT or MRI [4–6, 8, 12]. The three main types of vascular rings and sling are: double aortic arch, right aortic arch with an aberrant left subclavian artery, and pulmonary artery sling, which are discussed in the following sections.

Double Aortic Arch

The double aortic arch results from persistence of the right dorsal aorta and is the most common symptomatic vascular ring. In this aortic vascular anomaly, the ascending aorta bifurcates into the right and left aortic arches which encircle the trachea and esophagus and join together posteriorly to form a single descending aorta [4–6, 8, 12] (Fig. 8a). Each aortic arch gives rise to its own common ceratoid and subclavian arteries. The right aortic arch is usually larger in size and higher in position than the left aortic arch. Sometimes, an atretic segment of either right or left aortic arch is present. The double aortic arch is rarely associated with other congenital heart anomalies, which include TOF, VSD, and TGA. Affected patients typically present in the first 3 months of life.

On chest radiographs, bilateral paratracheal opacities representing two aortic arches and narrowing of the midline positioned trachea are typically seen. Bilateral indentations are seen on frontal esophagogram, and posterior compression of the esophagus on lateral esophagogram. CT and MRI with multiplanar and 3D reconstruction of the mediastinal vessels and large airway are useful for preoperative and postoperative assessments

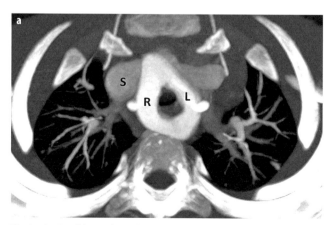

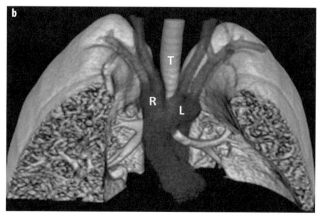

Fig. 8 a, b. Double aortic arch in a 4-month old male who presented with stridor and repeated apnea. **a** Axial maximum intensity projection image shows a double aortic arch (*R*, right arch; *L*, left arch; *S*, superior vena cava). **b** 3D volume-rendered image demonstrates a double aortic arch (*R*, right arch; *L*, left arch) surrounding the trachea (*T*)

[4–6, 8, 12, 13] (Fig. 8b). In particular, paired inspiratory and expiratory multi-detector CT should be considered as part of the routine preoperative evaluation of tracheomalacia (TM) in pediatric patients with double aortic arch because 33.3% of these patients have underlying concomitant TM [14].

The double aortic arch in symptomatic pediatric patients is currently treated with surgical division of the smaller of the two aortic arches. When concomitant TM is present, surgical repair of the trachea is also required [12, 13, 15].

Right Aortic Arch with an Aberrant Left Subclavian Artery

The right aortic arch with an aberrant subclavian artery is the second most common vascular ring in the pediatric population. Embryologically, it is due to persistence of the right dorsal aorta, regression of the left dorsal aorta, and regression at the left fourth aortic arch [4–6, 8, 12]. In this condition, the aorta is located on the right side of the spine and the left subclavian artery comes off the descending aorta, crosses the midline, and enters the left hemithorax (Fig. 9a). The ligamentum arteriosum (i.e., the remnant of the ductus arteriosus), which originates from a bulbous dilatation at the base of the left subclavian artery (the diverticulum of Kommerell) and attaches to the left pulmonary artery, is also present. The trachea and esophagus are encircled by the aortic arch on the right, the ligamentum arteriosum and the left pulmonary artery on the left, the ascending aorta anteriorly, and the descending aorta posteriorly [4–6, 12].

On the frontal chest radiograph, a right paratracheal opacity representing the right-sided aortic arch and an absent left-sided aortic arch shadow are characteristic. The right-sided compression or left-sided deviation of the trachea at the level of the right aortic arch and an aberrant left subclavian artery are also seen. Right-sided indenta-

tion of the esophagus is seen on frontal esophagogram, and oblique compression of the posterior esophagus on lateral esophagogram. The entire course of the right aortic arch, the aberrant left subclavian artery, and tracheal compression are best evaluated with CT and MRI with multiplanar and 3D reconstruction [4–6, 12, 15] (Fig. 9b). Surgical division of underlying vascular ring is the current management procedure of choice in symptomatic pediatric patients with right aortic arch with an aberrant left subclavian artery [4–6, 12].

Pulmonary Artery Sling

In pulmonary artery sling, also known as anomalous left pulmonary artery, the left pulmonary artery arises from the right pulmonary artery [16, 17] (Fig. 10). Embryologically, it is due to the regression or failure of devel-

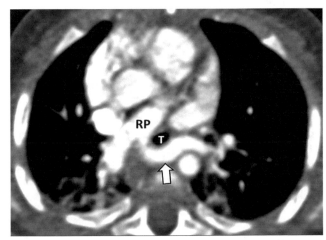

Fig. 10. Pulmonary artery sling in a 2-day-old female who presented with severe respiratory distress. Axial CT shows an anomalous left pulmonary artery (*arrow*) arising from the right main pulmonary artery (*RP*). *T*, Trachea

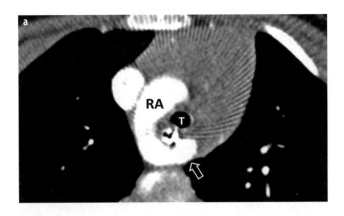

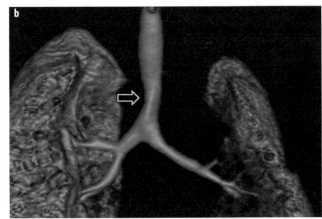

Fig. 9 a, b. Right aortic arch with an aberrant left subclavian artery in a 2-year-old female who presented with respiratory distress. **a** Axial CT shows a right aortic arch (*RA*) with an aberrant left subclavian artery (*arrow*). Note the nasogastric tube in the esophagus. *T*, trachea. **b** 3D volume rendered image demonstrates the exact location, degree, and extent of the tracheal compression (*arrow*) caused by a right aortic arch and an aberrant left subclavian artery

opment of the left pulmonary artery [4, 16, 17]. The anomalous left pulmonary artery courses between the trachea and esophagus on its way to the left side after arising from the right pulmonary artery. This can lead to extrinsic compression of the distal trachea and/or right main stem bronchus, and thus in respiratory distress. Intrinsic large airway anomalies such as TM and tracheal stenosis as well as right lung agenesis may also be present concomitantly [16, 17].

On frontal chest radiograph, either a hyperinflated or atelectatic right lung, depending on the degree of right main stem bronchial narrowing, is seen. On lateral chest radiograph or esophagogram, anterior displacement of the trachea and posterior displacement of the esophagus due to an anomalous left pulmonary artery are characteristically seen. CT and MRI with multiplanar and 3D reconstruction of the mediastinal vessels and large airway can demonstrate the entire course of an anomalous left pulmonary artery and an associated large airway narrowing or stenosis [4, 13, 15–17].

Surgical reimplantation of the left pulmonary artery and tracheal reconstruction in case of tracheal stenosis or TM are current treatment options in symptomatic patients [12, 15, 17].

Partial Anomalous Pulmonary Venous Return

In partial anomalous pulmonary venous return (PAPVR), some, but not all of the pulmonary veins have aberrant drainage into systemic veins or the right atrium [6, 16]. This condition results in a left-to-right cardiac shunt and the admixture of deoxygenated and oxygenated blood. PAPVR may be an isolated finding but it is often associated with other congenital cardiac or lung anomalies. Affected pediatric patients often present with respiratory distress, tachypnea, feeding intolerance, and failure to thrive. Depending on the degree of underlying shunting, the patient may also present with cyanosis. In addition, patients with associated lung anomalies may clinically present with recurrent lung infections.

PAPVR commonly involves the left superior, right inferior, and right superior pulmonary veins [6, 16]. In left superior PAPVR, the anomalous left superior pulmonary

vein drains into the left brachiocephalic or innominate vein, creating a vertical vein positioned lateral to the left superior mediastinum (Fig. 11). On chest radiographs, left superior mediastinal widening is seen. In case of the scimitar, or hypogenetic lung syndrome, which is a special form of anomalous pulmonary venous return from the lung that is associated with a hypoplastic lung, a vertically oriented, curvilinear opacity representing the scimitar vein, projecting over the lower hemithorax and ipsilateral hypoplastic lung, is seen on chest radiographs [6, 16] (Figs. 12, 13). In case of right superior PAPVR, CT and MRI can show an anomalous vein that usually drains into the SVC and an associated sinus venosus

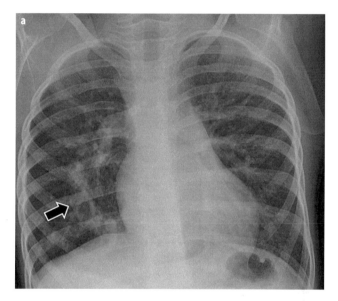

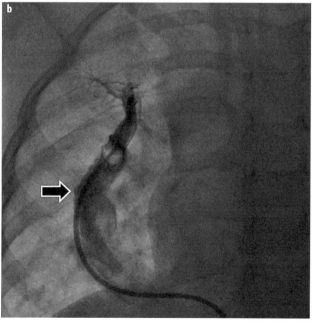

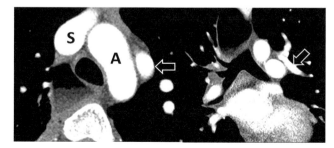

Fig. 11. Left upper lobe partial anomalous pulmonary venous return in a 17-year-old male. Axial (right) and coronal (left) CT show an anomalous left upper lobe partial anomalous pulmonary vein (*arrows*). *A*, aorta; *S*, superior vena cava

Fig. 12 a, b. Scimitar syndrome in a 3-year-old female. **a** Chest radiograph shows a curvilinear opacity (*arrow*) in the right lower lobe, representing the anomalous draining vein. **b** Angiography demonstrates an anomalous draining vein (*arrow*)

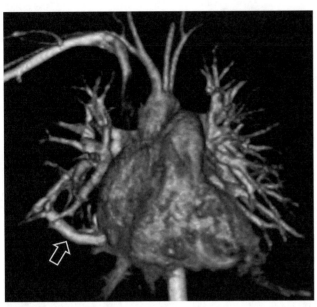

Fig. 13. Scimitar syndrome in a 2-year-old male. 3D volume rendered image shows the anomalous vein from the right lower lobe (*arrow*) draining into the inferior vena cava

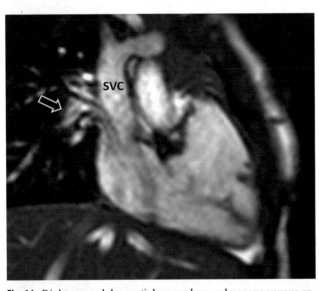

Fig. 14. Right upper lobe partial anomalous pulmonary venous return in a 7-year-old female who presented with exertional shortness of breath and mild hypoxia. Bright-blood MRA shows right upper lobe anomalous pulmonary venous return (*arrow*) into the superior vena cava (*SVC*)

ASD, which is often associated with right superior PAPVR [6] (Fig. 14).

The current management procedure of choice of PAPVR in symptomatic pediatric patients is surgical reconnection of the anomalous pulmonary vein with the atrium. Imaging plays an important role in the assessment of postoperative complications, including thrombosis or stenosis of the reimplanted anomalous vein [6, 15, 16].

Conclusion

A variety of congenital cardiovascular diseases can occur in the pediatric population. Clear knowledge of the underlying etiologies and their characteristic imaging appearances can help radiologists avoid potential pitfalls and render a more timely and accurate diagnosis in pediatric patients with cardiovascular diseases. This, in turn, will contribute to optimal pediatric patient care.

References

1. Browne LP, Krishnamurthy R, Chung T (2011) Preoperative and postoperative MR evaluation of congenital heart disease in children. Radiol Clin North Am 49:1011-1024.
2. Ferguson EC, Krishnamurthy R, Oldham SA (2007) Classic imaging sings of congenital cardiovascular anomalies. Radiographics 27:1323-1334.
3. Goo HW (2011) Cardiac MDCT in children: CT technology overview and interpretation. Radiol Clin North Am 49:997-1010.
4. Kondrachuk O, Yalynska T, Tammo R, Lee EY (2012) Multidetector computed tomography evaluation of congenital mediastinal vascular anomalies in children. Semin Roentgenol 47:127-134.
5. Lee EY, Browne LP, Lam W (2012) Noninvasive magnetic resonance imaging of thoracic large vessels in children. Semin Roentgenol 47:45-55.
6. Hellinger JC, Daubert M, Lee EY, Epelman M (2011) Congenital thoracic vascular anomalies: evaluation with state-of-the-art MR imaging and MDCT. Radiol Clin North Am 49:969-996.
7. Tawes RL Jr, Aberdeen E, Waterston DJ et al (1969) Coarctation of the aorta in infants and children. A review of 333 operative cases, including 179 infants. Circulation 39 (5 Suppl 1):l173-184.
8. Lee EY, Siegel MJ, Hildebolt CF et al (2004) MDCT evaluation of thoracic aortic anomalies in pediatric patients and young adults: comparison of axial, multiplanar, and 3D images. AJR Am J Roentgenol 182:777-784.
9. Lee EY, Siegel MJ, Chu CM et al (2004) Amplatzer atrial septal defect occlude for pediatric patients: radiographic appearance. Radiology 233:471-476.
10. Galea J, Ellul S, Schembri A et al (2014) Ebstein anomaly: a review. Neonatal Netw 33:268-274.
11. Woods RK, Sharp RJ, Holcom GW 3rd et al (2001) Vascular anomalies and tracheoesophageal compression: a single institution's 25-year experience. Ann Thorac Surg 72:434-438.
12. Lee EY, Boiselle PM, Shamberger RC (2010) Multidetector computed tomography and 3-dimensional imaging: preoperative evaluation of thoracic vascular and tracheobronchial anomalies and abnormalities in pediatric patients. J Pediatr Surg 45:811-821.
13. Lee EY, Siegel MJ (2007) MDCT of tracheobronchial narrowing in pediatric patients. J Thorac Imaging 22:300-309.
14. Lee EY, Zurakowski D, Waltz DA et al (2008) MDCT evaluation of the prevalence of tracheomalacia in children with mediastinal aortic vascular anomalies. J Thorac Imaging 23:258-265.
15. Lee EY, Greenberg SB, Boiselle PM (2011) Multidetector computed tomography of pediatric large airway diseases: state-of-the-art. Radiol Clin North Am 49:869-893.
16. Lee EY, Boiselle PM, Cleveland RH (2008) Multidetector CT evaluation of congenital lung anomalies. Radiology 247:632-648.
17. Lee EY (2007) MDCT and 3D evaluation of type 2 hypoplastic pulmonary artery sling associated with right lung agenesis, hypoplastic aortic arch, and long segment tracheal stenosis. J Thorac Imaging 22:346-350.

The Radiology of Diffuse Interstitial Pulmonary Disease in Children: Pearls, Pitfalls and Newly Recognised Disorders

Catherine M. Owens

Cardiothoracic Imaging Department, Great Ormond Street Hospital for Children NHS Trust, London, UK

Introduction

Diffuse interstitial lung disease (ILD) represents a heterogeneous group of disorders characterised by restrictive lung function and impaired gas exchange. As these diseases occur against a background of the developing lungs and immune system, the clinical presentation and disease progression are modified compared to their adult equivalents [1]. Thus, diffuse ILD often differs markedly in presentation, clinical features, and progress from ILD in adults, and it is not safe to extrapolate from adults to children. Rather, it is important to understand the normal growth and development of the lungs in children so as to understand the development of ILD [2].

Normal Growth and Development of the Lung and Immune System

ILD may present soon after birth, which suggests an antenatal onset in some cases. Thus, an understanding of the early changes in the morphology and biology of the primitive lung is important. The mature airway pattern is determined by week 16 of gestation [3] and is driven by growth factors produced by mesenchyme and extra- cellular matrix (including fibronectin, tenascin, the integrins, syndecans, and cadherins), and epimorphin and epidermal platelet-derived and insulin-like growth factors [4, 5]. Mature alveoli begin to develop late in foetal life, but most appear in the first 2 years of life [6]. Numbers increase more slowly in later childhood, and adult levels are attained by about 8 years of age [7, 8]. Treatment with steroids and oxygen in early life has been shown to interfere with alveolar development in the rat model [9]. Data from humans suggest that only limited catch-up growth may occur in later childhood following neonatal interference with lung growth [10]. Thus, ILD and its treatment, particularly early in life, may profoundly affect long-term function.

The immune system is immature at birth and the immune-pathogenesis of ILD therefore is different in children than in adults. Briefly, T-cell receptor activation is slow in the neonate and suppressor K cell activity higher [11]. The pattern of cytokine secretion is variable: levels of production of IL-2 (interleukin 2) are controversial [12], but secretion of IL-4 and interferon-gamma is markedly reduced [13].

B-cell function is reduced, but whether this is intrinsic or secondary to reduced T-cell function is unclear. Peripheral blood monocyte function, by contrast, seems relatively mature, although alveolar macrophages may be functionally deficient [14].

Morbidity and mortality associated with paediatric ILDs are high (range 14–39%), with a higher mortality in younger infants.

The diagnosis may be delayed, but once suspected the aim is to confirm the presence and severity of ILD, to uncover any predisposing factors, and to identify the dominant pathology. Although a diagnosis without biopsy is sometimes possible, the majority of patients will require histological studies using either open lung biopsy, video-assisted thoracoscopic biopsy, or high-resolution computed tomography (HRCT)-guided percutaneous biopsy.

The general classification includes disorders of known aetiology (aspiration, chronic infection, hyper-sensitivity pneumonitis, lipid storage diseases), un-known primary pulmonary disorders with lung involvement or systemic disorders with pulmonary involvement, and finally those diseases unique to childhood.

HRCT Technique

Because the chest radiograph is often non-specific, HRCT has been shown in adults and children to increase the accuracy at diagnosis of diffuse lung disease. The trade-off in sensitivity and specificity of HRCT over chest radiography is related to radiation dose, which is significantly higher with conventional spiral or volumetric CT. However, the use of low-dose (50 mA, 0.75 s) limited (1-mm slices every 15–20 mm) HRCT in inspiration, with three expiratory supplementary scans allows accurate assessment of the presence and extent of diffuse

Diseases of the Chest and Heart 2015-2018,
DOI: 10.1007/978-88-470-5752-4_31 © Springer-Verlag Italia 2015

lung disease at a dose equivalent to approximately ten chest radiographs. Images are reconstructed based on a high spatial resolution algorithm and displayed with a wide window setting, at a width of 1,500 Hounsfield units (HU) and at a level of –500 HU.

If a child is unable to breath-hold, the scans can be performed during quiet breathing, and decubitus scans can replace expiratory scans (the dependent lung behaving as the 'expiratory lung').

The role of HRCT in paediatric ILD is evolving. In adults, the diagnostic accuracy of HRCT has led to a decrease in the number of lung biopsies. The histospecific accuracy of HRCT compared with chest radiographs in making a correct first-choice diagnosis in an adult population with diffuse lung disease ranges from 46% to 75% for HRCT and from 38% to 63% for chest radiography [15–17]. HRCT had a diagnostic accuracy of 56% for a confident first-choice diagnosis in one series of 20 children with ILD [18]. This is comparable to a more recent series of 20 children with biopsy-proven ILD from a single institution [19]. A correct first-choice diagnosis was made in 61% of the cases on HRCT compared with 34% on chest radiographs.

The diseases that were correctly diagnosed on HRCT with a high degree of confidence were alveolar proteinosis, pulmonary lymphangiectasia and idiopathic pulmonary haemosiderosis. Differentiation between non-specific interstitial pneumonitis (NSIP), desquamative interstitial pneumonitis (DIP) and lymphocytic interstitial pneumonitis (LIP) was, however, less reliable.

There are several pitfalls in the interpretation of HRCT in children. One of the most important is in distinguishing diffuse ground glass infiltration from increased lung attenuation resulting from a suboptimal inspiration. In the upper zones, the position of the posterior tracheal membrane is helpful in distinguishing between the two. The posterior tracheal membrane is convex outwards in inspiration, and appears horizontal or slightly concave on expiration. The other difficulty that may be encountered is in determining which areas of the lung are abnormal when an investigation reveals a widespread 'mosaic' pattern of lung attenuation. Deciding on whether the areas of diminished attenuation represent, for example, small airways disease or whether areas of increased attenuation (ground glass opacity) represent diffuse infiltration can be challenging. Although expiratory images may be helpful, obtaining images at known phases of respiration is usually not achievable in children. Thus, the above-mentioned use of lateral decubitus imaging CT, with the dependent lung simulating expiration, is an important tool.

HRCT Features of Diffuse Interstitial Lung Disease

Idiopathic Interstitial Pneumonitis

NSIP, DIP and LIP in childhood appear to share common CT appearances. Widespread ground glass attenuation is the most frequent feature of interstitial pneumonitis/fibrosis [20]. There are no discriminating features for the radiological appearance of DIP, which includes widespread ground glass opacification; thus, it has a wide differential diagnosis, including subacute extrinsic allergic alveolitis, opportunistic infections such as *Pneumocystis jirovecii* pneumonia and, although it is rare in children, sarcoidosis. On HRCT, ground glass opacification is the dominant pattern and often has a lower zone predominance; long-term follow-up usually shows complete resolution

Based on the few reported cases of childhood NSIP, there is a distinct pattern of involvement. In a review of CTs of six cases of biopsy-proven NSIP [21], a distinct upper zone predominance of honeycomb pattern and parenchymal distortion on a background of diffuse ground glass opacification was seen in three children. The honeycomb pattern resembled emphysematous destruction with some cystic change.

Seely et al. described a similar HRCT appearance in their review of paediatric idiopathic interstitial fibrosis [20], but did not provide pathological correlation. Ground glass opacification, honeycombing and peripheral consolidation were features seen in three other cases of childhood NSIP. In the study by Copley et al. [19], one case of DIP resembled NSIP with predominant upper lobe involvement.

The existence of UIP (usual interstitial pneumonitis) in childhood is controversial and said to be exceedingly rare. The adult form of UIP has a poor prognosis. The HRCT findings of adult UIP include a subpleural reticular pattern of honeycombing that may result eventually in thick-walled cystic spaces and irregularity of the pleural surface with underlying traction bronchiectasis and bronchiolectasis.

LIP is characterised histologically by a diffuse interstitial infiltrate of polyclonal lymphocytes, plasma cells and histocytes. LIP is associated with viral infections including Ebstein Barr virus (EBV) and the acquired immunodeficiency syndrome. LIP is present in up to 30% of children with human immunodeficiency virus (HIV) disease, especially those from the sub-Saharan African continent, where EBV is endemic. This is unlike the situation in adult HIV disease, in which LIP is rare. Other associations include autoimmune diseases and lymphoproliferative disease secondary to underlying congenital immunodeficiency.

Chest radiographs show reticulonodular change with or without areas of consolidation. HRCT shows interstitial reticulonodular change of varying degrees There is usually marked resolution of the striking radiological appearances with therapy for HIV disease; however, if there has been chronic interstitial disease, fibrosis and ensuing traction bronchiectasis may result.

Follicular bronchiolitis is a term coined to described a form of LIP in which the lymphoid aggregates congregate around the small airways.

Chronic pneumonitis of infancy is a recently described pathological entity. Its HRCT appearance was reported based on a single biopsy-proven case, in which widespread ground glass opacification without focal areas of consolidation or cystic change was seen.

Connective Tissue Disorders

The prevalence of lung disease in paediatric patients with connective tissue disorders is high. In a study by Seely et al. [20], 10 of 11 children with systemic sclerosis who underwent HRCT had evidence of ILD. HRCT features included ground glass opacification, subpleural micronodules, linear opacities and honeycomb lung (consistent with UIP histologically). Aspiration pneumonitis secondary to abnormal oesophageal peristalsis may result in acute and chronic parenchymal change with bronchiectasis.

Systemic-lupus-erythematosus-induced vasculitis manifests as patchy areas of ground glass attenuation. Cryptogenic organising pneumonia with subsequent pulmonary fibrosis has been described.

Pulmonary Alveolar Proteinosis

Congenital pulmonary alveolar proteinosis (PAP) is an inherited autosomal recessive disorder caused by surfactant protein B deficiency. This condition presents early in a full-term neonate with clinical and radio- logical features indistinguishable from hyaline membrane disease. The differential diagnosis includes congenital viral infection and neonatal fibrosing alveolitis. The recently described chronic pneumonitis of infancy, characterised by alveolar septal thickening, alveolar pneumocyte hypoplasia and an alveolar exudate containing macrophages and cellular debris, has a similar appearance.

A later form of PAP usually occurs at between a few months to several years of age [22]. Chest X-rays show bilateral air space disease with ground glass opacification. Air space filling with low-attenuation proteinacious material and a superimposed 'crazy/paving' pattern, which represents thickened interlobular septa, are characteristic HRCT features enabling a confident diagnosis to be made in most cases.

Congenital Lymphangiectasia/Diffuse Pulmonary Lymphangiomatosis

Congenital lymphangiectasia and diffuse pulmonary lymphangiomatosis represent a minority of chronic ILDs in childhood and result from the abnormal proliferation and dilatation of lymphatic channels. The CT appearances of lymphangiomatosis can be easily predicted by knowing the distribution of the lymphatic system within the lungs. The constellation of smooth thickening of the interlobular septa, peribronchial thickening, patchy ground glass opacification and increased attenuation of the mediastinal

fat with bilateral pleural effusions and pleural thickening [23] is highly suggestive of the diagnosis. The condition is related to congenital lymphangiectasia, in which there is abnormal dilatation of the lymphatics. The CT findings of these two conditions are indistinguishable.

Idiopathic Pulmonary Haemosiderosis

Idiopathic pulmonary haemosiderosis (IPH) is a rare disease occurring in children and adults. It is characterised by recurrent episodes of pulmonary haemorrhage with haemoptysis. The aetiology is unknown. The childhood form of IPH usually presents before the age of 3 years, with no specific gender prevalence [24].

On HRCT, acute haemorrhage is characterised by ground glass opacification or consolidation. In the subacute/chronic phase, discrete pulmonary nodules of uniform size can be seen throughout the lung and are a characteristic feature. Interlobular septal thickening can also occur.

Sarcoidosis

Childhood sarcoidosis is rare. There appear to be two distinct types of sarcoidosis in children [25, 26]. The majority of these patients present at 13–15 years of age with a multisystem disease inseparable from the adult type. Lymphadenopathy and pulmonary involvement are common, with systemic symptoms of fever and malaise. The HRCT appearance of this form of childhod sarcoidosis is identical to that of the adult disease.

By contrast, children under 4 years of age [25, 26] present with a distinct form of the disease, characterised by rash, uveitis and arthritis/tenosynovitis. Although pulmonary involvement has been reported, it is rare in young patients.

Extrinsic Allergic Alveolitis

Extrinsic allergic alveolitis (hypersensitivity pneumonitis) is uncommon in children and is due to an immunological response to a variety of allergens. HRCT features are identical to those seen in adults. In the acute/subacute phase, diffuse ground glass shadowing is seen in the lungs, with small, poorly defined centrilobular nodules) [27, 28]. Patchy air trapping may also occur because of small airway inflammation [29]. In chronic phases, interstitial fibrosis develops [30].

Langerhans Cell Histiocytosis

Pulmonary involvement in children with LCH is usually part of a disseminated disease. Approximately 50% of children with multisystemic LCH will have pulmonary involvement, but this is not always associated with an adverse outcome [29, 30]. Isolated pulmonary LCH is extremely rare in children.

In children under 10 years of age, pulmonary involvement tends to regress spontaneously (V. Nandhuri, personal communication), but in older children the acute features resemble those seen in adults. HRCT shows multiple thin-walled cysts usually less than 1 cm in size and predominantly within the upper and mid-zones of the lungs.

Nodules show diffuse distribution throughout the lung, with relative sparing of the costophrenic angles. Multiple nodules measuring 1–3 mm in size occur and may be peribronchial in distribution. Nodules may cavitate and are the precursors of thin-walled cystic lesions. The distribution and profusion of the nodules correlates with disease activity [31].

Depositional Lung Diseases

Lipid Storage Diseases

Niemann-Pick disease is an inherited defect in sphingomyelinase production and has five clinical variants resulting in sphingomyelin deposition within the lung, liver, bone marrow and brain. HRCT shows a diffuse reticulonodular pattern with nodules 1–2 mm in size due to the accumulation of aggregates of large multi-vaculolated 'foam' cells deposited in the lungs.

Gaucher's disease is due to a deficiency of beta-glucosidase (the enzyme catabolizer of glucosylceramide), resulting in the accumulation of the latter in reticuloendothelial cells of the liver, spleen, lymph nodes, bones and the brain (especially in the infantile form of the disease). The Gaucher cells then accumulate in the alveolar interstitial and adjacent air spaces, leading to diffuse miliary or reticulo-nodular patterns that may be associated with lytic rib lesions.

Aspiration Pneumonitis

Children with chronic gastro-oesophageal reflux with silent or clinically overt aspiration of gastric contents can develop very severe pulmonary dysfunction with associated radiological changes. Chest X-ray initially shows air space disease, with subsequent interstitial fibrosis. In the infant, recurrent episodes of unexplained respiratory distress related to feeding, together with perihilar consolidations especially in the dependent right upper and superior segments lower lobe should suggest aspiration pneumonitis.

In the more chronic untreated forms, diffuse airway and interstitial changes with peripheral pulmonary fibrosis ensue. In these more advanced cases lung biopsy shows numerous fat-laden macrophages, confirming the diagnosis of aspiration-induced pulmonary fibrosis.

Newer Disorders and Mimics of ILDs of Childhood

Pulmonary Veno-occlusive Disease

Patients with this rare disorder present with the clinical picture of pulmonary hypertension. Chest X-ray shows enlarged pulmonary arteries, Kerley B lines, pleural effusions and mediastinal adenopathy. CT demonstrates pulmonary arterial enlargement, mediastinal lymphadenopathy and normal main pulmonary veins but shows smooth interlobular septal thickening due to peripheral pulmonary venous congestion. There is a mosaic pattern of lung attenuation.

Aetiological factors include the idiopathic type, inherited factors, post viral infections, autoimmune disorders and post bone marrow transplantation [32].

Pleuroparenchymal Fibroelastosis

Pleuroparenchymal fibroelastosis is a rare disorder, observed most often after allogenetic bone marrow transplantation, although it has previously been reported as an idiopathic, and related to dyskeratosis congenita. Fibrosis of the peripheral lung parenchyma with pleural thickening occurs often with pneumothorax. The lung apices are often more severely affected [33].

Filamin A Protein Deficiency Related Progressive Multilobar Emphysema

The role of the filamin proteins in lung growth was not previously recognized, but their importance for normal lung development and growth is crucial. Filamin protein A (FLNA) encodes actin-binding cytoskeletal scaffolding protein, which is involved in neuronal migration, cardiovascular development and connective tissue integrity.

Mutations of FLNA are associated with multisystemic disorders, including periventricular cerebral nodular heterotopia, cardiac valve dysplasia, aneurysms and Ehlers-Danlos variants. Infants normally present with progressive respiratory deterioration, sometimes complicated by pulmonary hypertension.

Chest X-ray and CT demonstrate hyperlucent lung parenchyma with peripheral pulmonary vascular attenuation, especially in the upper and middle lobes [34].

Conclusion

Diffuse ILD in children comprises a rare but heterogeneous group of conditions, many of which have no known cause. There is a clear need for definitive histological classification, which, along with the increasing experience in HRCT, will aid us in our ability to diagnose and follow these unusual, fascinating conditions.

References

1. Koh DM, Hansell DM (2000) Computed tomography of diffuse interstitial lung disease in children. Clin Radiol 55:659-667.
2. Bush A, du Bois R (1996) Congenital and paediatric interstitial disease. Curr Opin Pulm Med 2:347-356.
3. Reid L (1984) Lung growth in health and disease. BR J Dis Chest 74:113-139.
4. McGowan SE (1992) Extracellular matrix and the regulation of lung development and repair. FASEB J 6:2895-2904.
5. Minoo O, King RJ (1994) Epithelial-mesenchymal interactions in lung development. Annu Rev Physiol 56:13-45.
6. Hislop A, Wigglesworth JS, Desai R (1986) Alveolar development in the human fetus and infant. Early Hum Dev 13:1-11.
7. Thurlbeck WM (1982) Postnatal human lung growth. Thorax 37:564-571.
8. Dunnill MS (1982) The problem of lung growth. Thorax 37:561-563.
9. Thibeault DW, Heimes B, Rezaiekhaligh M, MabryS (1993) Chronic modifications of lung and heart development in glucocorticoid treated newborn rats exposed to hyperoxia or room air. Pediatr Pulmonal 6:81-88.
10. Chan KN, Noble-Jamieson CM, Elliman A et al (1989) Lung function in children of low birth-weight. Arch Dis Child 64:1284-1293.
11. Lawler SD, Ukaejiojo, Reeves BR (1975) Interaction of maternal and neonatal cells in mixed-lymphocyte cultures. Lancet 2:1185-187.
12. Miyawaki TH, Seki H, Taga K et al (1985) Dissociated production of interleukin-2 and immune gamma interferon by phytohaemagglutinen stimulated lymphocytes in healthy infants. Clin Exp Immunol 59:505-511.
13. Lewis DB, Yu CC, Meyers J et al (1991) Cellular and molecular mechanisms for reduced interleukin 4 and interferon gamma production by neonatal T cells. J Clin Invest 87:194-202.
14. McCarthy KM, Gong JL, Telford, Schneeberger EE (1992) Ontogeny of 1a+ accessory cells in fetal and newborn rat lung. Am J Respir Cell Mol Biol 6:349-356.
15. Grenier P, Valeyre D, Cluzel P et al (1991) Chronic diffuse interstitial lung disease: diagnostic value of chest radiography and high resolution CT. Radiology 179:123-132.
16. Padley SPG, Hansell DM, Flower CDR, Jennings P (1991) Comparative accuracy of high resolution CT and chest radiography in the diagnosis of diffuse infiltrative lung disease. Clin Radiol 44:222-226.
17. Copley SJ, Coren M, Nicholson AJ et al (2000) Diagnostic accuracy of thin-section computed tomography and chest radiograph in paediatric interstitial lung disease. AJR Am J Roentgenol 174:549-554.
18. Fan L (1998) Pediatric interstitial lung disease. In: Schawrz ML, King TE (eds) Interstitial lung disease. BC Decker, Hamilton, ON, pp 103-118.
19. Copley SJ, Coren M, Nicholson AG et al (2000) Diagnostic accuracy of thin-section CT and chest radiography of paediatric interstitial lung disease. AJR Am J Roentgenol 172:549-554.
20. Seely JM, Effmann EC, Muller NL (1997) High resolution CT of the paediatric chest: imaging findings. AJR Am J Roentgenol 168:1269-1275.
21. Fishback N, Koss M (1996) Update on lymphoid interstitial pneumonitis. Curr Opin Pulm Med 2:429-433.
22. Albafouille V, Sayegh N, Coudenhove SD et al (1999) CT scan patterns of pulmonary alveolar proteinosis in children. Pediatr Radiol 28:147-152.
23. Swensen SJ, Tashijian JH, Myers JL et al(1996) Pulmonary veno-occlusive disease. CT findings in eight patients. AJR Am J Roentgenol 167:937-940.
24. Cheah FK, Sheppard MN, Hansell DM (1993) Computed tomography of diffuse pulmonary haemorrhage with pathological correlation. Clin Radiol 48:89-93.
25. Fink CW, Cimaz R (1997) Early onset sarcoidosis: not a benign disease. J Rheum 24:174-177.
26. Tsagris VA, Liapi-Adamidou G (1999) Sarcoidosis in infancy: a case with pulmonary involvement as a cardinal manifestation. Eur J Paediatr 158:258-260.
27. Gurney JW (1992) Hypersensitivity pneumonitis. Radiol Clin North Am 30:1219-1230.
28. Hansell DM, Wells AU, Padley SP, Muller NL (1996) Hypersensitivity pneumonitis: correlation of individual CT patterns with functional abnormalities. Radiology 199:123-128.
29. Adler BD, Padley SP, Muller NL et al (1992) Chronic Hypersensitivity pneumonitis: high resolution CT and radiographic features in 16 patients. Radiology 185:91-95.
30. Ha SY, Helms P, Fletcher M et al (1992) Lung involvement in Langerhans' cell histiocytosis: prevalence, clinical features and outcome. Paediatrics 89:466-469.
31. Egeler RM, D'Angio GJ(1995) Langerhancellhistiocytosis. J Paediatr 127:1-11.
32 Heath D, Segel N, Bishop J (1966) Pulmonary veno occlusive disease: clinical manifestations. Circulation 34:242-248.
33 von der Thüsen JH, Hansell DM, Tominaga M et al (2011) Pleuroparenchymal fibroelastosis in patients with pulmonary disease secondary to bone marrow transplantation. Mod Pathol 24:1633-1639.
34. Guillerman RP, Metwalli ZA, Burrage LC et al (2013) Congenital multilobar pseudo-emphysema: a severe progressive lung growth disorder associated with filamin a gene mutations. Pediatr Radiol 43 (Suppl 2):S304.

Neonatal Medical and Surgical Lung Diseases

George A. Taylor

Department of Radiology, Boston Children's Hospital, Boston, MA, USA

Introduction

Respiratory distress is a common problem in the neonate, and imaging plays an important part in the initial diagnosis and management of these infants. This chapter discusses the most common medical and surgical conditions of the lung encountered in the newborn, with emphasis on the role of a multi-modal evaluation for surgical planning.

Medical Diseases

Approximately half of all premature infants suffer from some form of respiratory distress. The most common causes include surfactant deficiency (50%), transient tachypnea (4%), and sepsis (2%). In the full-term infant, transient tachypnea, meconium aspiration syndrome, and persistent pulmonary hypertension are the most frequently encountered etiologies of acute respiratory failure. Because there is a great deal of overlap in the radiographic appearance of several conditions, knowledge of the patient's gestational age and post-partum age, the clinical setting, and the degree of respiratory support is crucial in accurately assessing the underlying pathological process and its progression or resolution.

Surfactant Deficiency (Hyaline Membrane Disease)

Alveoli that are deficient in surfactant tend to collapse, resulting in generalized hypoinflation of the lungs, ventilation-perfusion mismatch, and poor gas exchange. Breathing causes overdistention of open alveoli and shear stresses on the fragile lung. As a result, there is leakage of proteinaceous fluid into the alveolar lumen (hyaline membranes), which further impairs gas exchange and worsens the respiratory distress.

The typical radiographic findings are hypoinflated lungs with a diffuse, reticulo-nodular appearance to the lungs and air bronchograms, caused by fluid-filled alveoli interspersed with air-filled sections of lung (Fig. 1).

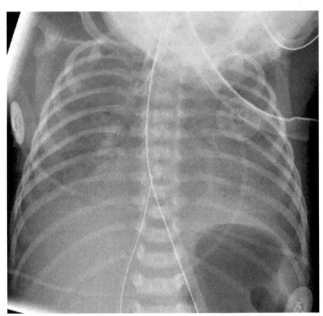

Fig. 1. Surfactant deficiency. A 27-week-gestation infant on the first day of life. Portable chest radiograph shows hypoinflated lungs with scattered air-bronchograms

Standard treatment regimens include positive pressure ventilation and endotracheal administration of exogenous surfactant. Treatment with surfactant typically results in symmetric central clearing of the lungs. However, the uneven distribution of surfactant may result in over-aeration of one lung or lung segment (Fig. 2). Uncomplicated surfactant deficiency typically resolves within the first week of life. However, high levels of inspired oxygen and inspiratory pressures may lead to prolonged respiratory difficulties, with eventual fibrosis and emphysema [1].

Pneumonia

The incidence of pneumonia in the newborn appears to be inversely proportional to gestational age, occurring in up

Diseases of the Chest and Heart 2015-2018,
DOI: 10.1007/978-88-470-5752-4_32 © Springer-Verlag Italia 2015

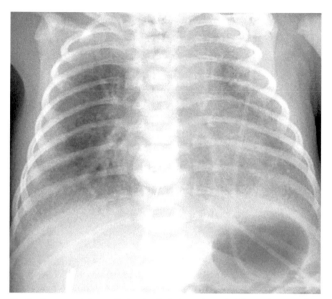

Fig. 2. Asymmetric surfactant administration. A 28-week-gestation infant on the first day of life. Chest radiograph obtained after intratracheal surfactant administration shows asymmetric central inflation of the right mid-lung due to asymmetric surfactant administration to the right lung

to 4% of premature infants <1000 g. The most common pathogens in this age group currently include *Escherichia coli*, group *B* streptococcus, and staphylococcus species. Although alveolar infiltrates may be seen in the premature infant with pulmonary infection (Fig. 3), both the clinical signs and the radiographic features of pneumonia may be indistinguishable from those of hyaline membrane disease.

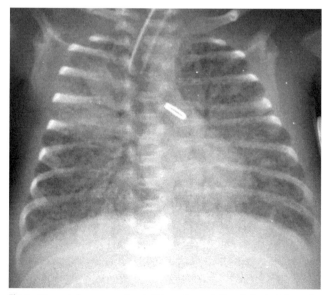

Fig. 3. Neonatal pneumonia. A 26-week-gestation infant at 2 weeks of life. Portable chest radiograph shows a focal right upper lobe pneumonia with air bronchograms superimposed on early chronic lung disease

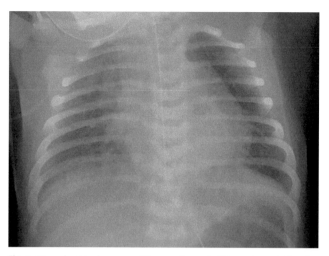

Fig. 4. Transient tachypnea of the newborn. A 36-week-gestation infant, born by cesarean section, on the first day of life. Chest radiograph shows increased central bronchovascular markings and a mild interstitial prominence

Transient Tachypnea of the Newborn

Transient tachypnea of the newborn is one of the most common causes of respiratory distress in the older premature and full-term infant. The basic underlying pathophysiology is one of delayed clearing of fetal lung fluid. Risk factors include prematurity and birth by cesarean section, usually without preceding labor. Respiratory difficulties begin within a few hours of birth, lasting between a few hours up to 2 days in uncomplicated cases. Chest radiographs typically show increased perihilar bronchovascular markings and fluid in the pulmonary fissures (Fig. 4). The lungs may vary in their degree of inflation, from normal to hyperinflated.

Meconium Aspiration

Meconium aspiration syndrome consists of fetal acidosis and subsequent hyperperistalsis, passage of meconium, fetal gasping, and aspiration of meconium into the trachea and lungs [2]. Thick meconium may cause physical obstruction of the distal airways, resulting in patchy, alternating areas of pulmonary overinflation and atelectasis. Meconium also inactivates surfactant and causes secondary surfactant deficiency and poor lung compliance. The clinical course of many patients with meconium aspiration syndrome is complicated by pulmonary hypertension, which increases illness severity and worsens clinical outcomes. The radiographic features of meconium aspiration vary widely, depending on the severity of aspiration. The mildest cases manifest as pulmonary hyperinflation with scattered interstitial pulmonary opacities, while in more severe cases patchy alveolar and interstitial infiltrates and more pronounced hyperinflation are seen, often together with pneumothorax and pneumomediastinum as complications (Fig. 5).

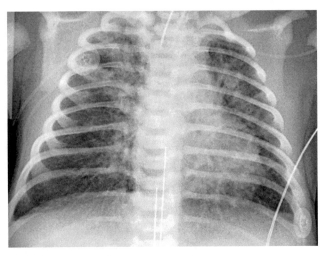

Fig. 5. Meconium aspiration. A 39-week-gestation infant on the first day of life. Heavy meconium staining and low APGAR scores at birth were recorded. Portable chest X-ray shows hyperinflated lungs with coarse bilateral interstitial opacities and focal right upper lobe atelectasis

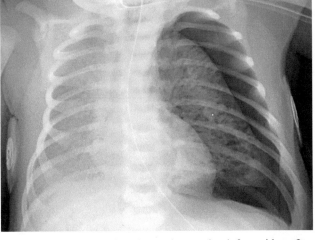

Fig. 6. Pulmonary air leak. A 27-week-gestation infant with surfactant deficiency requiring positive pressure ventilation. Chest X-ray shows tubular and flame-shaped lucencies throughout the left lung due to pulmonary interstitial emphysema. A large left pneumothorax is also present

Complications of Respiratory Support

Pulmonary air leaks are complications of greatest concern in newborns receiving positive pressure ventilation. They can manifest as pulmonary interstitial emphysema, pneumomediastinum, pneumothorax, and intravascular gas. As alveoli become overdistended and rupture, gas is forced into the connective tissues of the lung and can dissect along the interlobular septae toward the hilum of the lung. This pattern is of flame-shaped lucencies that may be bilateral or unilateral and is characteristic of pulmonary interstitial emphysema (PIE). Increasing distention can progress to plural or mediastinal air collections with or without PIE. In rare cases, gas is forced through lymphatic channels into the vascular tree, resulting in cardiovascular collapse (Fig. 6).

Surgical Diseases

Congenital anomalies of the lung that have surgical implications include a heterogeneous set of disorders of the lung parenchyma and of the vascular supply of the lung. They can occur alone or in various combinations that result in a wide range of clinical symptoms and outcomes. The most commonly occurring lesions, based on the Langston pathological classification system, include bronchial atresia, congenital pulmonary airway malformation (CPAM), bronchopulmonary sequestration, and congenital lobar hyperinflation, which together account for up to 90% of the congenital lesions encountered in the newborn [3, 4]. The majority of these lesions are now detected prenatally during routine screening, and while radiography still plays an important role in the day-to-

day management of these infants, cross-sectional imaging is the key to the accurate characterization of these lesions and to surgical planning [5]. Important goals for imaging evaluation include identifying the location of a lesion as well as its arterial and venous supply and the assessment of internal components and associated anomalies.

Bronchial Atresia

Bronchial atresia refers to complete atretic occlusion of a lobar or segmental bronchus close to its origin. The pathogenesis of bronchial atresia appears to be related to vascular accidents during organogenesis. While bronchial atresia may occur as a separate entity, it is often seen as a component of pulmonary sequestration and CPAMs. The upper lobes are most commonly affected, appearing hyperexpanded on prenatal sonography, radiography, and computed tomography (CT). A bronchocele with tubular or finger-like impacted mucus may also be present on imaging studies (Fig. 7).

Congenital Pulmonary Airway Malformation

These lesions reflect the overgrowth of lung parenchyma into micro- or macrocystic malformations. They may arise from acinar tissue (microcystic lesions), bronchioles (mixed types), or more proximal airways (macrocystic lesions). Most are unilateral, but multiple or bilateral lesions have been reported. While many communicate with the central airway, the communication is often abnormal, resulting in an initially fluid-filled pulmonary mass that gradually becomes air-filled and cystic (Fig. 8). Macrocystic (type I) CPAMs are the most frequently occurring. They are seen in approximately 65% of postnatal

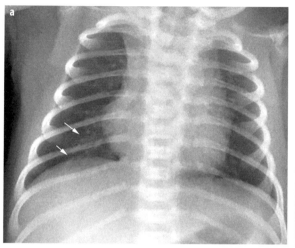
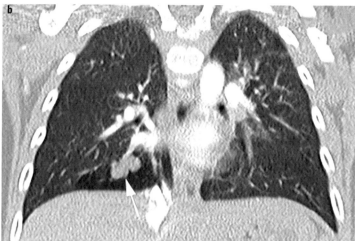

Fig. 7 a, b. Bronchial atresia and congenital pulmonary airway malformation. A 36-week-gestation infant at 2 weeks of life. Prenatal sonography had depicted a focal right lower lobe lesions (not shown). Chest radiograph (**a**) shows an ill-defined opacity in the right lower lobe (*arrows*). Coronal reconstruction of a contrast-enhanced chest CT (**b**) shows a hyperlucent segment of the right lower lobe with a lobulated, mucus-filled bronchocele (*arrow*) due to segmental bronchial atresia

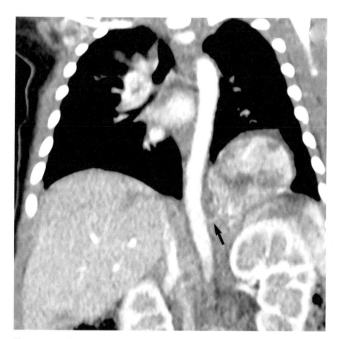

Fig. 8. Extralobar pulmonary sequestration. A full-term infant with a prenatally diagnosed lung mass. Coronal reconstruction of the contrast-enhanced CT shows a heterogeneous mass at the base of the left lung with a systemic arterial supply arising from the descending aorta (*arrow*)

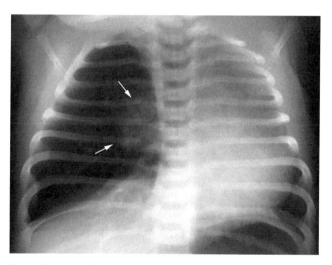

Fig. 9. Congenital lobar hyperinflation. A full-term newborn with a prenatally diagnosed hyperexpanded lung. Chest X-ray shows an overinflated, hyperlucent left lung with a centrally-placed atelectasis (*arrows*) and a contralateral mediastinal shift due to congenital lobar hyperinflation of the upper lobe

Bronchopulmonary Sequestration

Sequestrations are characterized by a lack of communication between the central airway and a systemic arterial supply, commonly arising from the descending thoracic aorta. There are two basic types of sequestration: intralobar sequestrations are part of the normal pulmonary lobe, are located within the visceral pleura, and their venous drainage is via the pulmonary artery. They are typically located in the lower lobes. Extralobar sequestrations are accessory lung tissue outside of the visceral pleura, drained by systemic or portal veins. They may be located within or below the diaphragm. Ultrasound can be used to identify the systemic arterial blood supply in solid or fluid-filled masses in the early postnatal period. CT arteriography is

cases, are typically located in the lower lobes, and involve a single lobe in over 95% of cases. Microcystic (type II) lesions comprise 15–20% of CPAMs and have a higher association with other congenital chest anomalies, such as sequestration, diaphragmatic hernia, and congenital heart disease. Mixed cystic and solid (type III) lesions account for about 10% of CPAMs and can involve an entire lobe or lung. CPAM lesions, even large ones associated with hydrops, regress prenatally in 50% of the cases.

very useful in fully characterizing the vascular connections prior to thoracoscopic removal of the lesion (Fig. 9).

Congenital Lobar Hyperinflation

Congenital lobar hyperinflation is primarily seen in the upper lobes and is caused by obstruction of the lobar bronchus. The obstruction may be intrinsic, due to malacia, stenosis, or atresia, or caused by extrinsic compression from mediastinal cysts or abnormal pulmonary vessels. On prenatal imaging, the affected lobe is typically overdistended. However, a specific prenatal diagnosis may be difficult because of the overlapping appearances of CPAM and bronchial atresia. On postnatal imaging, the affected lobe is distended and may exert a mediastinal shift. The cyst transitions from fluid-filled to air-filled over the first few days of life.

References

1. Jackson CJ (2012) Respiratory distress in the preterm infant. In: Gleason CA, Devaskar SU (2012) Avery's Diseases of the Newborn, 9th Ed. Elsevier, pp 633-646.
2. Parker TA, Kinsella JP (2012) Respiratory failure in the term infant. In: Gleason CA, Devaskar SU (2012) Avery's Diseases of the Newborn, 9th Ed. Elsevier, pp 647-657.
3. Langston C (2003) New concepts in the pathology of congenital lung malformations. Semin Pediatr Surg 12:17-37.
4. Epelman M, Daltro P, Soto G et al (2013) Congenital lung anomalies. In: Coley BD (2013) Caffey's Pediatric Diagnostic Imaging, 12th Ed, vol 1. Elsevier, pp 550-556.
5. Lee EY, Dorkin H, Vargas SO (2011) Congenital pulmonary malformations in pediatric patients: review and update on etiology, classification and imaging findings. Radiol Clin North Am 49:921-948.

BREAST IMAGING SATELLITE COURSE "PEARL"

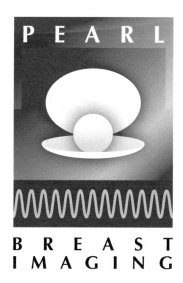

Scintimammography

Einat Even-Sapir

Sourasky Medical Center, Tel Aviv, Israel

Nuclear medicine has been i nvolved in the field of functional tumor imaging for decades. Its hallmark is the detection of viable tumor tissue based on functional and biological characteristics rather than on an altered tumor morphology. Scintigraphy has an important role in monitoring the response to therapy, by distinguishing active tumor mass, where the tumor-seeking tracer still accumulates, from residual mass composed of necrosis or scar, where tracer no longer accumulates. The use of scintigraphy in tumor detection depends on the mechanism of tracer uptake in the tumor, the pharmacokinetic and normal biodistribution of the tracer, and on the technology of the detecting system.

The detection of breast cancer using single-photon-emitting tracers with a gamma camera and positron-emitting tracers with PET technology has been an ongoing challenge of nuclear medicine [1]. The whole-body systems used originally in scintimammography were suboptimal for the detection of small lesions in the breast, as the distance from the collimator to the breast is approximately 15 cm and to the region of interest up to 25 cm. Instead, dedicated systems for breast imaging were needed, which are now commercially available.

Gamma-cameras dedicated to breast imaging may be single- or dual-headed cameras; in the latter, each breast is positioned between the two detectors in two views similar to the acquisition mode on mammography, with no pressure. Detectors can be the NaI (Tl) detectors routinely used in nuclear medicine, a technology referred to as breast-specific gamma imaging (BSGI), or the new generation of pixilated semiconductor [cadmium zinc telluride (CZT)] detectors with improved spatial resolution. A dual-headed system composed of CZT detectors, the molecular breast imaging system (MBI), was reported to have a high sensitivity in the detection of clinically relevant breast lesions as small as 3 mm [2-4].

Several dedicated breast imaging systems for positron-emitting tracers have been designed. The earliest one, positron emission mammography (PEM), uses two oppositely placed detectors, as in mammography. With another prototype, dedicated breast PET, the patient is prone and the breast hangs freely through a small ring of detectors. The first system to become commercially available was a stationary flat detector-based PEM scanner that used limited-angle tomosynthetic reconstruction with a spatial resolution of 2.4 mm [5]. A newer design is mammography with molecular imaging (MAMMI), a dedicated breast PET system that uses a complete ring of detectors for full tomographic image reconstruction with a spatial resolution of 1.6 mm [6]. Dedicated breast PET systems were shown to be significantly more sensitive for the detection of breast cancer than either whole-body PET or PET-CT [7].

The tracer used for breast imaging with a gamma-camera is ^{99m}technetium (Tc)-sestaMIBI. The mechanisms of the enhanced cellular uptake of ^{99m}Tc-sestaMIBI in cancer cells is the subject of ongoing investigation. ^{99m}Tc-sestaMIBI is a small lipophilic cation whose uptake is nine times higher in tumor tissue than in normal tissue, reflecting the high vascularity and mitochondrial activity of the former [8, 9]. The major advantage of ^{99m}Tc-sestaMIBI in breast cancer imaging is its wide availability in the routine practice of nuclear medicine departments, as it is also used in cardiac perfusion studies. Moreover, unlike PET tracers, it does not require cyclotron facilities for its production.

The most commonly used tracer for scintimammography with positron-emission technology is ^{18}F-fludeoxyglucose (FDG). As a rule of thumb, ^{18}F-FDG uptake is higher in breast tumors with prognostically unfavorable characteristics [10]. Primary tumor ^{18}F-FDG uptake was found to correlate with tumor size, histological type and grade, pleomorphism, lymphatic invasion, high Ki-67 level, and triple negativity (i.e., negative for the estrogen receptor, the progesterone receptor, and the human epidermal growth factor receptor 2) [11]. Yet, it should be borne in mind that ^{18}F-FDG avidity is a characteristic of the individual tumor and some tumor types, such as ductal carcinoma in situ and lobular carcinoma, may show only low-intensity uptake [7, 12]. Moreover, when dedicated PET systems are used for breast imaging, heterogeneous uptake in a large tumor probably reflects tumor heterogeneity within the mass [13].

Diseases of the Chest and Heart 2015-2018,
DOI: 10.1007/978-88-470-5752-4_33 © Springer-Verlag Italia 2015

Publications on the clinical use of scintimammography have explored its role in tumor detection in patients with no known malignancies and as a diagnostic tool in patients with diagnosed breast cancer. The reported sensitivity of BSGI for the detection of breast cancer is 78–100% for all tumor types, including lobular carcinoma [2, 14]. Using the MBI system, researchers at the Mayo Clinic were able to detect small malignant lesions of 3 mm and calculated a sensitivity of 90% for abnormalities 5–20 mm in size. Scintigraphy was found to be a valuable procedure when routinely used screening modalities, mainly mammography, were suboptimal, such as in the case of patients with dense breasts. Based on the screening of 936 at-risk women, Rhodes et al., of the Mayo Clinic, reported a sensitivity of 27% for mammography alone and 91% for combined mammography and MBI [15]. This group reported the good performance of MBI with a low-dose of 8 mCi ^{99m}Tc-sestaMIBI, with ongoing efforts aimed at dose-reduction to perform MBI with 4 mCi, with an effective dose twice that of a screening mammogram.

A recently published meta-analysis evaluated eight studies on the use of ^{18}F-FDG-PEM, comprising 873 women with breast lesions. The pooled sensitivity and specificity values of PEM were 85% and 79%, respectively, according to a per-lesion-based analysis [16]. Currently, however, scintigraphy is not recommended as a routine screening tool because of the higher total body radiation compared to routinely used breast imaging modalities.

Accurate assessment of disease extent in the breast is essential to optimize the treatment approach in patients with newly diagnosed breast cancer. As in the case of MRI, scintimammography can identify additional, unexpected sites of disease, resulting in a change in diagnosis from localized to multifocal, multicentric, or even bilateral disease. In a retrospective study of 159 women with one suspicious breast lesion on physical exam and/or mammography, BSGI detected additional suspicious lesions in 29% and occult cancer in 9%, both in the same breast as the index lesion (6%) and in the contralateral breast (3%) [12].

PEM and MRI were performed and compared in 388 patients with diagnosed cancer who were scheduled for surgery. Additional cancers were found in 21% of the women. PEM and MRI had comparable breast-level sensitivity, although MRI had greater lesion-level sensitivity and more accurately depicted the need for mastectomy. PEM had greater specificity at the breast and lesion levels. In 3.6% of the women, tumors were seen only on PEM [16]. In another study of 367 patients, 4% had contralateral cancer. The sensitivity and specificity of MRI in detecting these lesions was 93% and 89.5% respectively, compared to 73% and 95%, respectively, for PEM [17].

In patients with locally advanced disease receiving neoadjuvant therapy, monitoring response to therapy by morphologic imaging modalities reduces potential errors in interpretation due to findings of fibrosis or scar formation and tumor fragmentation rather than concentric shrinkage, which can lead to an underestimation of the patient's response to therapy, and to the antiangiogenic effects of the chemotherapeutic agent, which can alter the contrast kinetics thus leading to an overestimate of the response [1]. Assessing response to therapy by means of functional rather than anatomic changes is another indication for scintimammography. ^{99m}Tc-sestaMIBI is a substrate of the transmembrane P-glycoprotein (Pgp-170) present in cells overexpressing the multidrug resistance gene (MDR1). Pgp acts as a protective pump by extruding out of the tumor cells a wide range of molecules, including ^{99m}Tc-sestaMIBI. Studies performed in humans demonstrated that in tumors with high levels of Pgp, ^{99m}Tc-sestaMIBI efflux was significantly faster than in the control group or in tumors with no Pgp, suggesting a role for ^{99m}Tc-sestaMIBI scintigraphy in monitoring the response to chemotherapy [8, 9]. Serial ^{99m}Tc-sestaMIBI scintimammography was shown to accurately predict tumor response in patients with locally advanced breast carcinoma undergoing neoadjuvant chemotherapy. Patients with residual high uptake had poorer disease-free survival and overall survival, and uptake at completion of treatment was found to be an independent prognostic factor [18]. In a recent study, changes in the tumor to background ratio on MBI images performed at 3–5 weeks following the initiation of neoadjuvant chemotherapy were found to accurately predict the presence or absence of residual disease at the completion of treatment [19].

An MBI system was installed at our center in 2009. We approached our clinicians, breast surgeons, oncologists, and breast radiologists in conducting a registry research aimed at understanding the potential complementary role of MBI in the imaging algorithm of breast imaging. In patients with unknown cancer, indications for MBI included genetic and familial high-risk; equivocal findings on mammography, ultrasound (US), and/or MRI; nipple discharge with no suggested breast abnormality; contraindication for MRI or claustrophobia in patients with equivocal mammography and US assessment; and further assessment of the contralateral breast. In patients with diagnosed breast cancer, the indications for MBI were: assessment of the disease extent in the breasts of patients with newly diagnosed solitary breast cancer planned for lumpectomy, in which the surgeon was uncertain that disease was localized; in patients with locally advanced disease before and after neoadjuvant therapy; in assessing the presence of residual disease after surgery or of suspected recurrence; to search for a primary occult tumor in patients with metastatic axillary lymph nodes of breast cancer; and in follow-up.

Scintimammography technology and clinical cases reflecting the complementary role of scintimammography are discussed in the workshop for this chapter.

References

1. Fowler AM (2014) A molecular approach to breast imaging. J Nucl Med 55:177-180.

2. Sun Y, Wei W, Yang HW, Liu JL (2013) Specific gamma imaging as an adjunct modality to mammography for diagnosis of breast cancer: a systemic review and meta-analysis. Eur J Nucl Med Mol Imaging 40:450-463.

3. Brem RF, Shahan C, Rapleyea JA et al (2010) Detection of occult foci of breast cancer using breast-specific gamma imaging in women with one mammographic or clinically suspicious breast lesion. Acad Radiol 17:735-743.

4. Hruska CB, Phillips SW, Whaley DH et al (2008) Molecular breast imaging: use of a dual-head dedicated gamma camera to detect small breast tumors. AJR Am J Roentgenol 191:1805-1815.

5. MacDonald L, Edwards J, Lewellen T et al (2009) Clinical imaging characteristics of the positron emission mammography camera: PEM Flex Solo II. J Nucl Med 50:1666-1675.

6. Moliner L, Gonzalez AJ, Soriano A et al (2012) Design and evaluation of the MAMMI dedicated breast PET. Med Phys 39:5393-5404.

7. Kalinya JE, Berg WA, Schilling K et al (2014) Breast cancer detection using high-resolution breast PET compared to whole-body PET or PET/CT. Eur J Nucl Med Mol Imaging 41:260-275.

8. van Leeuwen FW, Buckle T, Kersbergen A et al (2009) Noninvasive functional imaging of P-glycoprotein-mediated doxorubicin resistance in a mouse model of hereditary breast cancer to predict response, and assign P-gp inhibitor sensitivity. Eur J Nucl Med Mol Imaging 36:406-412

9. Vecchio SD, Zannetti A, Salvatore B et al (2006) Functional imaging of multidrug resistance in breast cancer. Phys Med 21(Suppl 1):24-27.

10. Koolen BB, Vrancken Peeters MJ, Wesseling J et al (2012) Association of primary tumour FDG uptake with clinical, histopathological and molecular characteristics in breast cancer patients scheduled for neoadjuvant chemotherapy. Eur J Nucl Med Mol Imaging 39:1830-1838.

11. Ekmekcioglu O, Aliyev A, Yilmaz S et al (2013) Correlation of 18F-fluorodeoxyglucose uptake with histopathological prognostic factors in breast carcinoma. Nucl Med Commun 34:1055-1067.

12. Buck A, Schirrmeister H, Kühn T et al (2002) FDG uptake in breast cancer: correlation with biological and clinical prognostic parameters. Eur J Nucl Med Mol Imaging 29:1317-1323.

13. Koolen BB, Vidal-Sicart S, Benlloch Baviera JM, Valdés Olmos RA (2014) Evaluating heterogeneity of primary tumor (18)F-FDG uptake in breast cancer with a dedicated breast PET (MAMMI): a feasibility study based on correlation with PET/CT. Nucl Med Commun 35:446-452.

14. Brem RF, Ioffe M, Rapelyea JA et al (2009) Invasive lobular carcinoma: detection with mammography sonography MRI, and breast-specific gamma imaging. AJR Am J Roentgenol 192:379-383.

15. Rhodes DJ, Hruska CB, Phillips SW et al (2011) Dedicated dual-head gamma imaging for breast cancer screening in women with mammographically dense breasts. Radiology 258:106-118.

16. Berg WA, Madsen KS, Schilling K et al (2011) Breast cancer: comparative effectiveness of positron emission mammography and MR imaging in presurgical planning for the ipsilateral breast. Radiology 258:59-72.

17. Berg WA1, Madsen KS, Schilling K et al (2012) Comparative effectiveness of positron emission mammography and MRI in the contralateral breast of women with newly diagnosed breast cancer. AJR Am J Roentgenol 198:219-232.

18. Dunnwald LK, Gralow JR, Ellis GK et al (2005) Residual tumor uptake of [99mTc]-sestaMIBI after neoadjuvant chemotherapy for locally advanced breast carcinoma predicts survival. Cancer 103:680-688.

19. Mitchell D1, Hruska CB, Boughey JC et al (2013) 99mTc-sestaMIBI using a direct conversion molecular breast imaging system to assess tumor response to neoadjuvant chemotherapy in women with locally advanced breast cancer. Clin Nucl Med 38:949-956.

Breast MRI BI-RADS®: Second Edition Highlights

Elizabeth A. Morris

Department of Radiology, Breast Imaging Center, Memorial Sloan-Kettering Cancer Center, New York, NY, USA

Since the first edition of the magnetic resonance imaging (MRI) section of the illustrated BI-RADS® lexicon, the field of breast MRI has grown enormously. Understandably, certain terms have been added or deleted as better terms have been identified. Additionally, concepts such as background parenchymal enhancement (BPE) have been proposed and included. A section on nonenhancing findings has been added. A section devoted to implant description and assessment is new.

Focus

An enhancing focus is a tiny round pin-point "dot" of enhancement that is seen only on the postcontrast images. It is a round, homogeneously enhancing area with circumscribed margin. In general, foci are too small to exhibit internal enhancement characteristics. Foci can be found in women of any age and menopausal status. A focus can be benign or malignant.

In general, foci are a few millimeters in size; however, applying strict size criteria is not favored. It must be noted that cancers <5 mm can be identified in the breast on MRI. If margins and internal enhancement can be assessed, then the lesion would be considered a mass. As techniques improve, with higher resolution capabilities, fewer lesions will be described as a focus and more will be classified as a mass.

If a focus is not unique, it is likely to represent a component of the patient's background parenchymal enhancement (BPE). If it is unique and separate from the BPE, it may warrant evaluation. Margin analysis, kinetic analysis, internal enhancement and T2-weighted characteristics can be evaluated to determine whether a focus is likely to be benign or suspicious. Imaging features that favor benign etiology are circumscribed, persistent, homogeneous and very high signal intensity on bright fluid imaging. Imaging characteristics that favor malignancy are irregular, spiculated, wash out kinetics, rim or hetero-geneous enhancement, and not very high in signal on bright fluid imaging.

Mass

A mass is an area of enhancement with an epicenter and convex borders, existing as a three-dimensional (3D) structure. The committee decided not to assign a size requirement, recognizing that suspicious masses can be of all sizes. In general, as the mass size increases so does the likelihood of malignancy.

Mass descriptors for shape and margins have been adopted from the mammography BI-RADS® lexicon. In general, as with mammography, circumscribed oval or round masses are seen more with benign lesions, whereas irregular, spiculated masses are more likely to be malignant. Care should be taken with respect to morphology, as round circumscribed masses on MRI represent cancer more frequently than at mammography. There are several possible explanations for the presence of morphologically benign lesions representing cancer on MRI. First of all, MRI does not have the spatial resolution of mammography with current techniques and field strength so that margin analysis internal enhancement may suffer. Second, the cancers with benign morphology on MRI are usually small, and smaller than we might be used to detecting on mammography. As with most imaging techniques, the ability to resolve margins depends on the size of the lesion. Kinetic evaluation is important when considering these morphologically benign appearing lesions. As with other imaging techniques, the worst feature of the lesion under evaluation should be used to determine the need for biopsy.

A mass has internal enhancement that can be characterized. In general, homogeneous enhancement and nonenhancing internal septations indicate a possible benign process. While it is certainly possible to see classic appearances of certain lesions, morphologic overlap can occur between benign and malignant lesions; if there is any doubt, biopsy should be performed. The committee recognizes that when masses become large and ill-defined they might be described as regional enhancement.

This chapter was previously published in: Hodler J, von Schulthess GK, Zollikofer ChL (eds) Musculoskeletal Diseases 2013-2016. Springer-Verlag Italia, Milano 2013, pp. 275-281.

Diseases of the Chest and Heart 2015-2018,
DOI: 10.1007/978-88-470-5752-4_34 © Springer-Verlag Italia 2015

Mass analysis can benefit from bright fluid sequences [i.e., T2 weighted or short-tau inversion recovery (STIR)] in addition to the postcontrast sequences obtained. In general, benign mass lesions can be increased in signal relative to fibroglandular parenchyma on bright fluid imaging, particularly cysts, lymph nodes and fibroadenomas. Cancers may or may not exhibit increased signal on bright fluid imaging. Cancer can be heterogeneously high in signal on bright fluid imaging if the tumors are necrotic, cellular or mucinous. Mucinous carcinoma and liposarcoma classically demonstrate very high signal on bright fluid sequences; however, there are usually other suspicious features, such as irregular shape or noncircumscribed margins, that warrant biopsy.

Non-Mass Enhancement

In the first edition of the MRI section of the illustrated BI-RADS® lexicon, non-mass enhancement (NME) was used to describe BPE as well as areas that are still considered to be NME. With greater experience and understanding of BPE, some terms have been removed and the NME descriptors have been refined. NME describes enhancement in a pattern that does not have convex borders and may have intervening fat or normal fibroglandular tissue contained within the extent of the enhancement.

Clumped enhancement refers to enhancement that has the appearance of "cobble-stones" where there are small aggregates of enhancement that are variable in size and morphology. The term clumped refers to enhancement in a focal, linear or linear-branching, segmental or regional distribution. The term "clumped" on MRI is similar to the term "pleomorphic" on mammography, as it indicates enhancement in varying shapes and sizes. As ductal carcinoma in situ (DCIS) can present with this morphologic pattern, a description of clumped usually indicates a need for biopsy. The diagnosis of DCIS is usually made solely on lesion morphology, as many times the kinetic appearance does not meet minimal threshold and the time intensity curves are not typical for malignancy.

Report Organization

Amount of Fibroglandular Tissue

MRI is unique in that 3D volumetric data can be acquired from the image, and separation of fat and fibroglandular parenchyma is performed relatively easily. There are no data comparing mammographic density (breast composition) with MRI assessment of amount of fibroglandular tissue. Density is a term that should be applied only to mammography. The amount of fibroglandular tissue should be described as one of the following:
• Almost entirely fatty
• Scattered fibroglandular tissue
• Heterogeneous fibroglandular tissue
• Extreme fibroglandular tissue

As in the fifth edition of *BI-RADS® Mammography*, the amount of fibroglandular parenchyma is not described using percentages. Unlike mammography, where noncalcified breast lesions can be obscured by dense tissue, breast MRI is able to easily reveal an enhancing suspicious lesion independent of breast composition. Therefore, the amount of fibroglandular parenchyma does not adversely impact lesion detectability.

Background Parenchymal Enhancement

As MRI is performed with intravenous contrast, the fibroglandular breast parenchyma can demonstrate contrast enhancement. BPE refers to the normal enhancement of the patient's fibroglandular tissue on the first postcontrast image. BPE refers to both the volume of enhancement as well as the intensity of enhancement, and an evaluation of background enhancement should take both into consideration.

The background enhancement is described as one of the following:
• Minimal
• Mild
• Moderate
• Marked

Although these categories are roughly quartiles, assigning strict percentages to indicate the degree of enhancement is likely artificial, difficult to assess without automation, and should be avoided. In general, BPE might not be evenly distributed throughout the entire breast. Due to preferential blood supply, there is the probability of greater enhancement in the upper outer quadrant of the breast and along the inferior aspect of the breast (formerly described as "sheet-like" enhancement). BPE might be more prominent in the luteal phase of the cycle if the patient is premenopausal. Therefore, for elective examinations (e.g., high-risk screening), effort should be made to schedule the patient in the second week of her cycle (days 7-14) to minimize the issue of background enhancement. Despite scheduling the patient at the optimal time of her cycle, BPE will still occur and the BPE terms should be applied. Women in whom cancer has been diagnosed and MRI is performed for staging (i.e., diagnostic) should be imaged with MRI regardless of the timing of the menstrual cycle or menstrual status.

The pattern of BPE can be variable from patient to patient, though in general the pattern of BPE for an individual is fairly constant. It is uncertain what the patterns of enhancement mean, therefore description beyond the recommended descriptors is optional. There is some evidence that BPE might indicate a level of risk for the development of breast cancer, as therapeutic measures such as anti-estrogen therapy can decrease the level of BPE. However, BPE does not appear to affect the ability to detect breast cancer.

BPE can occur regardless of the menstrual cycle or menopausal status of the patient. BPE might not be directly related to the amount of fibroglandular parenchyma present. Patients with extremely dense breasts at mammography might demonstrate little or no BPE, whereas patients with mildly dense breasts might demonstrate marked BPE. Nevertheless, most of the time, younger patients with dense breasts are more likely to demonstrate BPE.

In general, BPE is progressive over time; however, significant and fast enhancement can occur on the first post-contrast image despite fast imaging techniques. BPE on MRI is unique to a patient as is breast density at mammography. A description of background enhancement should be included in the breast MRI report.

Patterns of BPE are under investigation, as there is wide variation in the appearance from woman to woman. BPE may present as multiple foci either uniformly scattered or more focal in one area, described previously as "stippled" enhancement. Stippled enhancement is a pattern of BPE; it is usually diffuse and symmetric, however it can present as a focal finding (particularly in an area where cysts are found) suggesting focal fibrocystic disease.

Non-Enhancing Findings

Non-enhancing findings seen on the precontrast or bright fluid images are benign. Examples include cysts, duct ectasia and some fibroadenomas and postoperative collections. Assessment of the absence of enhancement is best made on the subtraction image. Follow-up or biopsy of areas of non-enhancement is not necessary unless there are suspicious findings on another imaging modality, such as mammography or ultrasound.

Assessment Categories

The final assessment should be based on the most suspicious finding present in each breast. A separate BI-RADS® assessment for each breast should be stated after the impression text. If the interpretation is straightforward and the same for both breasts, an overall impression that includes both breasts may be used. The overall assessment should be based on the most worrisome findings present in each breast. For example, if benign findings, such as lymph nodes or cysts, are noted along with a more suspicious finding, such as a spiculated mass, the final assessment code should be reported category 4 or 5. Similarly, if immediate additional evaluation is needed for one breast for a suspicious finding (with targeted ultrasound, for example), and there is a probably benign finding in the breast as well, the final assessment code for that breast would be category 4. If a breast with a known cancer has an additional suspicious finding warranting biopsy, then the final assessment code for that breast is category 4, not category 6.

Category 0

Every effort should be made not to use category 0 in reading breast MRI. However, in the event that the examination is technically unacceptable (e.g., poor fat suppression, poor positioning) and would not be sufficient for interpretation, a meaningful report could not be issued and a category 0 may be issued. The MRI examination has characteristics that make it unique in comparison to mammography and ultrasound. The first and most obvious difference is the use of a contrast agent. This adds the parameter of blood flow to morphology with the associated flow metrics that may be calculated. The second is the acquisition of the exact same number and sequences whether the examination is for screening or diagnostic. As with mammography, BI-RADS® 0 should be used in the screening setting only. In interpreting breast MRI, there is enough information on the properly performed examination to decide to biopsy or recommend short-term follow-up of a specific finding. MRI, like mammography, can give a category 0 for prior MRIs before a report is issued that for auditing purposes will be replaced by the final assessment rendered in the addended report once prior examinations do become available – similar to a category 0 for technical reasons. This recommendation may change in the future when MRI screening becomes more commonplace.

A final assessment of 0 is helpful when a finding on MRI is suspicious but a benign corresponding finding on an additional study would prevent a biopsy. If a category 0 is given on MRI, then an explanatory note in the MRI report clarifying why this "suspicious" morphology is not immediately given a 4 or 5 is called for. For example, if a mass is suspicious on MRI but there is a possibility that it might represent a benign finding such as a lymph node, a targeted ultrasound that would prove that the lesion is benign would prevent a biopsy. In the case of an ultrasound recommendation following the MRI examination, the terms "MRI directed" or "MRI targeted" ultrasound are preferable to "second look" ultrasound, as it is not always certain that a "first look" ultrasound has been performed. Another example where category 0 would be useful is for a finding on MRI that is most likely fat necrosis, but the reader would like to confirm and correlate the findings to a mammogram that is not available.

When additional studies are compared or completed, a final assessment category attached to those additional studies would close out the MRI "0". When interpreting MRI it is extremely helpful to have all available imaging studies in order to give a complete report. If the additional studies can be reported in the same report, separate paragraphs indicating the pertinent findings from each imaging study can contribute to the final integrated assessment that takes into consideration the findings of all imaging studies.

Category 1

This is a normal examination. A description of the fibroglandular tissue and background parenchymal enhancement should be included.

Category 2

Benign findings are described in the report. Benign findings include intramammary lymph nodes, cysts, duct ectasia, postoperative collections, fat necrosis, scar, and masses, such as fibroadenomas, assessed as benign by morphology/kinetics or prior biopsy.

Category 3

We recognize that there are few data in defining types of lesions that can be followed. There are reports that support short-term follow-up of (1) a new unique focus that is separate from the BPE but has benign morphologic and kinetic features, and (2) a mass on an initial examination with benign morphologic and kinetic features. There are data to suggest that BPE should not be followed, therefore BPE is inappropriate for follow-up. Similarly, non-mass enhancement should be characterized as either benign or malignant and given a final assessment; it should not be recommended for surveillance imaging.

Category 4

Category 4 is used for the vast majority of findings prompting breast interventional procedures, ranging from diagnostic aspiration of complicated cysts to biopsy of fine linear and branching calcifications. According to BI-RADS® definitions expressed in terms of likelihood of malignancy, the cut points between category 3 versus category 4 assessments, and category 4 versus category 5 assessments, are 2% and 95%, respectively. Many institutions have, on an individual basis, subdivided category 4 to account for the vast range of lesions subjected to interventional procedures and corresponding broad range of likelihood of malignancy. This allows a more meaningful practice audit, is useful in research involving receiver-operating characteristic curve analysis, and is an aid for clinicians and pathologists.

Lesions that are appropriate to place in this category are: (1) suspicious non-mass enhancement such as clumped, linear, linear branching or segmental; (2) irregular, heterogeneous or rim enhancing masses; (3) foci with any suspicious morphology or kinetics. Specifically, a new focus with any suspicious feature warrants further evaluation by biopsy.

Suspicious findings on MRI warranting biopsy can be evaluated by targeted ultrasound. In general, masses are more likely to be seen on ultrasound than non-mass lesions. Biopsy of the finding should be performed with the modality that best illustrates the finding. If a correlate to the MRI finding can be reliably found on ultrasound, ultrasound biopsy might be preferable as it is usually more ubiquitous and cheaper than MR biopsy. Follow-up after both ultrasound and MRI biopsy is recommended, as missed lesions have been reported. Regarding the timing of follow-up, it has been recommended that a 6-month follow-up MRI is performed for all concordant nonspecific benign pathology to ensure adequate sampling of the lesion. Some authors have suggested a single non-contrast T1-weighted image following ultrasound-guided biopsy for a suspicious lesion to ensure adequate and accurate sampling.

Category 5

Category 5, highly suggestive of malignancy, was established at a time when most nonpalpable breast lesions underwent preoperative wire localization prior to surgical excision. Category 5 assessments were used for those lesions that had such characteristic features of cancer that one-stage surgical treatment might be performed immediately following frozen-section histological confirmation of malignancy. Today breast cancer diagnosis for imaging-detected lesions almost always involves percutaneous tissue sampling, so the current rationale for using category 5 assessment is to identify lesions for which any nonmalignant percutaneous tissue diagnosis is considered discordant, resulting in the recommendation for repeat (usually surgical) biopsy.

The likelihood of malignancy for category 5 assessments is ≥95%, so use of this assessment category is reserved for classic examples of malignancy. Note that there is no single MRI feature that is associated with a likelihood of malignancy of ≥95%. Just as it is found for mammography and breast ultrasound examinations, it takes a combination of suspicious MRI findings to justify a category 5 assessment.

Category 6

This assessment category was added to the fourth edition of *BI-RADS® Mammography* for use in the special circumstance when breast imaging is performed after a tissue diagnosis of malignancy but prior to complete surgical excision. Unlike the more common situations when BI-RADS® categories 4 and 5 are used, a category 6 assessment will not usually be associated with recommendation for tissue diagnosis of the target lesion because biopsy has already established the presence of malignancy. Category 6 is the appropriate assessment, prior to complete surgical excision, for staging examinations of previously biopsied findings already shown to be malignant, after attempted complete removal of the target lesion by percutaneous core biopsy, and for the monitoring of response to neoadjuvant chemotherapy.

However, there are other scenarios in which patients with known biopsy-proven malignancy have breast imaging examinations. For example, the use of category 6 is not appropriate for breast imaging examinations performed following surgical excision of a malignancy (lumpectomy). In this clinical setting, tissue diagnosis will not be performed unless breast imaging demonstrates residual or new suspicious findings. Therefore, if a postlumpectomy examination demonstrates surgical scarring but no visible residual malignancy, the appropriate assessment is benign (BI-RADS® category 2). On the other hand, if there are, for example, residual suspicious lesions, the appropriate assessment is category 4 or 5.

There is one other potentially confusing situation involving the use of assessment category 6. This occurs when, prior to complete surgical excision of a biopsy-proven malignancy, breast imaging demonstrates one or more possibly suspicious findings other than the known cancer. Because subsequent management should first evaluate them as yet undetermined finding(s), involving additional imaging, imaging-guided tissue diagnosis or both, it must be made clear that in addition to the known malignancy there is at least one more finding requiring specific prompt action. The single overall assessment should be based on the most immediate action needed. If a finding or findings are identified for which tissue diagnosis is recommended, then a category 4 or 5 assessment should be rendered. If at additional imaging for finding(s) other than the known malignancy, it is deter-

mined that tissue diagnosis is not appropriate, then a category 6 assessment should be rendered accompanied by the recommendation that subsequent management now should be directed to the cancer. As for any examination in which there is more than one finding, the management section of the report might include a second sentence that describes the appropriate management for the finding(s) not covered by the overall assessment.

Suggested Reading

American College of Radiology (ACR) (2013) ACR BI-RADS®, 5th Ed.

D'Orsi CJ, Mendelson EB, Morris EA et al (2012) Breast imaging reporting and data system: ACR BI-RADS. American College of Radiology, Reston, VA.

American College of Radiology (ACR) (2013) ACR BI-RADS® – Magnetic Resonance Imaging, 2nd Ed.

Morris EA, Ikeda DM, Lehman C et al (2012) Breast Imaging Reporting and Data System. American College of Radiology, Reston, VA.

Recent Developments in Breast Ultrasound with a Special Focus on Shear-Wave Elastography

Claudia Kurtz

Institute of Radiology, Cantonal Hospital Lucerne, Switzerland

Introduction

Since the first use of breast ultrasound by Wild and Reid [1] in 1953, it has taken half a century to achieve a level of ultrasound technology that allows it to be considered as a multimodality imaging tool for use at the highest level in breast diagnostics. Ultrasound has been described to detect mammographically occult breast cancer [2]. Indeed, mammography and ultrasound are complementary imaging tools for breast examination in everyday practice. The main indications for breast ultrasound are mammographically dense breasts, unclear or suspicious findings on mammography, patients with breast complaints, preoperative localization of breast cancer, aftercare of breast cancer patients, evaluation of high risk patients (familial history of BRCA 1 and 2 mutation), and second-look sonography after magnetic resonance imaging (MRI) [3].

Originally, in the early Breast Imaging Reporting and Data System version (BIRADS, 4th edition) of the American College of Radiology (ACR), mainly b-mode features of mass lesions were used to describe and classify the risk of a lesion's malignancy [4]. Masses were characterized according to their shape, orientation, margin, boundary, echo pattern, posterior acoustic features, surrounding tissue features, presence of calcifications, and the presence of vascularity. Over the last decade, however, improved spatial resolution with higher-frequency transducers and further technical developments, such as compound imaging, tissue harmonic imaging, color Doppler, 3D imaging, and elastography, have largely contributed to an increase in sonographic sensitivity and specificity [5]. These newer technical components play a vital role in lesion interpretation and have been integrated in the latest (5th) edition of BIRADS [6].

This chapter focuses on harmonic imaging, color Doppler, and elastography, describing the particular benefits and limitations of each approach. Elastography, a more recent method, is discussed in detail, including the possibilities to reduce false-positive and false-negative findings.

Tissue Harmonic Imaging

Despite technical advances, b-mode images with fundamental frequency contain artifacts that degrade image quality [7]. High-frequency imaging in particular is often responsible for the internal echo artifacts of otherwise simple cysts. By filtering (away) the fundamental frequency responsible for reverberations and speckle artifacts, artifact-reduced higher frequencies, so-called harmonics, are generated. In addition, tissue harmonic imaging (THI) helps to increase lesion conspicuity by improving image contrast and lateral resolution [8, 9], resulting in the following advantages :

1. Isoechoic lesions within fatty breast tissue on b-mode can be visualized with better contrast if THI is used (Fig. 1a, b)
2. Complicated cysts with internal echoes on b-mode appear anechoic on THI (Fig. 1c, d)
3. Echogenic parts (e.g., septal structures) are accentuated (Fig. 1c, d).

As a shortcoming, THI is not applicable to deeper regions and macromastia, since due to their physical properties harmonics can only be generated in more superficial layers.

Color Doppler

The development and growth of tumors is predominantly based upon neovascularization as a result of angiogenin production by the tumor cells [10]. This feature is used to visualize malignant lesions on MRI and color Doppler ultrasound. Numerous qualitative (morphological) and quantitative criteria, such as the resistance index (RI), the pulsatility index (PI), and systolic peak flow velocity (V_{max}) have been described with varying diagnostic significance [11-13]. A larger number of penetrating vessels and higher values of RI, PI, and V_{max} were considered as indicators of malignancy [14]. However, these flow-parameters are of less significance because of a large overlap between slowl-growing cancers with low vascularity and

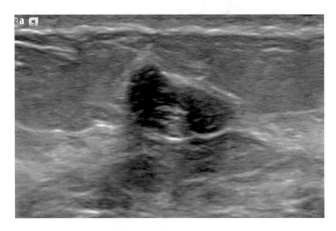
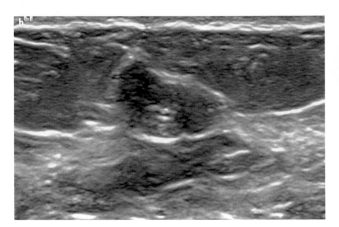
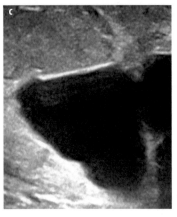
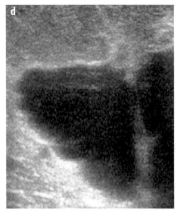

Fig. 1 a-d. Advantages of tissue harmonic imaging (THI) (**a, c**) compared to normal b-mode (**b, d**). Isoechoic fibroadenoma with lower visibility on normal b-mode (**b**) and better conspicuity on THI (**a**). Complicated cyst with internal echoes and less clearly visible septal structures (**d**); on THI, the internal part becomes anechoic and the septal structures more accentuated (**c**)

fast-growing cancers with higher vascularity. Moreover, they are not reproducible when the examination conditions differ (device, choice of flow parameter, location of measurement). Additionally, flow measurements are time-consuming and require vast experience. By contrast, morphological parameters are easier to assess, more reproducible, and of a higher diagnostic yield [15]. Thus, Madjar recommended simply observing the presence and number of vessels. Setting the cut-off for the depiction of vessels at >2, he was able to reach a sensitivity and specificity for the detection of malignancy of 90% and 93%, respectively [15]. Moreover, vascular pattern helps to predict the probability of a lesion's malignancy if used together with other criteria [14]. In this context, it can be helpful to consider the exact course of the vessels adjacent to the lesion, as performed by Svennson [16] (Fig. 2). Thus, benign vascular patterns, such as avascularity, higher vascularity in the periphery, and peripheral, marginal vessels connecting with internal vessels, significantly differed from malignant patterns. Typical of malignant lesions were radially aligned external vessels, radial internal vessels connected with radial external vessels, and a higher degree of internal than external vessels. It is worth mentioning that when using the Doppler function, it is essential to apply only a slight pressure on the probe and to keep the field of view (FOV) very small, thus obtaining better Doppler signals (Fig. 3).

To summarize, the essential features to be applied when evaluating a lesion with color Doppler are the presence of vascularity, the number of vessels, and the vessel pattern. However, vascular categorization is not always applicable due to poor vessel visualization and, even more importantly, vascular characterization can only be regarded as an adjunct to other b-mode features.

a   Benign
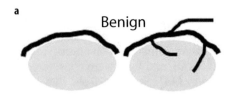

b   Malignant
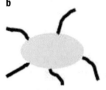

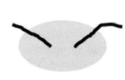

radial extern   radial intern   radial extern+intern

Fig. 2 a, b. Vascular pattern with color Doppler to estimate the risk of malignancy, according to Svennson: vessels in benign lesions tend to be more in the periphery, partially connecting with internal vessels (**a**), whereas vessels in malignant lesions have a radial pattern either in the outer or the inner part and a higher degree of internal than external vessels (**b**).

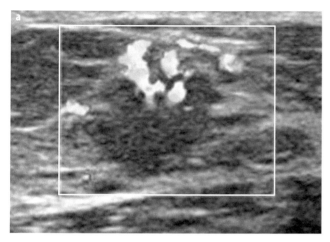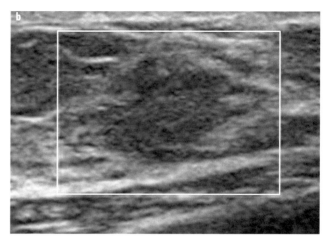

Fig. 3 a, b. Demonstration of the use of the color Doppler function in a strongly vascularized cancer lesion. A small region of interest, just around the lesions, should be chosen to achieve better Doppler signals. Only very slight pressure should be applied on the probe (**a**). If higher pressure is applied the Doppler signals, and thus vascularization, cannot be depicted (**b**)

Elastography

Ultrasound elastography is a recently introduced examination technique. In response to an external force, breast tissue is displaced, with stiff tissue being less displaced than soft tissue. Carcinomas exhibit an increased stiffness and thus less tissue displacement than normal breast tissue, and this mechanical characteristic is used to differentiate benign from malignant lesions. Thus, elastography is primarily a characterization rather than a detection tool, due to following physical properties: elasticity can generally be seen as the relation of necessary stress (pressure) to the relative change in length obtained (strain). It describes how much pressure has to be applied to elastically deform a tissue, which is dependent on its intrinsic elasticity (= Young`s modulus of elasticity) [17]. Young`s modulus of elasticity can therefore be considered as a description of tissue elasticity according to the formula: E = / (elasticity=pressure applied to the breast/ breast tissue deformation under pressure).

This differentiation criterion of absent strain (increased stiffness) has been evaluated in terms of its additional benefit to normal b-mode features in a series of studies, which demonstrated a general increase in specificity [18]. Nevertheless, the conditions of application and interpretation considerably vary between the different elastography software and devices. Essentially, two main elastography techniques can be distinguished: free-hand strain elastography and shear-wave elastography. Strain elastography can be further subdivided into real-time-elastography (e.g., Hitachi) and tissue-Doppler/ tissue strain imaging (e.g., Toshiba), whereas shear-wave elastography can be subdivided into genuine shear-wave elastography (e.g., Supersonic) and acoustic radiation force impulse (AFRI) technology (e.g., Siemens). In the following, only real-time elastography, as the most commonly applied form of strain elastography, and genuine shear-wave elastography are discussed in detail.

Free-Hand Strain Elastography

The manual compression applied on the probe can be described as rapid and sinusoidal movements of the hand. The induced tissue movements between the frames are calculated by a dedicated software, and the resulting signals registered before and after tissue displacement are transformed into b-modes images. Strain data are displayed as either a black/white elastogram, with black representing a stiff area and white a soft area, or a color map [19]. Color-coding is not uniform among the manufacturers, thus partially aggravating the interpretation. The most commonly applied color map, primarily used by the Hitachi ultrasound device, is the one developed by Itoh et al. [20]. This elasticity score (the Tsukuba score, named after the clinic where the work was conducted) has been validated in large series of histologically proven breast lesions and is based upon a 5-point scale (Fig. 4), with the risk of malignancy increasing from a score of 1 (=benign) to a score of 5 (=malignant). Numerous studies have shown that the additional use of an elasticity score increases specificity from 56–83% to 68–87% compared to normal b-mode images [21-23]. Another helpful tool is to compare the b-mode image with the elastographic image: benign lesions on the elastographic display are typically identical in size or smaller than on b-mode display, whereas malignant lesions appear to be larger on elastography than on b-mode display.

Nevertheless, the main disadvantage of strain elastography is that it is strongly operator-dependent such that large images may vary widely [23, 24]. Attempts have been made to reduce the interobserver variability by implementing semi-quantitative region of interest (ROI) measurements, such as the strain-ratio (strain of surrounding fat tissue/ strain of the lesion to be investigated). Lesion assessment was further improved by the additional use of a cut-off value, which can vary between 2.27 and 4.3 [21, 25, 26]. Values below the cut-off value

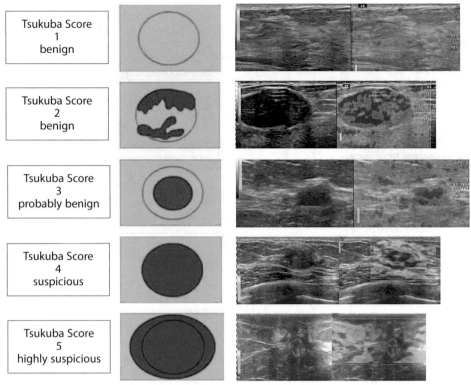

Tsukuba Score
1
benign

Tsukuba Score
2
benign

Tsukuba Score
3
probably benign

Tsukuba Score
4
suspicious

Tsukuba Score
5
highly suspicious

Fig. 4. Tsukuba elasticity score to estimate the risk of a lesion of being malignant. 1: lesion entirely green (same elasticity throughout the lesion). 2: blue and green mosaic (most of the lesion deformable). 3: deformability only in the periphery of the lesion. 4: blue lesion (no deformability throughout the entire lesion). 5: lesion and adjacent tissue are blue (no deformation of the lesion or the adjacent tissue).

indicate a benign lesion whereas values above the cut-off indicate a suspicious lesion. Although a certain improvement in interobserver agreement [21] and accuracy [25] has been obtained by the strain-ratio compared to the basic Tsukuba-elastography scoring, the difficulty in accurately assigning a lesion to a certain category remains, since strain-ratio measurements are based upon the individually generated elastography image.

Moreover, free-hand elastography requires a certain training phase to learn the adequate manual skills to be applied [19]: pressure on the probe, frequency of compression/decompression, and angulation of the probe. Hence, misinterpretations are possible by improper compression, deeply located lesions (>3 cm), large lesions (especially lesions larger than the FOV), non-perpendicular orientation of the probe, and if the lesions slides out of the FOV. When drawing the FOV, it is essential that the lesion is surrounded by sufficient adjacent tissue to avoid images of poor quality and misleading color coding; thus, it is advisable to draw the FOV as large as possible (from the subcutaneous fat layer to the superficial fascia of pectoral muscle) (Fig. 5).

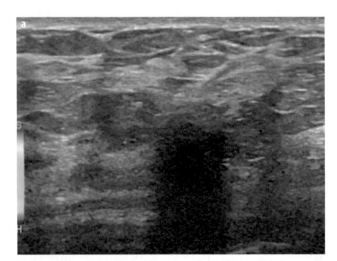
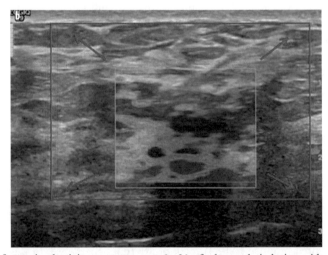

Fig. 5 a, b. Demonstration of improper field of view (FOV) placement for strain elasticity measurements (**a, b**) of a hypoechoic lesion with posterior shadowing on b-mode (**a**). The originally placed FOV covers only the lesion; thus, its estimation using the obtained color map remains difficult (**b**). For correct calculations, the lesion has to be surrounded by enough adjacent tissue. Therefore, the size of the FOV should reach from the subcutaneous fat layer to the superficial fascia of pectoral muscle (red rectangle in **b**)

Shear-Wave Elastography

In shear-wave elastography, unlike the method described above, mechanical vibrations are generated by an acoustic radiation impulse induced by the ultrasound probe itself. This push impulse generates slowly propagating shear waves at a low-frequency (~50 Hz) and at different depths. The ultrasound probe is equipped with an ultrafast acquisition frequency (5000 frames/s) and captures the propagation of shear waves. The propagation speed is used to calculate Young's modulus of elasticity according to the formula: E=acoustic radiation impulse/strain=3 μ=3 p v^2 (m/s) where μ is the shear wave, p is a constant and v the shear wave speed.

Stiffness information can be displayed in kPa based upon ROI measurements (e.g., maximum elasticity, E_{max}, in kPa). Additionally, images can be evaluated on a real-time color map linked to the value in kPa, ranging from 0 to 249 kPa (=E_{col}) (Fig. 6).

Given that the probe is constantly held using only a light pressure, interobserver agreement is good, or at least much better than strain imaging [27]. As shear waves propagate quickly in stiff tissue and slowly in soft tissue, higher shear-wave speeds are typical of cancer (red color=highly suspicious). The color indicating shear-wave speed can be located either in the center or at the margin of the lesion. There are two theories explaining the absence of shear waves in the lesion's center: (1) the shear-wave speed is too high to be captured by the probe and (2) the ultrasound beam to capture the shear waves cannot penetrate the deeper parts of scirrhous cancer [28]. It is worth mentioning that there are different modes of lesion visualization (Fig. 6b, c). Thus, in penetration rather than standard mode, the amplitude of the signal and the signal-to-noise ratio (SNR) are increased based upon constructive interfaces and color-coding of the lesion can thus be modified, e.g., from no shear waves in the center of the lesion with standard mode to a certain color-coding assigned with penetration mode.

Interpretation

Benign lesions (viscous cysts, fibroadenomas) and normal soft tissue are generally displayed in blue, but interpretation difficulties may occur, as non-viscous cysts do not support shear waves (Fig. 7a, b). Thus, absent shear waves in the center of a lesion have to be carefully assessed, as both malignancy and benign findings are possible (Figs. 6, 7).

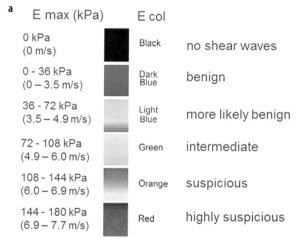

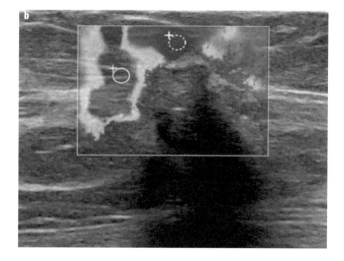

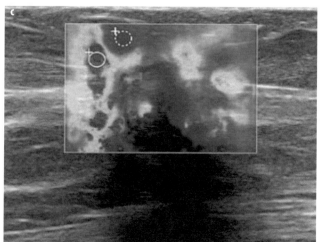

Fig. 6 a-c. Color spectrum of shear waves with quantitative parameters of maximum elasticity E_{max} (kPa) and qualitative parameters of elasticity color E_{col} (**a**) to characterize the depicted cancer lesion. The red color at the margin of the cancer lesion along with the measured E_{max} of 156 kPa (region of interest within the red area) indicates increased stiffness. With standard mode (**b**) no shear waves are visible in the center of the lesion, which suggests that their shear wave speed is extremely high. When penetration mode (**c**) is used, shear-wave signals are increased and shear waves become visible even in the center of the lesion, even though the stiffest part is still at the margin of the lesion

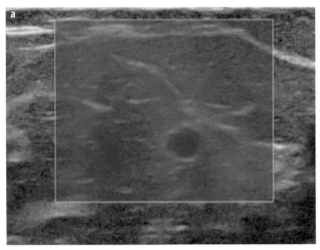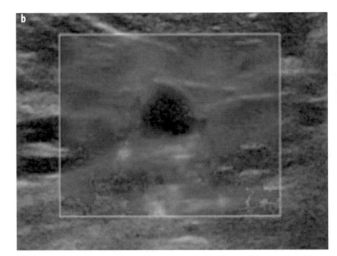

Fig. 7 a, b. Visualization of shear waves in cystic lesions. Viscous cysts (**a**) support shear waves, thus demonstrating a blue color. Non-viscous cysts (**b**) do not support shear waves, resulting in a black/absent shear-wave signal. As no increased stiffness is observed at the margin of the lesion, it can still be classified as benign

Although shear-wave images can be interpreted more reliably than strain elastography, difficulties remain in image generation and assessment.

False-Positives and Strategies to Avoid Them

False positives can be generated by: (1) poorly deformable lesions (e.g. scar, larger calcifications, fibrous fibroadenoma, focal strong fibrosis); (2) too-strong compression; and (3) insufficient "normal tissue" surrounding the lesion (too-small FOV).

Poorly deformable lesions: This feature is peculiar to the lesion and thus other imaging modalities, including mammography, b-mode, Doppler function, and comparisons to a preceding imaging study of the same lesion have to be taken into account.

Stronger (pre-)compression: Overly strong pressure applied on the probe will cause the peak in the generated shear waves to occur at an earlier time, thus simulating a higher shear-wave speed, as observed in cancers (Fig. 8). Therefore, it is crucial to use only slight pressure, except the lesion is small (≤5 mm), since small lesions might be missed if insufficient pressure is used.

Insufficient FOV: As with strain imaging, the FOV should be as large as possible, with sufficient adjacent "normal tissue" surrounding the lesion. This is important because the propagation of shear waves in the surrounding tissue is more visible such that misinterpretation will be unlikely. In particular, artifacts (from too-strong pre-compression) arising between the subcutaneous fat layer and the lesion are easier to perceive (vertical-cord artifact). The 4-pattern visual evaluation system described by

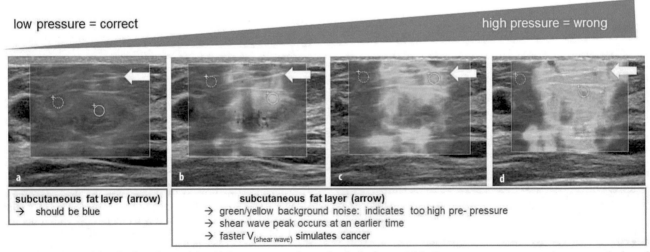

Fig. 8 a-d. False positive findings by applying high pressure on the probe. Left picture (**a**) indicates correct pressure, since no vertical-cord artifacts within the subcutaneous fat layer are seen. The subcutaneous fat layer is blue (*white arrow*). **b-d** With increasing pressure on the probe, higher shear wave speed is simulated thus producing a color coding typical of cancer. The green-yellow background noise within the subcutaneous fat layer indicates the artifact induced by too strong (pre-)compression (*white arrow*)

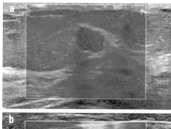

Pattern 1: homogeneously blue (no findings)

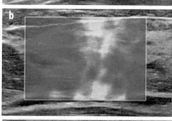

Pattern 2: color, that differs from the color around the lesion, observed at the margin or the interior of the lesion and extends in vertical cords beyond the lesion (artifact)

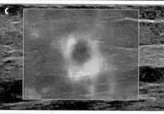

Pattern 3: localized colored area at the margin of the lesion (positive finding)

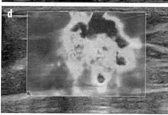

Pattern 4: colored areas in the interior of the lesion and heterogeneous (positive finding)

Fig. 9 a-d. Four-pattern visual evaluation of shear waves according to Tozaki as a method to avoid misinterpretations. **a** Pattern 1: homogeneously blue (no findings). **b** Pattern 2: color that differs from the color around the lesion observed at the margin or interior of the lesion and extending in vertical cords beyond the lesion (artifact). **c** Pattern 3: localized, colored area at the margin of the lesion (positive finding). **d** Pattern 4: colored areas in the interior of the lesion and heterogeneous (positive finding)

Tozaki [29] is very helpful in better differentiating between real positive findings and artifacts (Fig. 9).

If a "pattern-2 vertical- cord artifact" (Fig. 8 b-d) is observed during real-time elastography, then less pressure should be applied until the artifact disappears (Fig. 8a). Only if a colored area at the lesion's margin persists can the lesion be assumed to have increased stiffness.

False-Negatives and Strategies to Avoid Them

False negatives occur due to the following: (1) deeply located lesions (<2.5–3 cm); (2) as a reflection of the cancer type (high stiffness in scirrhous cancer, less stiffness in mucinous cancer or ductal carcinoma in situ); (3) lesions larger than the FOV (large single lesion, diffusely infiltrating cancer); (4) small lesions (<5 mm)

Deep lesions: At a depth of approximately 2.5–3 cm, shear waves are hardly visible. Better visibility can sometimes be gained by rotating the patient, so that the lesion under investigation is possibly displaced to a more superficial layer.

Cancer type: If shear waves are absent on the standard mode, they are more likely to be visualized using the penetration mode (increased amplitude of the shear waves) (Fig. 6). Nevertheless, in certain cancer types abnormal shear waves cannot be depicted; in such cases, other imaging modalities or further ultrasound techniques/features have to be considered.

Lesions larger than the FOV: Although the reasons are still unclear, it seems to be related to the fact that the lesion is not surrounded by sufficient "normal tissue" such that only differences in the elasticity the lesion and the surroundings are too small [18].

Small lesions: Normal (pre-)compression can be insufficient to generate abnormal shear waves, given that the area of stiffness is too small. Applying a higher (pre-)compression on the probe often allows the visualization of shear waves [19], even if the degree of stiffness is subtle.

Diagnostic Value of Shear-Wave Elastography

A previous large multicenter trial [30] evaluated diverse parameters of shear-wave elastography in terms of highest diagnostic value if used in addition to the normal BIRADS classification. The results showed that the qualitative parameter E_{col} (observed color in or around the lesion) had the highest accuracy ($AUC-BIRADS+E_{col}$ 0.971), followed by the quantitative parameter of maximum elasticity E_{max} (kPa) ($AUC-BIRADS+E_{col}$ 0.962). For this reason, only the observation of the displayed color is of major significance and might be sufficient for lesion assessment. The same study found that masses with $E_{max}>30–80$ kPa had a malignancy rate of 8.9% and those with $E_{max}>80$ to <160 had a malignancy rate of 39.9%. At an $E_{max} \geqslant 60$ kPa, 74.1% of the masses were malignant. In a preceding multinational study, shear-wave elastography

Table 1. Shear wave parameters for upgrading BIRADS 3 respectively downgrading BIRADS 4 a lesions whith an increase in specificity and no change in sensitivity according to Berg [30]

BIRADS 3+ parameters for BIRADS upgrading	BIRADS 4+ parameters for BIRADS downgrading	Increase in specificity
E_{col} red	E_{col} black to light blue	61.1→78.5
Irregular shape on SW elastography	oval shape on SW elastography	61.1→69.4
$E_{max} \geq 160$ kPa	$E_{max} \leq 80$ kPa	61.1→77.4

was shown to be particularly helpful in borderline lesions (between benign and malignant) according to b-mode criteria. By using these elastographic features as an adjunct to b-mode features, these lesions could be more accurately assigned to either BIRADS 3 or 4 [30]. Initially classified BIRADS 4a lesions with a lack of stiffness were more frequently benign, and initially classified BIRADS 3 lesions with increased stiffness were more often malignant. With the use of certain parameters for upgrading BIRADS 3 lesions and downgrading BIRADS 4a lesions, specificity could be increased while maintaining sensitivity (Table 1). The conclusion would be that unclear findings, e.g., a complicated cysts planned for biopsy, could be more frequently sent to follow-up, and initially classified BIRADS 3 lesions with an increased stiffness but in fact malignant could be sent earlier to biopsy. However, shear-wave elastography should not be used to change the strategy in typical BIRADS 2 , BIRADS 4c and BIRADS 5 lesions, as it might lead to misguided decisions.

Another study [31] was performed to exactly determine the benefit of shear-wave elastography in ultrasound-characterized BIRADS 3 lesions (primarily characterized without elastographic features). The aim was to search for features that would help to not send the patient to follow-up but rather to reclassify the lesion to a "new BIRADS 2" without downgrading a malignant lesion to "new BIRADS 2." Only the color (black to dark blue) and $E_{max} \leq 20$ kPa were sufficiently safe and helpful criteria to downgrade a benign-appearing BIRADS 3 lesions to a "new BIRADS 2," thus sparing patients from short-term follow-up.

Further advantages of shear-wave elastography currently being investigated or still to be evaluated are its apparent ability to more precisely depict the extent of invasive lobular carcinomas compared to b-mode ultrasound, and to better visualize small satellite lesions in the surroundings of the index cancer, irrespective of the tumor entity (ductal or lobular cancer).

Summary

Nowadays, breast diagnostics have to be considered as a complementary multimodality approach, one that is mainly based on mammography and ultrasound and supplemented by MRI, whenever required. However, ultrasound on its own has emerged as a complex examination modality, offering diverse technical features to characterize a lesion (THI, compound imaging, color Doppler, 3D imaging, elastography). But depending on the chosen ultrasound device, only a certain number of technical features will be available with different diagnostic value. Irrespective of the technical component is utilized, ultrasound always has to be considered in the context of further imaging modalities or technical components. This chapter has focused on THI, color Doppler, and elastography, as fast and easy methods that are also very helpful in lesion detection and differentiation. In particular, shear-wave elastography is considered a promising method because it is less operator-dependent than strain elastography and has a significant increase in specificity. The major benefit is seen in lesions primarily categorized as BIRADS 3 or 4a, which can be more accurately assessed based on their elastographic features. In this regard, patients with suspicious lesions (BIRADS 4a characterization without shear-wave elastography) with benign features on elastography (dark blue color within the lesion and its surroundings) could be spared from biopsy and instead be sent to follow-up. Conversely, unclear lesions (BIRADS 3 characterization without shear-wave elastography) with suspicious elastographic features could be sent for biopsy with higher confidence. To reduce misinterpretations and avoid misguided decisions, it is essential to be familiar with the reasons for false-positives and false-negatives. It is also important that every imaging finding be evaluated in a larger context, such as clinical complaints, findings in previous examinations, age of the patient, individual risk situation, and comparison with other imaging methods.

References

1. Woo J (2004) A short history of the development. Radiol Clin N Am 42:845-851.
2. Berg WA, Blume JD, Cormack JB et al (2008) Combined screening with ultrasound and mammography vs mammography alone in women at elevated risk of breast cancer. JAMA 299:2151-2163.
3. Mundinger A, Wilson ARM, Weisman C et al (2008) Breast ultrasound- update. EJC Supplements 9:11-14.
4. ACR BI-RADS – Ultrasound (2003). In: ACR Breast Imaging Reporting and Data System, Breast Imaging Atlas. American college of Radiology, Reston, VA.
5. Candelaria RP, Hwang L, Bouchard RR et al (2013) Breast ultrasound: current concepts. Semin Ultrasound CT MR 34:213-225.
6. Mendelson EB, Böhm-Vélez M, Berg WA et al (2013) ACR BI-RADS® Ultrasound. In: ACR BI-RADS® Atlas, Breast Imaging Reporting and Data System. American College of Radiology, Reston, VA,

7. Sehgal CM, Weinstein SP, Arger PH et al (2006) A review of breast ultrasound. J Mammary Gland Biol Neoplasia 11:113-123.
8. Rosen EL, Soo MS (2001) Tissue harmonic imaging sonography of breast lesions: improved margin analysis, conspicuity, and image quality compared to conventional ultrasound. Clin Imaging 25:379-384.
9. Szopinski KT, Pajk AM, Wysocki M et al (2003) Tissue harmonic imaging: utility in breast sonography. J Ultrasound Med 22:479-487.
10. Hartmann A, Kunz M, Köstlin S et al (1999) Hypoxia-induced up-regulation of angiogenin in human malignant melanoma. Cancer Res 59:1578-1583.
11. Milz P, Lienemann A, Kessler M et al (2001) Evaluation of breast lesions by power Doppler sonography. Eur Radiol 11:547-554.
12. Gokalp G, Topal U, Kizilkaya E (2009) Power Doppler sonography: anything to add to BI-RADS US in solid breast masses? Eur J Radiol 70:77-85.
13. Carpentier GL, Roubidoux MA, Fowlkes JB et al (2008) Suspicious breast lesions: assessment of 3D Doppler US indexes for classification in a test population and fourfold cross-validation scheme. Radiology 249:463-470.
14. Raza S, Baum JK (1997) Solid breast lesions: evaluation with power Doppler US. Radiology 203:164-168.
15. Madjar H, Sauerbrei W, Hansen L (2011) Multivariate analysis of flow data in breast lesions and validation in a normal clinical setting. Ultraschall Med 32:511-517.
16. Svensson WE, Pandian AJ, Hashimoto H (2010) The use of breast ultrasound color Doppler vascular pattern morphology improves diagnostic sensitivity with minimal change in specificity. Ultraschall Med 31:466-474.
17. Krouskop TA, Wheeler TM, Kallel F et al (1998) Elastic moduli of breast and prostate tissues under compression. Ultrason Imaging 20:260-274.
18. Fischer T, Sack I, Thomas A (2013) Characterization of focal breast lesions by means of elastography. Rofo 185:816-823.
19. Barr RG, Destounis S, Lackey LB 2nd et al (2012) Evaluation of breast lesions using sonographic elasticity imaging: a multicenter trial. J Ultrasound Med 31:281-287.
20. Itoh A, Ueno E, Tohno E et al (2006) Breast disease: clinical application of US elastography for diagnosis. Radiology 239:341-350.
21. Fischer T, Peisker U, Fiedor S et al (2012) Significant differentiation of focal breast lesions: raw data-based calculation of strain ratio. Ultraschall Med 33:372-379.
22. Thomas A, Degenhardt F, Farrokh A et al (2010) Significant differentiation of focal breast lesions: calculation of strain ratio in breast sonoelastography. Acad Radiol 17:558-563.
23. Thomas A, Kümmel S, Fritzsche F et al (2006) Real-time sonoelastography performed in addition to B-mode ultrasound and mammography: improved differentiation of breast lesions? Acad Radiol 13:1496-504.
24. Yoon JH, Kim MH, Kim EK et al (2011) Interobserver variability of ultrasound elastography: how it affects the diagnosis of breast lesions. AJR Am J Roentgenol 196:730-736.
25. Zhi H, Xiao XY, Yang HY et al (2010) Ultrasonic elastography in breast cancer diagnosis: strain ratio vs 5-point scale. Acad Radiol 17:1227-1233.
26. Mansour SM, Omar OS (2012) Elastography ultrasound and questionable breast lesions: does it count? Eur J Radiol 81:3234-3244.
27. Cosgrove DO, Berg WA, Doré CJ et al (2012) Shear wave elastography for breast massesis highly reproducible. Eur Radiol 22:1023-1032.
28. Cosgrove D, Piscaglia F, Bamber et al (2013) EFSUMB guidelines and recommendations on the clinical use of ultrasound elastography. Part 2: Clinical applications. Ultraschall Med 34:238-253.
29. Tozaki M1, Fukuma E (2011) Pattern classification of Shear-Wave™ Elastography images for differential diagnosis between benign and malignant solid breast masses. Acta Radiol 52:1069-1075.
30. Berg WA, Cosgrove DO, Doré CJ et al (2012) Shear-wave elastography improves the specificity of breast US: the BE1 multinational study of 939 masses. Radiology 262: 435-449.
31. Schäfer FK, Hooley RJ, Ohlinger R et al (2013) ShearWave™ Elastography BE1 multinational breast study: additional SWE™ features support potential to downgrade BI-RADS®-3 lesions. Ultraschall Med 34:254-259.

Magnetic Resonance Imaging of Breast Implants and the Reconstructed Breast

Isabelle Thomassin-Naggara[1], Michael Atlan[2], Jocelyne Chopier[1], Emile Darai[3]

[1] Department of Radiology, Hopital Tenon - APHP, Paris, France
[2] Plastic Reconstructive and Aesthetic Surgery Unit, Hopital Tenon - APHP, Paris, France
[3] Department of Gynecology and Obstetrics, Hopital Tenon - APHP, Paris, France

Introduction

For many years, breast augmentation was exclusively obtained by the use of breast implants. However, during the last 20 years, the multiplication of plastic surgical treatments has been such that several different methods of breast augmentation are now available. In asymptomatic women with breast implant abnormalities detected with conventional imaging, as well as in symptomatic women with breast implants or a reconstructed breast, magnetic resonance imaging (MRI) may be the best imaging technique in the absence of a consensus on imaging follow-up.

Breast Implants

General Considerations

There are two main types of breast implants: saline implants and silicone implants, which are used in similar proportions according the U.S. Food and Drug Administration (FDA) (FDA Update on the Safety of Silicone Gel-Filled Breast Implants. http://www.fda.gov/). Most breast implants have a single compartment that is filled with a saline solution or with silicone, or two such compartments. During the last 50 years, the breast implant industry has evolved. Silicone of the first generation was dense and viscous, with a very thick shell, and did not accurately mimic breast tissue. In the second generation of implants, the filler material was a less viscous gel (with less cross-linking) and the shell was thinner. However, because of a high rate of rupture and leakage, the need for a third generation implant soon became obvious. In this attempt, the gel was more viscous and the envelope was thicker (textured or smooth), with a barrier within the shell to avoid perspiration of the gel [1]. The last generation of implants, still in use today, is a stable implant, with a variety of shapes (anatomic or round implant) and

shells (textured or smooth). The silicone used is cohesive, to maintain the shape of the implant in the body and to avoid silicone migration in case of rupture.

Saline- or silicone-containing gel breast prostheses are still the two main types of implants, although there are other, albeit rarely used, implant materials, such as hydrogel. The silicone used to fill the envelope comes mainly from two manufacturers. More than 25% of poly-implant prostheses (PIP) are filled with non-medical-grade silicone, which is less "cohesive" at body temperature and do not include an anti perspiration barrier; thus in case of rupture they have a higher risk of an uncontrolled dispersion [2-4].

Different surgical approaches are used to place the implant in the breast (hemi-areolar, sub-mammary, or axillary incisions), with three possible locations, or pockets, relative to the position of the pectoralis major muscle: pre, retro-pectoral, or dual plane (the upper half of the implant under the muscle and the lower half under the gland). When the implants are positioned in the breast, a foreign-body reaction is induced and a fibrous capsule corresponding to a second, frequently very soft, envelope is created. However, this capsule may undergo capsular contracture, thereby becoming rigid and sometimes painful and causing a deformation of breast shape. For reconstruction, surgeons typically use the previous scar of the mastectomy, placing the implant under the pectoralis major or, in some cases, under the pectoralis minor or serratus anterior muscle. New devices such as biologic matrix are used to cover the implant in the lower aspect that is not covered by muscle [5].

Patients with breast implants are vulnerable to a vast array of complications that should be familiar to the radiologist, including hematoma, infection, implant rotation, pain, change of breast size or shape, capsular contracture, implant rupture, and the extrusion of soft-tissue silicone. The two most frequent complications are capsular contracture and implant rupture. The physiopathology of capsular contracture is unclear but probably involves sub-clinical infections with, e.g., *Staphyloccus epidermidis* or *Pseudomonas acnei* [3, 6], silicone fluid bleed, hema-toma, glove-talc reaction, implant rupture, and foreign body reaction to the silicone elastomer shell. Capsular contracture may occur within the first month after surgery or several years later. Its occurrence usually cor-relates with the age of the implant and it is most fre-quently observed after 10 years. In 2011, the FDA re-ported a possible association of breast implants with anaplastic large cell lymphoma [7], but the relationship has yet to be confirmed in a prospective study.

To enhance the cosmetic results of implant-based re-constructions, a fat graft procedure can be performed in the subcutaneous plane above the gland, to avoid ripples and implant visibility.

MR Findings

MRI of breast implants has the highest sensitivity and specificity for the detection of silicone implant rupture and is thus considered the gold standard in this specific setting. MRI is not performed systematically in the fol-low-up of patients with breast implants. Rather, it is in-dicated if the patient is symptomatic (including pain, burning, or a mass in the implant-bearing breast or the surrounding tissue). The patient may note hardening or softening of the implant [8] with the degree of hardness defined according to the Baker classification [9]. MRI is also usually a second-line technique after ultrasonogra-phy, as recommended by the FDA, because of its high sensitivity (73–97%) and specificity (73–97%) in diag-nosing implant rupture. In patients with silicone breast implants, an implant rupture should be diagnosed as soon as possible so as to limit the risk of capsular con-tracture.

Acquisition Technique

Using MRI, both the axial and the sagittal planes should be imaged because every rupture suspected in one plane must be confirmed in its perpendicular plane [10]. Spe-cial attention must be paid to ensure that the field of view includes the axillary regions. The imaging protocol must include sequences that suppress or emphasize the signal from water, fat, or, especially, silicone, i.e. T2-weighted fast spin-echo, T1-weighted sequences, and, if the implant contains silicone, a water-fat suppression se-quence (silicone only), to differentiate water from sili-cone since both appear bright on T2-weighted sequences (Fig. 1).

MR Analysis

In the Breast Imaging-Reporting and Data System (BI-RADS) lexicon published in 2013, Chapter IV is devoted to describing breast implants, in the section on MRI. The MRI report should include implant type (silicone or saline content), location (pre or retropectoralis), contour (regular, focal budge, ruptured), and the location of the silicone. Intra-capsular rupture is observed in 80% and extra-capsular rupture in 20% of patients with silicone gel implants The combination of five different features needs to be analyzed to diagnose a rupture: (a) the fi-brous capsule, (b) the implant envelope, (c) the signal of the periprosthetic fluid, (d) the location of the detected silicone, and (e) the overall implant shape (Table 1).

The radial folds are illustrated in Fig. 2. Water droplets inside breast implants are seen on water-specific images; they may be normal (due to the injection of silicone gel during surgery, for example) or associated with implant rupture. The presence of silicone within axillary lymph nodes does not necessarily imply implant rupture.

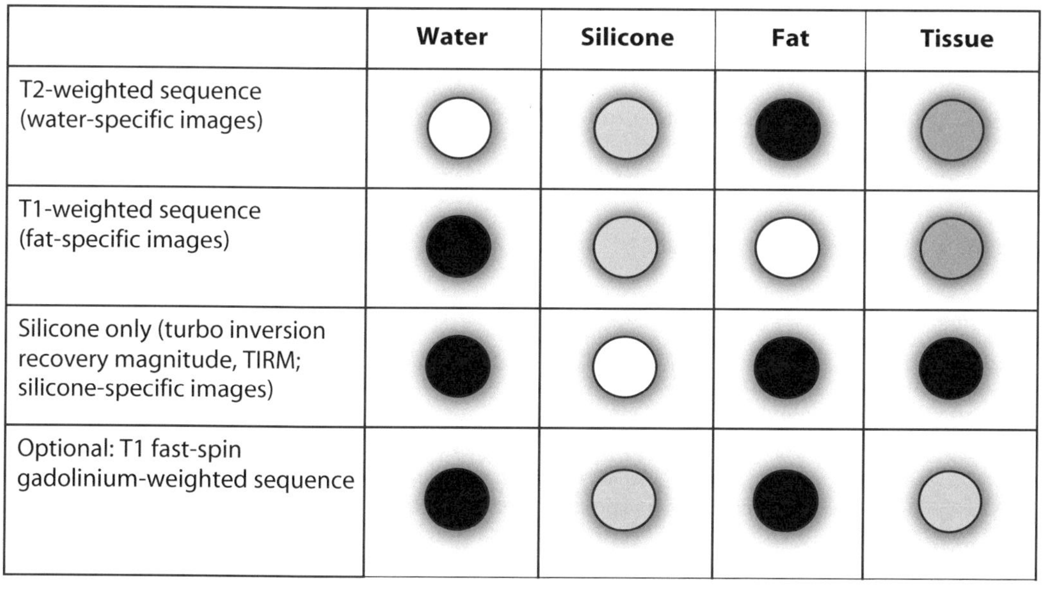

	Water	Silicone	Fat	Tissue
T2-weighted sequence (water-specific images)	○	◔	●	◑
T1-weighted sequence (fat-specific images)	●	◔	○	◑
Silicone only (turbo inversion recovery magnitude, TIRM; silicone-specific images)	●	○	●	●
Optional: T1 fast-spin gadolinium-weighted sequence	●	◔	●	○

Fig. 1. MRI standard proto-col and findings according to tissue characteristics

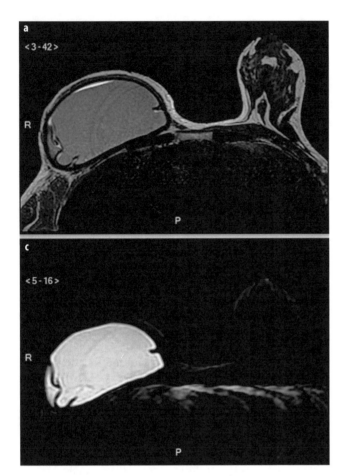
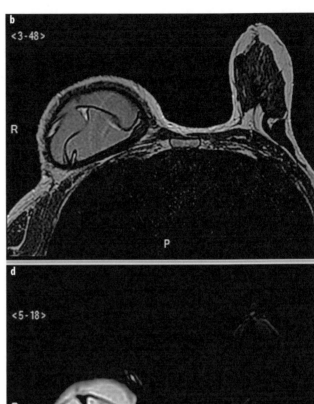

Fig. 2 a-d. Radial folds. **a**, **b** T2-weighted sequence showing dark lines with different signal intensities inside and outside the implants. Periprosthetic fluid displays a high T2-weighted signal intensity. **c**, **d** Silicone-only sequence shows the absence of silicone outside the prosthesis

Table 1. Implant analysis using magnetic resonance imaging

	Intact implant		Rupture	
	Normal	Capsule contraction	Intracapsular	Extracapsular rupture
Fibrous capsule	Not seen	Focal bulge	Undisrupted	Seen Disrupted
Implant envelope	Smooth, or radial fold (with dark ball end)	Smooth, or radial folds (with dark ball end)	Key-hole, tear drop, noose (with white ball end) Linguine sign	Linguine sign
Periprosthetic fluid Signal	Thin Water	Thin or thick Water	Thick Silicone*	Absent Silicone*
Silicone location*	Only inside the implant envelope	Only inside the implant envelope	Outside the implant envelope Inside fibrous capsule	Outside the implant envelope and fibrous capsule
Overall implant shape	Normal	Abnormal	Normal	Abnormal (extruded silicon globe separated by a dark line)

*In the case of silicone breast implants

Autologous Reconstruction

During the last 20 years, oncological, reconstructive, and cosmetic surgery techniques have evolved considerably, with the development of novel surgical approaches and skin-and nipple-sparing mastectomies that can be completed with silicone-filled implants, an autologous flap (pedicled or free flaps), or by autologous fat grafting. In certain oncological or prophylactic cases, a skin-sparing or nipple-areola-complex-sparing mastectomy may allow enhanced cosmetic results by conserving most of the skin envelope. The need for systematic imaging follow-up of these patients is unclear, including for patients with oncological indications [11, 12]. Normal mammary gland is found in about 60% of patients after a skin-sparing mastectomy, according to Tokin et al. [13]. In skin- and nipple-sparing mastectomy performed in oncology patients, it should be noted that the risk of local recurrence correlates with the margin status and the type of mastectomy. According to Kroll et al. [14], regardless of the reconstruction technique, this risk is 4–6% at 5 years, similar to that in the group of patients not undergoing reconstruction. Depending on the location of the recurrence, the patient may or may not be symptomatic. In 50–70% of cases, the recurrence develops in the anterolateral part of the reconstructed breast and is easily detected by the clinician, but in 30% of cases the recurrence may be in the axillary region or within the thoracic wall, which in either case is very difficult to diagnose clinically. When the patient is symptomatic, the radiologist must be able to distinguish normal imaging features from features of malignancy, which as a prerequisite requires an awareness of the different types of breast reconstruction options.

Autologous Flaps

General Considerations

The two most common types of conventional pedicled flaps are the latissimus dorsi myocutaneous (LDM) flap and the transverse rectus abdominis myocutaneous (TRAM) flap; the latter is harvested from excess abdominal tissue. These autologous breast reconstruction methods allow the insertion of a muscle with a skin island and are mainly indicated when there is a lack of skin after conservative mastectomy. The LDM flap is vascularized by the thoracodorsal pedicle whereas the epigastric superior vessels supply the TRAM flap. These flaps include the muscle to insure good vascularization of the skin and fat. By contrast, free flaps, such as the deep inferior epigastric perforator (DIEP) flap, are becoming increasingly popular because they are muscle-sparing. Autologous tissue transfer involves complete separation of the donor tissue. In the case of the abdominal excess transferred in the DIEP flap, a pedicle is dissected in the muscle, and there is absolutely no muscle within the flap (hence the name perforator flap). The harvested tissue is then connected to the recipient site by an anastomosis, with microsurgical sutures performed under the microscope: the deep inferior vessels are ligated to the internal mammary vessels lying under the cartilage of the third or fourth rib [15]. The techniques required for perforator flaps are more complex, with a significantly longer operating time, than those involved in the placement of a conventional pedicled flap [16, 17]. Other flaps that may be used are the superior inferior epigastric perforator (SIEP) flap, the superior gluteal artery perforator (SGAP) flap, and the inferior gluteal artery perforator (IGAP) flap.

The potential complications of autologous reconstruction include partial or total necrosis, pulmonary embolism, edema, hematoma, and seroma. After 1–2 years, steatonecrosis (including potential sclerosing retraction and calcification) may occur, with the risk depending on the quality of the anastomosing pedicle. According to Garvey et al., the rates of fat necrosis are higher for the TRAM flap (58.5%) than for the DIEP flap (17.7%) [16]. Moreover, abdominal hernias occur more frequently in patients receiving a TRAM flap (16%) than a DIEP flap (1%). Together, these considerations account for the preference for and further refinement of DIEP rather than TRAM reconstructions [18, 19].

MR Findings

In the follow-up of patients with a reconstructed breast(s), MRI is not systematically performed except in patients who are at high risk of breast and ovarian cancer. The radiologist may have to analyze the autologous reconstruction if the patient undergoes MRI for the contralateral breast or if there is a suspicion of recurrence in the reconstructed breast. At MRI, the volume of the flap decreases over time such that eventually it is composed only of fat or muscle or of a fatty component, depending on the type of autologous reconstruction. The radiologist should examine the remaining mammary gland and its location to help the clinician to orient the sites of normal tissue and/or correlate normal tissue with a potential abnormality at clinical examination.

Autologous Fat Grafting

This technique of breast augmentation consists of harvesting the fat by classic liposuction followed by treatment of the harvested tissue (centrifugation, washing, and/or filtration) to enhance the viability of the adipocytes and mesenchymal stem cells, before their injection into the breast. Autologous fat grafting can be used as the sole technique in a reconstruction or it may be combined with autologous-tissue- or implant-based breast reconstructions. If the autologous fat graft technique is used by itself, e.g., in breast augmentation, all the layers of the breast can be injected: pectoralis major muscle, the retropectoral space, above the gland, and within the gland. When it is combined with another technique of breast augmentation, the lipoaspirate is mainly injected into the subcutaneous space above the gland.

Imaging Features

The classic MRI findings of a fat-injection site include hyperintensity on non-fat-saturated T1-weighted images, hypointensity on fat-saturated images, and hypointensity on T2-weighted images [15]. Three types of abnormalities as seen on MRI have been described:
1. Oil cyst without any enhancement after gadolinium injection (BI-RADS 2) (Fig. 3)

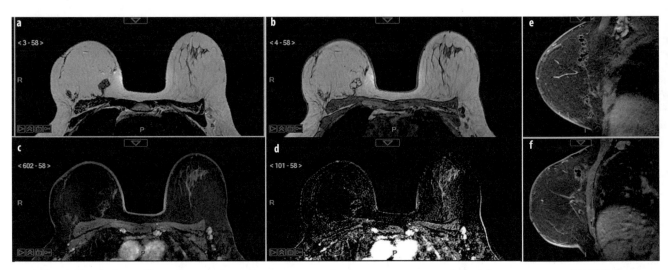

Fig. 3 a-f. Autologous fat grafting, oil cyst. Primary breast augmentation by transverse rectus abdominis myocutaneous (TRAM) flap combined with autologous fat grafting. **a** Axial TSE T2-weighted sequence. **b** Axial EG T1-weighted sequence. **c** Axial Native EG T1 DCE MR weighted sequence after the 24' after injection. **d** Axial Substracted EG T1 DCE MR weighted sequence after the 24' after injection. **e, f** Sagittal Native EG T1-weighted sequence (upper and lower right). Magnetic resonance imaging shows the presence of a high T1 signal intensity without any wall enhancement in the posterior part of the breast corresponding to the location of autologous fat grafting

2. Complex cyst of fat necrosis that displays rim enhancement (BI-RADS 3)
3. Granuloma appearing as a heterogeneous mass containing inflammatory and fibrous tissue (BI-RADS 4). In the third case, the detection of a small fatty component inside may help in the diagnosis.

Cancer Recurrence Risk

According to the Society of Plastic Surgeons, in a report based on a multicenter European study, the use of autologous fat grafting does not affect radiologic follow-up and is not associated with an increased risk of breast cancer [20]. Long-term follow-up of these patients is ongoing.

References

1. Calobrace MB, Capizzi PJ (2014) The biology and evolution of cohesive gel and shaped implants. Plast Reconstr Surg 134:S6-11.
2. Beretta G, Panseri S, Manzo A et al (2014) Analytical investigations on elastomeric shells of new Poly Implant Prothèse (PIP) breast and from sixteen cases of surgical explantation. J Pharm Biomed Anal 98:144-152.
3. Del Pozo JL, Tran NV, Petty PM et al (2009) Pilot study of association of bacteria on breast implants with capsular contracture. J Clin Microbiol 47:1333-1337.
4. Oulharj S, Pauchot J, Tropet Y (2014) PIP breast implant removal: a study of 828 cases. J Plast Reconstr Aesthetic Surg JPRAS 67:302-307.
5. Spear SL, Sher SR, Al-Attar A, Pittman T (2014) Applications of a cellular dermal matrix in revision breast reconstruction surgery. Plast Reconstr Surg 133:1-10.
6. Cordeiro PG, McCarthy CM (2006) A single surgeon's 12-year experience with tissue expander/implant breast reconstruction: part II. An analysis of long-term complications, aesthetic outcomes, and patient satisfaction. Plast Reconstr Surg 118:832-839.
7. Adrada BE, Miranda RN, Rauch GM et al (2014) Breast implant-associated anaplastic large cell lymphoma: sensitivity, specificity, and findings of imaging studies in 44 patients. Breast Cancer Res Treat 147:1-14.
8. Tolhurst DE (1978) "Nutcracker" technique for compression rupture of capsules around breast implants. Plast Reconstr Surg 61:795.
9. Baker JL, Bartels RJ, Douglas WM (1976) Closed compression technique for rupturing a contracted capsule around a breast implant. Plast Reconstr Surg 58:137-141.
10. Ikeda DM, Borofsky HB, Herfkens RJ et al (1999) Silicone breast implant rupture: pitfalls of magnetic resonance imaging and relative efficacies of magnetic resonance, mammography, and ultrasound. Plast Reconstr Surg 104:2054-2062.
11. Yoo H, Kim BH, Kim HH et al (2014) Local recurrence of breast cancer in reconstructed breasts using TRAM flap after skin-sparing mastectomy: clinical and imaging features. Eur Radiol 24:2220-2226.
12. Helvie MA, Bailey JE, Roubidoux MA et al (2002) Mammographic screening of TRAM flap breast reconstructions for detection of nonpalpable recurrent cancer. Radiology 224:211-216.
13. Tokin C, Weiss A, Wang-Rodriguez J, Blair SL (2012) Oncologic safety of skin-sparing and nipple-sparing mastectomy: a discussion and review of the literature. Int J Surg Oncol 2012:921821.
14. Kroll SS, Schusterman MA, Tadjalli HE et al (1997) Risk of recurrence after treatment of early breast cancer with skin-sparing mastectomy. Ann Surg Oncol 4:193-197.
15. Margolis NE, Morley C, Lotfi P et al (2014) Update on imaging of the postsurgical breast. Radiogr Rev Publ Radiol Soc N Am Inc 34:642-660.
16. Garvey PB, Buchel EW, Pockaj BA et al (2006) DIEP and pedicled TRAM flaps: a comparison of outcomes. Plast Reconstr Surg 117:1711-1719.
17. Granzow JW, Levine JL, Chiu ES, Allen RJ (2006) Breast reconstruction with the deep inferior epigastric perforator flap: history and an update on current technique. J Plast Reconstr Aesthetic Surg JPRAS 59:571-579.
18. Yueh JH, Slavin SA, Adesiyun T et al (2010) Patient satisfaction in postmastectomy breast reconstruction: a comparative evaluation of DIEP, TRAM, latissimus flap, and implant techniques. Plast Reconstr Surg 125:1585-1595.

19. Chun YS, Sinha I, Turko A et al (2010) Comparison of morbidity, functional outcome, and satisfaction following bilateral TRAM versus bilateral DIEP flap breast reconstruction. Plast Reconstr Surg 126:1133-1141.

20. Petit JY, Lohsiriwat V, Clough KB et al (2011) The oncologic outcome and immediate surgical complications of lipofilling in breast cancer patients: a multicenter study – Milan-Paris-Lyon experience of 646 lipofilling procedures. Plast Reconstr Surg 128:341-346.

Printed in the United States
By Bookmasters